Vascular Surgery: Current Questions

Vascular Surgery: Current Questions

Edited by

A. A. B. Barros D'Sa
Vascular Surgery Unit, Royal Victoria Hospital, Belfast, UK

P. R. F. Bell
The Leicester Royal Infirmary, Department of Surgery, Leicester, UK

S. G. Darke
Department of Surgery, Royal Bournemouth Hospital, Bournemouth, UK

P. L. Harris
Vascular Surgery Unit, Broadgreen Hospital, Liverpool, UK

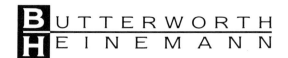
BUTTERWORTH
HEINEMANN

Butterworth-Heinemann Ltd
Linacre House, Jordan Hill, Oxford OX2 8DP

PART OF REED INTERNATIONAL BOOKS

OXFORD   LONDON   BOSTON   MUNICH
NEW DELHI   SINGAPORE   SYDNEY   TOKYO
TORONTO   WELLINGTON

First published 1991

British Library Cataloguing in Publication Data
Vascular Surgery: Current questions.
  I. Barros D'Sa, A. A. B.   II. Bell, P. R. F.
  617.4

ISBN 0 7506 1381 5

Library of Congress Cataloging in Publication Data
A CIP catalogue record for this book is available from the
Library of Congress.

Filmset by Latimer Trend & Company Ltd.
Printed and bound in Great Britain by
Bath Press Ltd, Bath, Avon.

Foreword

Vascular surgery is a relatively young speciality and the whole scope of its widespread clinical application is easily encompassed within the career of one surgeon. The pioneers of vascular surgery, in the 1930s particularly, and during its rapid growth during the late 1950s, established a speciality which will continue to expand until atheroma can be prevented or treated by medical means rather than by surgery. The first generation of vascular surgeons was sustained by the excitement of technical advances and increasingly successful operations. With mounting expertise and familiarity the duration of operations decreased, mortality fell and results improved. Advances in surgical technique were paralleled by considerable evolution in anaesthetic service, intensive care and the investigation of vascular disease using improved forms of angiography and, in particular, non-invasive assessment.

The second generation of vascular surgeons needs to take a colder, harder look at their chosen speciality. There are very few controlled trials available in the vast literature on the results of vascular surgical operations and adjuvant treatment. When compared with the established specialities of gastroenterology and oncological surgery, vascular surgery seems a poor and unscientific relation. The reasons for the lack of good objective scientific data to support our clinical decisions are not hard to find. Each individual vascular surgeon does not perform sufficient operations per annum to achieve an adequate controlled trial within a limited period. The trial which runs on for several years tends to be abandoned through a general waning of interest and the natural feeling that the answer will have been found by some other means before the trial is completed. The casual, multicentre trial has equally serious problems: it is very difficult to persuade surgeons to co-operate on an ad hoc basis, data collection is usually incomplete, many surgeons fail to co-operate having shown an initial willingness to participate and the final collection and follow-up of patients is usually less than ideal.

After preliminary discussions, a group of thirteen British consultant vascular surgeons, who also happen to be friends, held a meeting hosted by Tony Chant in Southampton on 25 March 1983 to form the Joint Vascular Research Group of the United Kingdom. The concept of the JVRG UK was originally attributable to Simon Darke who must be congratulated for his foresight. The prime objective of this collaborative group is to try to enter as many patients as possible into multicentre controlled trials of vascular operations and their complications, as well as studies of the natural history of vascular disease. Their success may be judged from the contents of this book. The members agreed to attempt to standardize their collection of data, to meet twice a year and at these meetings to propose new protocols and reassess the

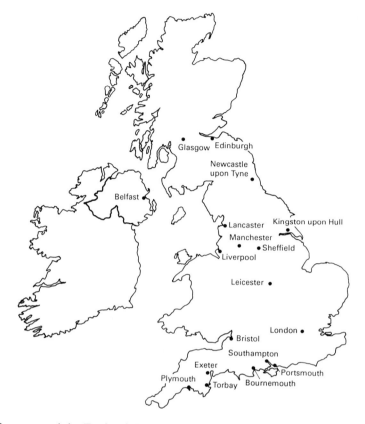

results of current trials. Each trial becomes the responsibility of one member of the group, but that member is assisted by a full-time research co-ordinator.

JVRG UK is a registered charity, which is entirely self-supporting and relies upon donations to cover the cost of research assistance and trial analysis. The group has grown, with some minor changes in membership, to a total of twenty-one members to date and the principles involved in its original inception have been very successful. The agreed format of common recording techniques and a general co-ordinator greatly facilitate the collection of accurate data during a rapid controlled clinical trial and the speed with which the trial can be completed maintains the interest and enthusiasm of the members. The membership is not static and younger surgeons join older ones, who drop out as they become less productive members of the group, and it is hoped that the current enthusiasm and productiveness of this research will continue.

Crawford Jamieson

Preface

'... but when we have stuffed
These pipes and these conveyances of our blood
With wine and feeding, we have suppler souls
Than in our priest-like fasts ...'

Coriolanus V.1

Over a period of approximately three decades vascular surgery has matured within
the broad spectrum of general surgery into a speciality responsible for the treatment
of serious vascular diseases. It is a field which has grown enormously, not only in the
numbers of patients receiving surgical treatment, but also in the range and complexity
of procedures undertaken. A large proportion of this patient population is burdened
by intercurrent and sometimes generalized arterial and other diseases, the care of
which calls for participation by clinicians in other medical disciplines. Invariably,
some operations carry a risk of complications, a few of which are potentially fatal.

Amidst the proliferating volumes and reference texts covering a multitude of
vascular surgical subjects there appears to be a need to explore specific topics which
are not only of practical interest but also arouse controversy and provoke debate. In
an attempt to fulfil this end, the path chosen here is one which endeavours to avoid a
didactic approach or an indulgence in restating well-worn answers. This book does
not aim to be a comprehensive review of every conceivable subject within the arena of
vascular surgery. Rather, its purpose is to raise current questions in a manner which
will induce the reader to scrutinize established and newer modes of therapy, and to reexamine surgical practices in order to develop fresh perspectives in management.
Prompted by such objectives, a number of surgeons actively involved in teaching,
training and collaborative research, and representing the membership of the Joint
Vascular Research Group UK, were called upon to make a contribution. Inevitably,
each of the topics covered in this book will bear the personal stamp of the author
concerned. The subjects were presented at a major vascular symposium held in Belfast
on 9 May 1991.

The areas addressed are those which confront us all – in outpatient clinics, on the
wards, in the operating theatre and in the intensive care unit. Throughout the book,
attention is focused on diagnostic accuracy, judgement in challenging clinicopathological situations, selection of patients for various modalities of treatment,
assessment of surgical techniques and interventional procedures, prevention of
serious complications, and finally, an objective appraisal of outcome. The contents

are of interest to consultant and trainee vascular and general surgeons and other specialists who share in the overall management of patients with vascular problems.

On behalf of the editors, I would like to place on record my appreciation to the membership of the Joint Vascular Research Group UK for their contributions, my co-editors for their assistance, Mrs Andrea Chetcuti, our research co-ordinator, for her initial help, Dr June Greig-Smith and Miss Deena Cook of Butterworth-Heinemann for their expertise in processing this book through to publication in the limited time available, and above all Miss May Weller for secretarial excellence which became evident in so many ways throughout the preparation of this book.

Aires A.B. Barros D'Sa

Contributors

Roger N. Baird, BSc ChM FRCS FRCS(Ed)
Consultant Surgeon, Royal Infirmary, Bristol; Senior Clinical Lecturer in Surgery, Department of Surgery, University of Bristol

Aires A. B. Barros D'Sa, MD FRCS FRCS(Ed)
Consultant Vascular Surgeon, Vascular Surgery Unit, Royal Victoria Hospital, Belfast; Honorary Lecturer in Surgery, The Queen's University of Belfast

Jonathan D. Beard, ChM FRCS
Consultant Vascular Surgeon, Department of Surgery, Royal Hallamshire Hospital, Sheffield; Honorary Clinical Lecturer in Vascular Surgery, University of Sheffield

Peter R. F. Bell, MD FRCS
Professor of Surgery, Department of Surgery, Leicester Royal Infirmary, Leicester; Professor of Surgery and Head of Department, University of Leicester

W. Bruce Campbell, MS MRCP FRCS
Consultant in Vascular and General Surgery, Department of Surgery, Royal Devon and Exeter Hospital, Exeter

John Chamberlain, FRCS(Ed)
Consultant Surgeon, Department of Surgery, Freeman Hospital, Newcastle-upon-Tyne; Clinical Lecturer in Surgery, University of Newcastle-upon-Tyne

Anthony D. B. Chant, BA BSc MS FRCS
Consultant Vascular Surgeon, Department of Vascular Surgery, Royal South Hants Hospital, Southampton; Honorary Clinical Lecturer, University of Southampton

Charles A. C. Clyne, MS FRCS(Ed) FRCS(Eng)
Consultant Vascular and General Surgeon, Torbay Hospital, Torquay

Simon G. Darke, MS FRCS
Consultant Vascular and General Surgeon, Royal Bournemouth Hospital, Bournemouth; Honorary Lecturer, University of Southampton

John M. D. Galloway, ChM FRCS(Ed)
Consultant Surgeon, Department of Surgery, Hull Royal Infirmary, Hull

Peter L. Harris, MD FRCS
Consultant Vascular Surgeon, Vascular Surgery Unit, Broadgreen Hospital, Liverpool; Lecturer in Surgery, University of Liverpool

Michael Horrocks, MS FRCS
Consultant Surgeon, Surgical Unit, Bristol Royal Infirmary, Bristol; Honorary Lecturer in Surgery, University of Bristol

Paul Lieberman, FRCS
Consultant Surgeon, Department of Surgery, Glasgow Royal Infirmary, Glasgow

John A. Murie, MA BSc MD FRCS
Consultant Vascular Surgeon, Department of Surgery, The Royal Infirmary, Edinburgh; Honorary Senior Lecturer in Surgery, University of Edinburgh

Simon D. Parvin, MD FRCS
Consultant General and Vascular Surgeon, Department of Surgery, Royal Bournemouth Hospital, Bournemouth

P. Michael Perry, MS FRCS
Consultant Surgeon, Department of Surgery, Queen Alexandra Hospital, Portsmouth; Honorary Clinical Lecturer, University of Southampton

C. Vaughan Ruckley, ChM FRCS(Ed)
Consultant Vascular Surgeon, Vascular Surgery Unit, Royal Infirmary, Edinburgh; Reader in Surgery, University of Edinburgh

Denis C. Wilkins, MD FRCS
Consultant Vascular Surgeon, Department of Surgery, Derriford General Hospital, Plymouth

Colin C. Wilmshurst, MRCS LRCP
Associate Specialist in General and Vascular Surgery, Torbay Hospital, Torquay

John H. N. Wolfe, MS FRCS
Consultant Vascular Surgeon, Department of Vascular Surgery, St Mary's Hospital, London; Honorary Senior Lecturer, St Mary's Medical School and Royal Postgraduate Medical School, Hammersmith, London

Contents

Foreword   v

Preface   vii

List of Contributors   ix

 1 The clinical vascular laboratory – requirements and recommendations   1
   Michael Horrocks
 2 Risk factors in peripheral vascular disease and their modification   11
   Charles A. C. Clyne
 3 Carotid endarterectomy – a pragmatic viewpoint   21
   Anthony D. B. Chant
 4 Carotid body tumours – the premise of the vascular surgeon   31
   Aires A. B. Barros D'Sa
 5 Should we operate on thoracoabdominal aneurysms?   50
   John H. N. Wolfe
 6 Abdominal aortic aneurysms – a topic of enlarging interest   62
   Roger N. Baird
 7 How can we prevent complications from elective aortic surgery?   70
   W. Bruce Campbell
 8 Mesenteric ischaemia – recognition reaps rewards   85
   Paul Lieberman
 9 Renal artery disease – when should it be treated surgically?   100
   John A. Murie
10 Iliac artery occlusive disease – what is the role of surgery?   116
   Simon D. Parvin
11 Selection of patients for and assessment of femorodistal bypass   127
   Peter R. F. Bell
12 Operative techniques and adjuvant measures influencing outcome in
   femorodistal bypass   141
   Peter L. Harris
13 Vascular surgical sepsis – challenges in prevention   155
   Jonathan D. Beard and **Colin C. Wilmshurst**
14 The popliteal artery – sinister harbinger of pathology   165
   P. Michael Perry
15 The diabetic foot – how can it be saved?   177
   John Chamberlain

16 Lower limb amputation – time for critical appraisal   190
   C. Vaughan Ruckley
17 Chronic venous insufficiency – should the long saphenous vein be
   stripped?   207
   Simon G. Darke
18 Deep vein thrombosis and its sequelae – how can they be averted?   219
   John M. D. Galloway
19 How do I audit my general/vascular surgery?   233
   Denis C. Wilkins

Appendix   **248**

Index   **253**

Chapter 1

The clinical vascular laboratory – requirements and recommendations

Michael Horrocks

Clinical vascular laboratories have gradually appeared over the last 30 years and are now an established department in many hospitals. They arose originally in teaching hospitals where there was interest in non-invasive measurement of blood flow and blood pressure in patients with vascular disease. In the last decade new techniques have evolved, necessitating the purchase of very expensive equipment. With the increase of new technology and enthusiasm it becomes increasingly important to reflect on the value of these investigative techniques and to attempt to assess the cost-effectiveness of many of the procedures advocated. As long ago as 1976 the Intersociety Commission for Heart Disease Resources issued a report on medical instrumentation in peripheral vascular disease and stated that a vascular laboratory is desirable in any institution which is performing angiography of the peripheral vascular, coronary or cerebral vessels[1]. The report also emphasized the value of vascular laboratory assessment in the management of trauma patients, in those undergoing arterial reconstruction and in the care of patients suffering from venous thromboembolic disease. It was clear from that time that vascular laboratories would be required in most large hospitals but this has not come about, largely because of the failure to provide the necessary finance.

Different hospitals vary in their requirements such as their need for personnel and equipment. Where the laboratory should be sited and how it should be financed are other unanswered problems. In recent years the vast majority of young vascular surgeons who have been trained in teaching hospitals where vascular laboratories are available have become familiar with the techniques and the advantages that vascular laboratories can offer. They are therefore understandably dissatisfied on appointment to a definitive consultant post to find neither the facilities nor the funding to provide even the minimum equipment and staffing for a vascular laboratory. It is the author's opinion that this question needs to be addressed urgently so that minimum standards of non-invasive diagnostic support are available for all surgeons practising arterial reconstruction.

The purpose of the clinical vascular laboratory

The primary purposes are clinical and research. Although most laboratories provide a wide variety of diagnostic services they are also a good source of clinical research. The two are usually inseparable. Although most vascular laboratories are located at the core of a hospital there are a few which can be found in outpatient facilities or interdisciplinary clinics which, for instance are shared by diabetic physicians, neurologists and vascular surgeons. The hospital-based laboratory appears to offer the best compromise of availability and access to multiple disciplines. The primary function of the laboratory is to provide objective physiological measurements to facilitate the diagnosis of all kinds of vascular disease. Basic requirements are the ability to assess occlusive disease in the legs, to evaluate extracranial cerebrovascular disease, to diagnose deep venous thrombosis and to study vasospastic syndromes of the upper arm. Other functions may include investigation of normal structures such as veins prior to bypass and more sophisticated evaluation of mesenteric and renal blood flow. In addition there may be facilities for intraoperative blood flow measurement and for postoperative evaluation and monitoring following reconstruction[2].

In addition the vascular laboratory may give important information about the natural history of the disease which in turn could lead to a change in management policy. Vascular laboratories have taken on the responsibility of postoperative surveillance of grafts, particularly femoropopliteal and femorodistal grafts as these have a high early attrition rate and lend themselves to such a programme. Furthermore, the database acquired may be the basis of a full audit of the outpatient and inpatient functions of a unit or hospital, providing precise information on the results of surgery or demographic data as required.

A few of the more well equipped laboratories can study the pathophysiology of vascular disease and give information about blood flow in normal and diseased vessels.

Which studies?

A large number of different tests have been described for the diagnosis of vascular disease. For the sake of brevity and clarity only those which the author feels are likely to be helpful in a general vascular laboratory are considered here.

Peripheral occlusive disease of the legs

All vascular laboratories should be capable of measuring ankle pressures at rest and after exercise if required. The measurement of resting ankle pressures provides an excellent screen for patients with pain in the legs on walking and the addition of some form of stress test, usually in the form of walking on a treadmill, is ideal for identifying those patients who have a non-vascular cause for their leg pain. In the vast majority of patients this is all that is required to make the diagnosis and to confirm the severity of the disease. In those patients with rest pain or gangrene stress tests are unhelpful.

In patients where the diagnosis is less certain waveform analysis, segmental plethysmography, and segmental pressures may all be helpful in delineating the site and extent of disease. Many laboratories have set up sophisticated methods to try and quantify and localize disease but my own feeling is that the decision to proceed to angiography can be made on the basis of resting ankle pressures, distance walked and post-exercise ankle pressures where any doubt remains. In patients with rest pain or gangrene Doppler studies are often of little value as flow in the peripheral arteries of the ankle is exceedingly poor. In these cases even angiography may seriously underestimate the extent of disease, and the vascular laboratory can play a valuable role in identifying patent arteries which have minimal flow at rest. The recent introduction of pulse-generated runoff has shown that in most patients with gangrene patent vessels can be identified even when invisible on intra-arterial digital subtraction arteriography[3].

Carotid artery disease

A large number of investigations have been advocated for the diagnosis of extracranial carotid artery stenosis with a view to identifying those patients suitable for carotid endarterectomy[4]. These tests include periorbital Doppler examination, ocular plethysmography and phonoangiography[4,5]. The diagnostic technique of choice now firmly established is duplex scanning which not only gives an image of the carotid bifurcation but also gives information about the blood flow through spectral analysis[6]. In good hands duplex scanning has a sensitivity and specificity of greater than 90% in the diagnosis of extracranial carotid artery stenosis. The one area where uncertainty remains is in distinguishing an extremely tight stenosis from an occlusion. The recent introduction of colour duplex scanning has made the identification of the carotid vessels much easier and quicker but has not increased the sensitivity or specificity of the technique. Those who are familiar with duplex scanning and comfortable with simple black and white machines have found no advantage with the addition of colour. This has obvious financial implications when buying new equipment. Duplex scanning also has the ability to delineate plaque morphology which may be important in deciding on surgical treatment. Echolucent soft plaques are thought to be more dangerous than calcified smooth lesions.

Vasospastic disease

Most of the information required in the evaluation of the upper limb for vasospastic disease is provided by pressure measurements. Doppler velocimetry and digital plethysmography. The diagnosis of stenosis or the identification of embolic disease can usually be made by these techniques and patients then subjected to angiography and appropriate treatment.

Venous thromboembolic disease

The vascular laboratory should ideally have a duplex scanner for detecting deep venous thrombosis. Duplex scanning has now superseded simple Doppler velocity detectors or venous occlusion plethysmography. It has been shown to have a sensitivity and specificity for diagnosing deep vein thrombosis exceeding 90%, the only area of uncertainty being the iliac veins which are difficult to scan. In a situation where the deep veins are apparently normal and there is deep suspicion of thrombosis, venography should be performed to outline these vessels. Duplex scanning of the deep veins will probably displace routine venography in the diagnosis of leg vein thrombosis and has become the diagnostic technique of choice.

Equipment

The minimum equipment required for a vascular laboratory is a Doppler flow velocimeter and it is surprising what can be achieved with this simple item. With a pneumatic cuff and a sphygmomanometer or aneroid manometer the detection of arterial and venous flow can be combined with pressure measurements. Ankle pressure at rest can be supplemented by exercise or reactive hyperaemia to give further information. Segmental pressures give a good idea of the site of major occlusive disease and localized stenoses can be detected by the trained ear.

A simple Doppler velocimeter is also very useful in the assessment of varicose veins. Venous incompetence can easily be recognized and reflux demonstrated. Similarly, incompetent deep veins can be identified and abnormalities of deep venous flow can be noted in the presence of deep venous thrombosis. The Doppler velocimeter may also be used in the operating theatre to measure ankle pressures before operation and again, following reconstruction, to assess the efficacy of the graft. The graft itself can be insonated in the ward in order to assess patency and simple parameters such as diastolic blood flow can be estimated. If a slightly more sophisticated Doppler flow velocimeter is used directional flow, which may be useful in the extracranial arterial circulation, can be assessed with particular reference to reversed flow in the periorbital vessels. Directional Doppler is very useful for venous work, and the addition of a strip chart recorder allows a permanent record to be made of flow characteristics.

More sophisticated Doppler velocimeters may incorporate wave form analysis and sonography to give quantitative information about the wave form itself. Many of the commercially available pieces of equipment are expensive and their value in a busy vascular laboratory is questionable. Sonogram analysis has been scrutinized for over 20 years and in my opinion little of clinical value has emerged from such sophisticated technology.

Photoplethysmography has been strongly advocated as a relatively cheap and simple technique for recording digital pulses, measuring digital and penile pressures, and for studying cerebrovascular and venous reflux. While the strongest advocates are very much in favour of this technique it has not met with widespread approval.

The use of a treadmill for standardizing exercise tests has many advantages – it allows the patient to be exercised within the vascular laboratory or in the outpatient clinic and provides a reproducible stress test. Treadmills are relatively inexpensive pieces of equipment which are highly serviceable and provide a simple way of studying a large number of patients in a relatively short period of time. For patients with critical ischaemia or those who are unable to exercise because of degenerative joint disease a post-hyperaemia stress test is more appropriate. A treadmill should ideally be capable of speeds of up to 4 km/h and be inclined up to 10° to compensate for the lack of forward motion. It is also possible to add an ECG to patients being stressed on a treadmill. Segmental plethysmography, particularly air plethysmography, has been strongly advocated. It is a relatively expensive technique and gives semi-quantitative results. Its principal value is in peroperative evaluation of vascular reconstructions where it can immediately distinguish between success and failure of a reconstruction. The technique can then be repeated in the recovery area and the ward if required. It is a more sensitive and reliable method than simple ankle pressure measurement but remains a great deal more expensive.

In those laboratories where cerebrovascular disease is assessed a duplex scanner is essential for the diagnosis of extracranial carotid artery stenosis. The combination of real-time imaging (which gives information about the morphology of the arterial wall) and spectral analysis of the waveform (which gives information about the flow of blood) is unrivalled for non-invasive diagnosis of extracranial carotid disease. Considerable experience is required to produce reliable results with a duplex scanner but once this experience has been gained the technique is reliable and reproducible. The addition of colour coding has been disappointing particularly in carotid artery disease where many experts prefer to use black and white.

Other techniques such as ocular plethysmography, while advocated by many, do not approach the sensitivity of duplex scanning and add little even in the best hands.

Duplex scanners have the additional useful function of being ideal for preoperative assessment of veins before insertion of a femoropopliteal or femorodistal graft. The long saphenous vein and the short saphenous and arm veins can be assessed for patency, size, wall thickness, compliance, and therefore their suitability for use as an arterial graft. Furthermore, identification of the vein helps in planning the surgical approach and in making an accurate incision over the vein thereby averting the undermining of skin flaps and reducing wound necrosis and infection. If a vein is not available on the same leg veins can be marked on other limbs and composite long grafts can be planned before surgery. This is a particularly useful technique and one which is rapidly gaining popularity.

The identification of patent distal vessels using the pulse generated runoff apparatus is a recently developed technique which is very useful (Figure 1.1). A cuff is placed around the limb above or below the knee and rapidly inflated and deflated. Patent vessels can then be identified using a simple hand-held Doppler velocimeter. Analysis of the waveform produced can give further information about the quality of that vessel, and by tracing the signal into the foot information about the patency of the pedal arch is also obtained. Thus patients who were previously deemed inoperable because patent vessels could not be identified on angiography can now undergo reconstructive surgery.

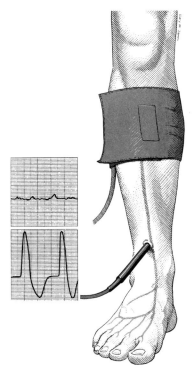

Figure 1.1 Pressure generated runoff to demonstrate patent distal vessels

The relatively high failure rate of femorodistal bypass grafts and the recognition of graft stenosis proceeding to graft occlusion has heralded an era of postoperative graft surveillance for femoropopliteal and femorodistal grafts. Many clinical vascular laboratories have advocated duplex scanning for this purpose but it has proved to be expensive, time consuming and stenoses can only be detected within the graft itself and not in the runoff vessels. A new technique of non-invasive impedance (Figure 1.2) has been investigated which is cheap, simple and appears to be an excellent screening technique for grafts at risk. A high impedance value warns the vascular surgeon that the graft may be in danger of occlusion and is an indication for urgent angiography. Other methods of graft surveillance such as ankle pressures before and after stress testing may reveal the presence of some graft stenoses but will unfortunately miss a proportion which will go on to occlude unless surgically corrected.

A computer program for use in the vascular laboratory is essential for record keeping, retrieving and reporting data. Ideally a record should be kept for statistical analysis of all the important functions of the laboratory and the system should be able to talk to the mainframe computer of the hospital. It is highly desirable that this system be linked to a vascular audit program so that all information about vascular surgical problems going through the hospital can be annexed using the vascular laboratory computer. While it is possible to use the same computer for various non-invasive devices such as spectrum analysis of Doppler signals it is probably best to have designated small computers for these individual components and to keep the main vascular laboratory computer for records and data processing. In a vascular laboratory which is involved in clinical research the same computer should be capable

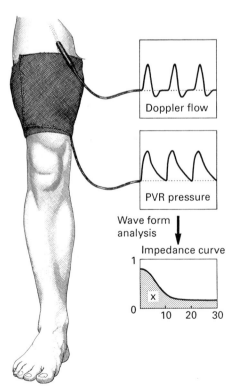

Figure 1.2   Non-invasive impedance to assess the 'at risk' femorodistal graft

Table 1.1   Desirable basic equipment for clinical vascular laboratory

---

Simple Doppler velocimeter
Pneumatic cuff and manometer
Treadmill
Dedicated computer
Duplex scanner
Pulse generated runoff equipment
Non-invasive impedance
Air plethysmography

---

of dealing with graphics programs for word processing and for analysing all the data. Ideally it should have multiple entry points with terminals in the outpatient department, the operating theatre and with the clinical secretaries in addition to the vascular laboratory.

Currently there are large numbers of manufacturers producing a huge array of instruments designed for the vascular laboratory. Before purchasing any of these the exact requirements of a vascular laboratory should be analysed and advice sought about the appropriate equipment to buy. It is possible to spend a large amount of money buying equipment, most of whose functions are not required. Careful analysis of the range of requirements can lead to an economical purchase of instruments which will fulfil all the desired functions with a minimum of wasted capital (Table 1.1). Most companies will allow short-term loans for evaluation before purchase. In a highly competitive world it pays the purchaser to be cautious before parting with any money. In addition to special instruments for measuring blood flow such basic equipment as a couch, trolleys on which to place the instruments, filing cabinets and desks for the computer and for reporting results will be required.

The couch should be one on which the patient can sit up, lie flat or be placed in the Trendelenberg position, and ideally should be of an adjustable height to allow patients to climb on and off with ease. A modern hospital outpatient couch is an ideal compromise.

Siting of the clinical vascular laboratory

While it is perfectly possible to study many patients at the bedside or in the outpatient department the ideal set up is a designated vascular laboratory. Ideally the laboratory should be sited some distance from the crowded outpatients' or inpatient facility but it must be easily accessible and conveniently placed in proximity to lifts, the minimum requirements being a waiting area, an office area, a clinical investigation area, changing rooms and toilets. The waiting area should allow room for chairs, a wheelchair and a trolley for patients who cannot be transferred in any other way. The clinical area requires a couch and sufficient room for all the instruments that have been selected and it should be possible to wheel a hospital trolley or bed into the laboratory and transfer the patient onto the couch if necessary. There should be sufficient floor space around the couch to allow easy movement of staff in and out of the room and to move equipment as required. It is preferable to have the couch away from a wall so that the patient can be approached easily from either side. If changing rooms are not available and the clinical area is shared mobile screens are essential for privacy when changing or when several patients are being studied simultaneously. There should be easy access to facilities for emergency resuscitation if required. The laboratory should be well lit, preferably by natural light, and amply supplied with electrical sockets. A sink for washing is essential and the general decor of the room should be designed to make the patient feel comfortable and at ease. Although a temperature-controlled room is ideal some simple device to keep the ambient temperature at approximately 23°C will avoid troublesome vasoconstriction. Patients may feel intimidated by large amounts of electronic equipment and instruments which are not in use ought to be kept out of sight. The office space should contain sufficient space for a desk, filing cabinet, dictaphones and other equipment for day-to-day running of the vascular laboratory. The computer can be accessed here for research purposes. In a large hospital the size of the facility should reflect the number of patients being examined each day. When two or more clinical areas are identified specialist functions can be ascribed to each room; for example one area may be used for peripheral vascular and another for carotid artery disease. In laboratories with elaborate research programmes further space will be required.

Personnel

The clinical vascular laboratory should be run by a consultant with a major interest in the diagnosis and treatment of vascular disease. In many centres, however, for historical or other reasons this arrangement does not pertain and a clinical scientist is the effective director. Whosoever runs the vascular laboratory should have a good understanding of the pathophysiology and natural history of vascular disease, and a sound knowledge of the clinical problems being investigated. An awareness of the management options available and the nature of investigations most helpful in coming to a decision as well as an appropriate sense of urgency are necessary for the more serious clinical problems. A lack of rapport or poor liaison between clinician and the laboratory staff can lead to failure. The director should have a firm grasp of the accuracy and reproducibility of all investigation and should constantly reexamine standards. This means taking an interest in the day-to-day organization of laboratory studies and bearing the responsibility for the supervision of training of staff. There should be a formalized training scheme for all staff employed in the laboratory. Vascular surgeons in training should spend some time in the vascular laboratory and should be familiar with the various techniques being used. It is advisable that surgical trainees should learn to use all the equipment themselves and thereby understand the weaknesses, difficulties and drawbacks of each technique employed.

Most consultant vascular surgeons have little enough time to supervise standards of work, training and research but it is essential that time is set aside each week for this purpose.

Training of vascular technicians and nurses

Currently in the United Kingdom there are no formalized training programmes or agreed qualifications for vascular laboratory technicians and nurses. A society of Noninvasive Vascular Technologists has been set up in the US and an examination is held to certify competence in Vascular technology. It is desirable that all full-time technicians and nurses who work in a vascular laboratory should attend a course on the physics and electronics of the equipment they use and have a good understanding of the pathophysiology of arterial disease and the problems which are being studied.

It is also highly desirable that there be an agreed examination to allow certification of competence in vascular technology.

Currently recruitment into vascular laboratories is rather haphazard and may be via a hospital physics department, nursing or by direct recruitment into the laboratory. If appropriate funding were given to vascular laboratories throughout the UK then appropriate courses and examinations could be set up, resulting in an overall improvement in standards. Currently a laboratory technician can perform up to ten examinations per day, not counting the time spent interviewing patients, preparing equipment just before a study, travelling between the laboratory and the ward, completing reports and on occasions communication with referring physicians about unexpected findings. In order to make a vascular laboratory work well at least two technicians are required to provide an overlap for holidays and courses. Additional help such as a secretary for typing and filing and a receptionist to organize patient transfer would improve the overall efficiency of the unit. If the laboratory is placed in a diagnostic services area then one receptionist may be shared between several clinical areas.

Clearly the number of patients studied and the complexity of the tests will dictate the number and qualifications of employees required. If research and development work is undertaken then the addition of a pure scientist such as a physicist or engineer would be highly desirable.

Reporting

The principal function of the laboratory will be to communicate the measured vascular data and their significance to the referring consultant. All reports may be transmitted immediately but formal reports are ideally produced by the computer and printed out for despatch to the referring physician within 24 hours. Standard forms should be developed for specific areas of study, namely lower limb assessment, carotid artery disease, venous thromboembolic disease and vasospastic disease. In addition to documenting the results of the tests the forms must record the patient's demographic data including cross-reference numbers and computer numbers for the vascular unit.

Other data may be included such as medical history, physical signs and relevant medication. It is essential that a copy of all the reports be retained within the vascular laboratory, and preferably recorded on the laboratory computer. All reports should be checked before despatch from the laboratory to make sure that the data are correct and complete. Complex reports such as those for cerebrovascular disease should ideally be accompanied by a photocopy of the scan obtained and some comment as to the confidence levels achieved by the operating technician. It has been my experience that since the introduction of confidence levels the reliability of scans has improved considerably, allowing the referring clinician more insight into the value of the scan before proceeding to invasive investigations.

It is important that all information despatched from the clinical vascular laboratory is in a form that the referring physician can understand. It is desirable that a part of the form be set aside for conclusions in which the findings of the investigations and recommendations for further investigation are summarized. It is possible that the laboratory can provide a service by offering carefully worded opinions as to whether further investigation is indicated or, for instance, if pain in a foot is likely to be vascular in origin or not. Clearly this depends to an extent on the experience of the technicians involved, but with careful monitoring this can be a very useful additional function of the laboratory.

Data storage

All data recorded in the clinical vascular laboratory should be kept in a form allowing easy retrieval. All reports should be filed under the patient's name and cross-reference according to the hospital number, the vascular studies number and the principal diagnosis. A well-designed computer system would allow correlations to be made and statistical analyses to be performed. It is helpful to keep the hard copy records of the salient features of the report as a back-up, particular for medicolegal reasons.

Finance

Under the present financial arrangements in the UK no financial provisions exist for the establishment of clinical vascular laboratories. The practice of peripheral vascular surgery is increasingly dependent on non-invasive information and those of us fortunate enough to have a clinical vascular laboratory realize how much we rely on the technological backup in the management of our patients. The time has come for proper recognition of this essential service in the hospital management structure and clinical laboratories under the directorship of vascular surgeons should be established in all major hospitals where peripheral vascular surgery is undertaken. Just as in the past it was impossible to practise vascular surgery without vascular radiology I believe the time has come to state unequivocally that we cannot practise vascular surgery without the backup of a clinical vascular laboratory.

References

1. Bergan, J. J., Darling, R. C., De Wolfe, V. G., Raines, J. K., Strandnese, D. E. Jnr. and Yao, J. S. T. (1976) Report of the Inter-Society Commission of Heart Disease Resources. Medical Instrumentation in Peripheral Vascular Disease Circulation. S4, A–1
2. Bergan, J. J. and Yao, J. S. T. (1980) Invited Overview. Role of the Vascular Laboratory. *Surgery*, **88**, 9
3. Scott, D. J. A., Beard, J., Farmilo, R. W., Poskitt, K. R., Evans, J. M., Skidmore, R. and Horrocks, M. (1988) Non-invasive assessment of calf vessels by pressure generated run off – (PGR). *Br. J. Radiol.*, **61**, 543–544
4. Horrocks, M., Rocberts, V. C. and Cotton, L. T. (1980) *Diagnosis and monitoring in arterial surgery.* (eds. Woodcock and Baird) John Wright, Bristol, pp. 88–90
5. Baker, J. D., Barker, W. F. and Machlader, H. I. (1978) Ocular pneumophlethysmography in the evaluation of carotid stenosis. *Am. J. Surg.*, **136**, 206
6. Blackshear, W. M., Phillips, D. J., Thiele, B. L., Hirsch, J. H., Chikos, P. M. *et al.* (1979) Detection of carotid occlusive disease by ultrasound imaging and pulsed Doppler spectrum analysis. *Surgery*, **86**, 698
7. Wyatt, M. G., Tennant, W. G., Baird, R. N. and Horrocks, M. (1991) Impedence analysis to identify the 'at-risk' femoro-distal vein graft. *J. Vasc. Surg.* (in press)
8. Strandness, D. E. Jr. (1979) The use and abuse of the vascular laboratory. *Surg. Clin. N. Am.*, **59**, 707

Chapter 2

Risk factors in peripheral vascular disease and their modification

Charles A. C. Clyne

As all vascular surgeons are aware, the separation of occlusive peripheral vascular disease from vascular disease occurring in the coronary vessels and the carotid arteries is frequently impossible. Hence any dissertation on the risk factors for peripheral vascular disease (PVD) necessarily embraces studies not always dedicated to the peripheral distribution of atheroma, but more frequently to coronary heart disease (CHD). An assumption must be made then that in general terms PVD and CHD coexist more often than not and that separation of empirical data regarding degree of risk is not possible (see Figure 2.1). Patients with intermittent claudication (IC) are up to four times more likely to have CHD and about half will die from a heart attack, whereas patients with CHD have at least a five-fold risk of developing IC[1].

The Framingham study

Without doubt the most useful database available to the current generation of physicians and surgeons regarding the origins of vascular disease derives from the longitudinal prospective study set up in 1949 by the National Heart Institute in Framingham, Massachussetts. The study still continues[2–4], and the risk factors for the development of PVD have become clear (see Table 2.1).

Age, systolic blood pressure, cigarette smoking, obesity, serum cholesterol and blood sugar all have a significant effect. Diabetes *per se* exerted a profound influence on the development of IC although measurement of casual blood sugars and their relationship to IC was not significant.

Most other studies on risk factors for PVD are cross-sectional in design and give slightly differing weight to individual variables, but essentially they support the results from Framingham. Cross-sectional studies will tend to suffer from case selection and bias from such occurrences as early death from both related and unrelated cases, i.e. CHD mortality during evolving PVD development or lung cancer. The major risk factors however can be discussed individually against this background.

Age and sex

The male predominance of symptomatic PVD persists at all ages but latterly a great increase in prevalence in females at and beyond the menopause has appeared. Indeed, the mortality from CHD in females approaches that of the male around the age of 60,

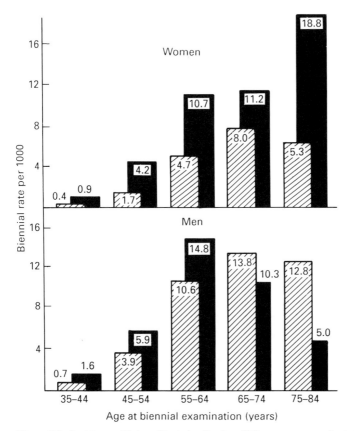

Figure 2.1   Incidence of intermittent claudication (IC) versus uncomplicated angina pectoris. (Data from 26-year follow-up of the Framingham study.) ■, Angina; ▨, IC

and becomes equal by the age of 80[5]. In the Framingham study uncomplicated angina in females beyond the age of 75 had doubled or trebled in comparison with that in males[3]. The assumption from these data is that endogenous oestrogens protect the pre-menopausal female from CHD and PVD, but no clear message from the research to date exists on the effects of exogenous oestrogen administration to the ageing female[6]. The Framingham study showed an increased risk of CHD amongst oestrogen users after the menopause, especially smokers[7,8], whereas a back-to-back publication (reference 8 in the same journal) concludes that post-menopausal oestrogen administration reduces the risk of severe CHD[9]! Exogenous oestrogen given to men who appear at risk after myocardial infarction does, however, give rise to increased cardiovascular mortality and therefore cannot be regarded as protective[10]. The situation is complicated by other factors, such as the apparent protective effect from the administration of oestrogens, which improve the serum lipid profile by lowering low-density lipoprotein cholesterol and raising the protective high-density lipoprotein cholesterol[11,12].

Age and sex therefore should probably be regarded as unmodifiable risk factors, but as the development of atherosclerosis is multifactorial there is still more to be learnt. The epidemiology of peripheral vascular disease shows similar prevalence in

Table 2.1 Net effect and ranking of risk factors for intermittent claudication

| | Multivariate standardized regression coefficient | |
	Men	Women
Age	0.410***	0.271*
Systolic pressure	0.317***	0.478***
Cigarettes	0.295**	0.379***
Relative weight	−0.199*	0.038†
Serum cholesterol	0.194**	0.185**
Blood sugar	0.184**	0.189**
Vital capacity	−0.183*	−0.271**
Hematocrit	0.182*	0.125†
Heart rate	−0.066†	−0.127†
ECG-IVB	0.062†	−0.030†
ECG-LVH	−0.007†	0.068†
Number of cases	152	103

Data from 26-year follow-up of the Framingham study; subjects aged 35–84 years.
† not significant
*   ** $P < 0.01$ ***$P < 0.001$

the western world – perhaps with the exception of rural Finland[13] – but the separation of single risk factors such as age is fraught with problems. For instance, systolic and diastolic blood pressures relate to the presence of vascular disease for both coronary and peripheral distribution; this in itself is age related and may simply be no more than an association[14].

Cigarette smoking

It must now be beyond dispute that cigarette smoking is the single most preventable cause of PVD[15]. From the Framingham study it is suggested that cigarettes are third only to age and systolic pressure in the ranking of risk factors for intermittent claudication, the risk apparently being relatively greater for women[3]. In the Oxford study[14] cigarette smoking was associated with a higher relative risk than any other factor studied in the development of IC. It is probable also that risk tends to rise with the number of cigarettes smoked, although this may be a simplification and risk may well relate more accurately to carbon monoxide intake (which can only be monitored by appropriate testing)[15,16]. Much has been written about the association of smoking and arterial disease and there are many ways in which smoking appears to harm arteries although the ultimate noxious factor still remains unidentified – it is probable that this too is multifactorial[17]. Smoking exerts its influence on the blood cells, the blood serum and the blood vessel walls – particularly the vascular endothelium, which may become more permeable and allow increased deposition of fibrinogen and lipids in the subintimal layers in response to smoking damage[18]. It is likely that smoking does not affect every individual to the same degree and that the vessel wall response to the acute changes resulting from smoking may also differ between individuals[19]. Smoking continues to exert its noxious effects on reconstructive operations in patients with PVD and manifests itself as reduced graft patency at follow-up in those who continue to smoke. This occurs in both autologous and prosthetic reconstructions and probably represents disease progression in general as well as specific effects on the dynamics of graft performance[20,21]. What, then, are the effects of cessation of smoking? Almost without exception the data reported confirm the benefits on mortality, amputation and claudication distance[22] of giving up smoking. As most of those with PVD will succumb to CHD, cessation of smoking appears to improve life expectancy of this group, as seen in the Framingham study, where it is believed that the improvement in cardiovascular risk factors in the male cohorts studied was associated with reductions in blood cholesterol, hypertension and smoking[4]. A prevalence of smoking of 56% in the 1950 cohort dropped to 34% in the 1970 group. Similar cardiovascular data suggest that the increased risk of a first myocardial infarction in women also declines within 2–3 years after stopping smoking[23].

The effect on mortality of stopping smoking appears then to be great – Jonason showed a reduction in mortality from 27% to 12% in those patients with IC who managed to give up[24]. The classic study of Juergens et al.[25] showed the total avoidance of amputation in a series of patients with IC from the Mayo Clinic who gave up smoking, but such figures have never been repeated.

Stopping smoking also appears to improve claudication distance but is so frequently combined with other risk factor modifications such as exercise and diet that it is difficult to assign a specific figure to the improvement to be expected[26]. One problem is the poor compliance of those patients asked to give up smoking in spite of the dire warnings given to them about limb loss etc.[27]. Probably less than 30% of patients actually do give up smoking when instructed so to do by their physicians[28], and this low incidence, combined with a certain degree of deception by the patients, makes accurate data collection on the effects of smoking cessation very difficult[16].

There can be no dispute however that death from CHD is 3 times more common in men with IC than in men without[29], and that continued smoking is associated with an adverse prognosis in all patients with IC[26].

Diabetes

The Framingham study confirmed clinical experience that diabetes was a powerful risk factor for the development of PVD (see Table 2.1), and every indicator of impaired glucose tolerance including elevated blood sugar and glycosuria was associated with increased risk[3] (see Table 2.2). In spite of this resounding evidence

Table 2.2   Risk of intermittent claudication by indicators of glucose intolerance

	Glucose intolerance		Glycosuria status		Hyperglycaemia status	
Abnormality	Men	Women	Men	Women	Men	Women
Absent	6.4	3.0	6.8	3.3	5.5	3.1
Present	15.1	11.9	24.0	28.5	10.0	4.9
Risk ratio	2.4*	4.0*	3.5*	8.6*	1.8*	1.6*

Data from 26-year follow-up of the Framingham Study; subjects aged 35–84 years. Values are given as the age-adjusted two-year rate per 1000.
   * $P < 0.001$

there is still no answer to the question 'does good control of blood sugar lessen the macrovascular complication of diabetes?' The answer to this question should be forthcoming in this decade when two longitudinal studies (The UK Prospective Diabetes Study and The Diabetes Control and Complications Trial), commenced several years ago, will report.

Intermittent claudication is four times more common in the diabetic patient than in comparable patients without diabetes[30,31], and the risk of developing gangrene and undergoing amputation is also increased[32,33]. A prevalence rate of 15.9% of macrovascular disease in diabetes has been reported[34], and its distribution has been widely researched, with a tendency to more calcification[8] and more distal disease than in the non-diabetic[32,35]. Intriguingly, there is no answer to the question of the importance of the role of the microcirculation in the development of vascular complications in the foot[36,37], although microvascular disease elsewhere appears to be decreased when diabetic control is good[38].

Cross-sectional data confirm the increased prevalence of vascular disease in diabetics[39], but it is only the longitudinal studies such as Framingham, Whitehall[40], and Basle[41] that attempt to identify specific risk factors associated with glucose intolerance, and the results are confusing. Whether the risk factor can be assessed by fasting blood glucose, postprandial hyperglycaemia or longer term control, is still controversial[42,43]. It has even been suggested that insulin itself and hyperinsulinism (seen in some types of diabetes) may be atherogenic[44]! There is also evidence that, even in those patients without overt diabetes, some form of glucose intolerance may be present and increase the likelihood of developing PVD[45,46].

Whatever the pathogenesis even at the time of initial diagnosis most non-insulin dependent diabetics already have apparent PVD[47], and those with retinopathy as well as a 'diabetic foot' at presentation (the 'eye-foot' syndrome) have a particularly poor prognosis for life and limb[48]. Diabetics have a higher incidence of premature death, gangrene and rest pain than their non-diabetic colleagues with PVD, and a higher frequency of aorto-iliac and multiple stenoses[30,49].

Lipids and cholesterol

Probably the most fruitful and rewarding area of research in the management of vascular disease lies in the understanding and modifying of blood lipids and cholesterol. In the Framingham study total serum cholesterol as a risk factor ranked ahead of blood sugar in men with claudication and just behind blood sugar in women (see Table 2.2). What has also become clear since Framingham is that total cholesterol itself may be an inadequate marker for the development of cardiovascular disease, and that once broken into high-density lipoprotein (HDL) and low-density lipoprotein (LDL) fractions, risk factors become more marked[3,50]. There is now general acceptance that an inverse relationship exists between HDL levels and the development of PVD, i.e. raised HDL may protect against PVD, and indeed may determine both the site and severity of that disease[51–54]. Those with the lowest HDL seemed to have the most stenoses. The ratio of HDL cholesterol to the total cholesterol has also been shown to relate to PVD[55], and also to vascular disease at other key sites[56]. Cholesterol levels, like other risk factors, do not stand alone however and the complex relationship between lipids, diabetes and vascular disease is well reviewed elsewhere[56,57]. Smoking reduces HDL levels[56,58,59], and reasonably strenuous exercise appears to raise HDL[60].

Hypertriglyceridaemia presents an uncertain risk factor for patients with PVD[51], and although the perceived wisdom suggests that it is important, longitudinal studies supporting this hypothesis are lacking[13], although the link with PVD seems stronger than that with CHD[1].

A full assessment of lipid status then is mandatory, and new markers of the risk of vascular disease are emerging. The classification of primary hyperlipidaemias is still valuable[57] as described by Fredrickson, but further analysis of the LDL structure reveals a genetically determined atherogenic marker, lipoprotein (a), which carries a strong independent risk factor for CHD in patients with familial hypercholesterolaemia, which affects native vessels and coronary artery vein grafts[61,62]. Its effect on PVD is as yet unknown.

Haematological factors

There exists a body of research into the effects of the number and nature of red blood cells, platelets, and various constituents of serum such as viscosity and fibrinogen that relate to the presence of PVD. After two decades however it remains totally unclear whether they are simply disease markers or whether they operate separately as risk factors. In general it is believed that they arise secondarily to primary risk factors such as smoking and the effects of the disease process itself[13,63] and any treatment of them appears to be of little importance.

Modification of risk factors

Faced with this information on the aetiology of PVD can the surgeon advise a patient in any useful way to modify his or her lifestyle? The answer, based on less definitive information than most realize, is probably 'yes'.

First, patients must choose their parents wisely to avoid hypercholesterolaemia, obesity, hypertension and diabetes. Atherosclerosis originates in childhood and risk modifications should begin then[64]. One should also avoid being male and growing old. Women should probably avoid the pill and an early menopause, and in some cases take hormone replacement therapy[6,65,66]. Hypertension should be treated for, in addition to being a risk factor for the development of IC, it is a significant cause of mortality in any patient with vascular disease due to stroke and CHD[3].

Secondly, one should attempt to correct any metabolic defects and their secondary effects. Obesity may well relate to diet, or possibly diabetes, and empirically these should be treated and screened for where possible, although as already stated the development of macrovascular complications in diabetes has not yet been firmly linked to tight blood sugar control. The most fruitful area for metabolic screening (and possibly PVD prevention, control and possibly regression) may be in the management of hyperlipidaemia[65]. All patients at presentation should have their fasting blood lipids including triglycerides and HDL fully assessed[67], but clearly common sense should be exercised in the management of the elderly frail patient with irreversible PVD. The European Atherosclerosis Society has issued a clear statement on the recognition and management of hyperlipidaemia[68] which includes screening of the patient's family where necessary. The implications of their recommendations are important, time-consuming, and will require personnel and financial investment which will be best achieved in a dedicated Lipid Clinic where accurate assessment of a patient's lipids and diet can be followed by correct advice and drugs where necessary. Most hyperlipidaemic states can be treated in this way and the apparent reduction in cardiovascular risk is beginning to show its effect[4]. Evidence for reduction in peripheral atherosclerosis is also accruing; firm control of hyperlipidaemic states appears to prevent the angiographic progression of disease, and in some cases gives rise to documented cases of regression[69–71]. It may, then, be possible to undo some of the cardiovascular damage resulting from hyperlipidaemia[72].

Thirdly, we should advise our patients with vascular disease to stop smoking – indeed we should probably expend more time, energy and money in preventing our children from ever smoking at all, because for the most part cessation of smoking in the patient with advanced symptomatic PVD is, for practical purposes, too late. At best, according to one much quoted paper, they may avoid amputation by stopping smoking, at worst they may avoid dying of a myocardial infarct[24,25,26].

Finally, what other areas should be explored? Exercise benefits both the psyche and the physical and metabolic status of the patient with moderate PVD and so should be positively encouraged. Many of the antiplatelet trials carried out in PVD show beneficial trends, possibly by risk-factor modifications in the long term, and further prostaglandin research may yield useful data[73]. It is however only by clearer documentation of the natural outcome of PVD[74], preferably using longitudinal studies (such as Framingham), and the subsequent use of those data, that adequately funded population-based education will make any impact on the reduction of cardiovascular mortality[75].

References

1. Foukes, F. G. R. (1989) Aetiology of peripheral atherosclerosis. *Brit. Med. J.*, **298**, 405–406
2. Kannel, W. B., Skinner, J. T., Schwartz, M. J. and Shurtleff, D. (1970) Intermittent claudication: incidence in the Framingham Study. *Circulation*, **XLI**, 875–883
3. Kannel, W. B. and McGee, D. L. (1985) Update on some epidemiologic features of intermittent claudication: the Framingham Study. *J Am. Ger. Soc.*, **33**, 13–18
4. Sytkowski, P. A., Kannel, W. B. and D'Agostino, R. B. (1990) Changes in risk factors and the decline in mortality from cardiovascular disease: The Framingham Heart Study. *New Engl. J. Med.*, **322**, 1635–1641
5. Ryan, K. J. (1976) Oestrogens and Atherosclerosis. *Clin. Obs. Gynaecol.*, **19**, 805–825
6. Huppert, L. C. (1987) Hormonal replacement therapy. *Med. Clin. N. Am.*, **71**, 23–39
7. Gordon, T., Kannel, W. B., Hjortland, M. C. and McNamara, P. M. (1978) Menopause and coronary heart disease: The Framingham Study. *Ann. Int. Med.*, **89**, 157–161
8. Wilson, P. W. F., Garrison, R. J. and Castelli W. P. (1985) Post-menopausal oestrogen use, cigarette smoking and cardiovascular morbidity in women over 50: The Framingham Study. *New Eng. J. Med.*, **313**, 1038–1043
9. Stampfer, M. J., Willett, W. C., Colditz, G. A., Rosner, B., Speizer, F. E. and Hennekens, C. H. (1985) A prospective study of post-menopausal oestrogen therapy and coronary heart disease. *New Eng. J. Med.*, **313**, 1044–1049
10. The Coronary Drug Project Research Group (1970) The Coronary Drug Project: initial findings leading to modifications of its research protocol. *J. Am. Med. Ass.*, **214**, 1303–1313
11. Miller, G. J. and Miller, N. E. (1975) Plasma high-density lipoprotein concentration and the development of ischaemic heart disease. *Lancet*, **i**, 16–19
12. Gordon, T., Castelli, W. P., Hjortland, M. C., Kannel, W. B. and Dawber, T. R. (1977) High density lipoprotein as a protective factor against coronary heart disease: The Framingham Study. *Am. J. Med.*, **62**, 707–714
13. Foukes, F. G. R. (1988) Epidemiology of atherosclerotic arterial disease in the lower limbs. *Eur. J Vasc. Surg.*, **2**, 283–291

14. Hughson, W. G., Mann, J. I. and Garrod, A. (1978) Intermittent Claudication: Prevalence and risk factors. *Br. Med. J.*, **1**, 1379–1381
15. Lord, J. W. (1965) Cigarette smoking and peripheral atherosclerotic occlusive disease. *J. Am. Med. Ass.*, **191**, 249–251
16. Clyne, C. A. C., Arch, P. J., Carpenter, D., Webster, J. H. H. and Chant, A. D. B. (1982) Smoking, ignorance and peripheral vascular disease. *Arch. Surg.*, **117**, 1062–1065
17. Greenhalgh, R. M. (ed.) 1981 *Smoking and arterial Disease*. Pitman Medical
18. Allen, D. R., Browse, N. L., Rutt, D. L., Butler, L. and Fletcher, C. (1988) The effect of cigarette smoke, nicotine and carbon monoxide on the permeability of the arterial wall. *J. Vasc. Surg.*, **7**, 139–152
19. Lusby, R. J., Bauminger, B., Woodcock, J. P., Skidmore, R. and Baird, R. N. (1981) Cigarette Smoking: acute main and small vessel haemodynamic responses in patients with arterial disease. *Am J. Surg.*, **142**, 169–173
20. Myers, K. A., King, R. B., Scott, D. F., Johnson, N. and Morris, P. J. (1978) The effect of smoking on the late patency of arterial reconstructions in the legs. *Brit. J. Surg.*, **65**, 267–271
21. Wiseman, S., Powell, J., Greenhalgh, R. M., McCollum, C., Kenchington, G. *et al.* (1990) The influence of smoking and plasma factors on prosthetic graft patency. *Eur. J. Vasc. Surg.*, **4**, 57–61
22. Porter, J. M. (1989) Basic data underlying decision making in clinical vascular surgery. *Ann. Vasc. Surg.*, **3**, 273–277
23. Rosenberg, L., Palmer, J. R. and Shapiro, S. (1990) Decline in the risk of myocardial infarction among women who stop smoking. *New Eng. J. Med.*, **322**, 213–217
24. Jonason, T. and Bergstrom, R. (1987) Cessation of smoking in patients with intermittent claudication: effects on the risk of peripheral vascular complications, myocardial infarction and mortality. *Acta Med. Scand.*, **221**, 253–260
25. Juergens, T. L., Barker, N. W. and Hines, E. A. (1960) Arteriosclerosis obliterans: review of 520 cases with special references to pathogenic and prognostic factors. *Circulation*, **21**, 188–195
26. Hughson, W. G., Mann, J. I., Tibbs, D. J., Wood, H. F. and Walton, I. (1978) Intermittent claudication: factors determining outcome. *Br. Med. J.*, **1**, 1377–1379
27. Jelnes, R., Gaardsting, O., Jensen, K. H., Baekgaard, N., Tonnesen, K. H. and Schoroeder, T. (1986) Fate in intermittent claudication: outcome and risk factors. *Br. Med. J.*, **293**, 1137–1140
28. Wilson, S. E., Schwartz, I., Williams, R. A. and Owens, M. L. (1980) Occlusion of the superficial femoral artery: what happens without operation. *Am. J. Surg.*, **140**, 112–118
29. Reunanen, A., Takkunen, H. and Aromaa, A. (1982) Prevalence of intermittent claudication and its effect on mortality. *Acta Med. Scand.*, **211**, 249–256
30. Kannel, W. B. and McGee, D. L. (1979) Diabetes and cardiovascular risk factors: The Framingham Study. *Circulation*, **59**, 8–13
31. Kannel, W. B. and McGee, D. L. (1979) Diabetes and cardiovascular disease: The Framingham Study. *J. Am. Med Ass.*, **241**, 2035–2038
32. Strandness, D. E., Priest, R. E. and Gibbons, G. E. (1964) Combined clinical and pathologic study of diabetic and non-diabetic peripheral arterial disease. *Diabetes*, **13**, 366–372
33. Most, R. S. and Sinnock, P. (1983) The epidemiology of lower extremity amputation in diabetic individuals. *Diabetes Care*, **6**, 87–91
34. Janku, H. U., Standl, E. and Mehnert, H. (1980) Peripheral vascular disease in diabetes mellitus and its relationship to cardiovascular risk factors: screening with doppler ultrasound technique. *Diabetes Care*, **3**, 207–212
35. Ferrier, T. M. (1967) Comparative study of arterial disease in amputated lower limbs from diabetes and non-diabetics. *Med. J. Aust.*, **1**, 5–11
36. Tooke, J. E. (1987) The Microcirculation in diabetes. *Diabetic Med.*, **4**, 189–196
37. Logerfo, F. W. and Coffman, J. D. (1984) Vascular and microvascular disease of the foot in diabetics. *New Eng. J. Med.*, **311**, 1615–1619
38. Godine, J. E. (1988) The relationship between metabolic control and vascular complications of diabetic mellitus. *Med. Clin. N. Am.*, **72**, 1271–1284
39. Paisey, R. B., Arredondo, G., Villalobos, A., Lozano, O., Guevara, L. and Kelly, S. (1984) Associations of differing dietary, metabolic and clinical risk factors with macrovascular complications of diabetes. *Diabetes Care*, **7**, 421–427
40. Fuller, J. H., Shipley, M. J., Rose, G., Jarret, R. J. and Keen, H. (1980) Coronary heart disease and impaired glucose tolerance: The Whitehall Study. *Lancet*, **i**, 1373–1376
41. Da Silva, A., Leo, K. W., Ziegler, H. W., Nissen, C. and Schweizer, W. (1979) The Basle Longitudinal Study: report on the relation of initial glucose level to baseline ECG abnormalities, peripheral artery disease, and subsequent mortality. *J. Chron. Dis.*, **32**, 797–803

42. Keen, H. and Ashton, C. E. (1989) Mechanisms of excess cardiovascular mortality in diabetes. *Postgrad. Med. J.*, **65** (suppl. 1), S26–S29
43. Fuller, J. H. and Shipley, M. J. (1989) Hyperglycaemia as a cardiovascular risk factor. *Postgrad. Med. J.*, **65** (suppl. 1), S30–S32
44. Jarrett, R. J. (1988) Is insulin atherogenic? *Diabetologia*, **31**, 71–75
45. Kingsbury, K. J. (1966) The relationship between glucose tolerance and atherosclerotic vascular disease. *Lancet*, **ii**, 1374–1379
46. Clyne, C. A. C., Shandall, A., Webster, J. H. H. and Chant, A. D. B. (1980) Glycosylated Haemoglobin in non-diabetic peripheral vascular disease. *J. Cardiovasc. Surg.*, **21**, 578–580
47. Keen, H., Rose, G., Pyke, D. A., Boyns, D., Chlouverakis, C. and Mistry, S. (1965) Blood sugar and arterial disease. *Lancet*, **ii**, 505–508
48. Walsh, C. H., Fitzgerald, M. G., Soler, N. G. and Malins, J. M. (1975) Association of foot lesions with retinopathy in patients with newly diagnosed diabetes. *Lancet*, **i**, 878–880
49. Jonason, T. and Ringqvist, I. (1985) Diabetes mellitus and intermittent claudication. *Acta Med. Scand.*, **218**, 217–221.
50. Gordon, T., Kannel, W. B., Castelli, W. P. and Dawber, T. R. (1981) Lipoproteins, cardiovascular disease and death. *Arch. Int. Med.*, **141**, 1128–1131
51. Bradby, G. V. H., Valente, A. J. and Walton, K. W. (1978) Serum high density lipoproteins in peripheral vascular disease. *Lancet*, **ii**, 1271–1274
52. Horby, J., Grande, P., Vestergaard, A. and Grauholt, A. M. (1989) High-density lipoprotein cholesterol and arteriography in intermittent claudication. *Eur. J. Vasc. Surg.*, **3**, 333–337
53. Vogelberg, K. H., Berchtold, P., Berger, H., Gries, F. A., Klinger, H. *et al.* (1975) Primary hyperlipoproteinaemias as risk factors in peripheral artery disease documented by arteriography. *Atherosclerosis*, **22**, 271–285
54. Schneider, J. (1980) High-density lipoproteins and peripheral vascular disease in octo and nonagenerians. *J. Am. Ger. Soc.*, **28**, 215–219
55. Trayner, I. M., Mannarino, E., Clyne, C. A. C. and Thompson, G. R. (1980) Serum lipids and high density lipoprotein cholesterol in peripheral vascular disease. *Br. J. Surg.*, **67**, 497–499
56. Bihari-Varga, M., Szekely, J. and Gruber, E. (1981) Plasma high density lipoproteins in coronary, cerebral and peripheral vascular disease. *Atherosclerosis*, **40**, 337–345
57. Betteridge, D. J. (1989) Lipids, diabetes and vascular disease: the time to act. *Diabetes Med.*, **6**, 195–218
58. Garrison, R. J., Kannel, W. B., Feinleib, M. *et al.* (1979) Cigarette smoking and HDL cholesterol: The Framingham Offspring Study. *Atherosclerosis*, **30**, 17–25
59. Berg, K., Borrensen, A. L. and Dahlen, G. (1979) Effect of smoking on serum levels of HDL apoproteins. *Atherosclerosis*, **34**, 339–344
60. Enger, S. C., Herbjornsen, K., Erikssen, J. and Fretland, A. (1977) High-density lipoproteins (HDL) and physical activity – the influence of physical exercise, age and smoking on HDL-cholesterol and the HDL/total cholesterol ratio. *Scand. J. Clin. Lab. Invest.*, **37**, 251–255
61. Litermann, G. (1989) The mysteries of lipoprotein (a). *Science*, **246**, 904–910
62. Seed, M., Hoppichler, F., Reaveley, D. *et al* (1990) Relation of serum lipoprotein(a) concentrations and apolipoprotein(a) phenotype to coronary heart disease in patients with familial hypercholesterolaemia. *New Eng. J. Med.*, **322**, 1494–1499
63. Dormandy, J., Hoare, E., Colley, J., Arrowsmith, D. E. and Dormandy, T. L. (1975) Clinical, haemodynamic, rheological and biochemical findings in 126 patients with intermittent claudication. *Br. Med. J.*, **4**, 576–581
64. Evans, G. R. and Taylor, K. G. (1988) The paediatric origins of atherosclerosis. *Br. J. Hosp. Med.*, **39**, 132–137
65. Thompson, G. R. (1989) Current management of hyperlipidaemia. *Br. J. Hosp. Med.*, **42**, 268–274
66. Meerloo, J. M. and Billimoria, J. D. (1979) High density lipoprotein choleterol levels in peripheral vascular disease and in women on oral contraception. *Atherosclerosis*, **33**, 267–269
67. Neil, H. A. W., Mant, D., Jones, L., Morgan, B. and Mann, J. I. (1990) Lipid screening: is it enough to measure total cholesterol concentration? *Br. Med. J.*, **301**, 584–587
68. Study Group, European Atherosclerosis Society (1988) The recognition and management of hyperlipidaemia in adults: a policy statement of the European Atherosclerosis Society. *Eur. Heart J.*, **9**, 571–600
69. Malinow, M. R. (1984) Regression of atherosclerosis in humans. In *Recent Advances in Cardiology, 9*, (ed. D. J. Rowlands). Churchill Livingstone, pp. 227–239
70. Duffield, R. G. M., Miller, N. E., Brunt, J. N. E., Lewis, B., Jamieson, C. W. and Colchester, A. C. F.

(1983) Treatment of hyperlipidaemia retards progression of symptomatic femoral atherosclerosis. *Lancet*, **ii**, 639–642

71. Glueck, C. J. (1986) Role of risk factor management in progression and regression of coronary and femoral artery atherosclerosis. *Am. J. Cardiol.*, **57**, 35G–41G

72. Thompson, G. R. (1989) Lipid lowering therapy and its effect on atherosclerosis. *Postgrad. Med. J.*, **65** (suppl. 1), S22–S25

73. Anti-Platelet Trialists Collaboration. (1990) Second meeting. Christ Church, Oxford, U.K. March 23–25

74. Lassila, R., Lepantalo, M. and Lindfors O. (1986) Peripheral arterial disease—natural outcome. *Acta Med. Scand*, **220**, 295–301

75. Leeder, S. and Gliksmam, M. (1990) Prospects for preventing heart disease. *Br Med. J.*, **301**, 1004–1005

Chapter 3

Carotid endarterectomy – a pragmatic viewpoint

Anthony D. B. Chant

Introduction

As most strokes are associated with atherosclerosis or embolism, it would seem to follow that surgical intervention has a large part to play in stroke prevention. Sadly for those of us who believe this, the case has yet to be proved, despite the fact that the first successful carotid artery endarterectomy by Eastcott, Pickering and Robb was described nearly 30 years ago[1]. Even more sadly, because of the manner in which our understanding has increased, it seems likely that the role of the operation in stroke prevention may well remain obscure for several more years to come!

Knowledge about any subject comes from three main sources. Carotid endarterectomy illustrates these *par excellence*: knowledge by argument from first principles (so called *a priori* knowledge); knowledge by experiments (empirical) and so-called pragmatic knowledge (you do it because it works). Our European colleagues tend to value the first approach highly. Their argument proceeds thus . . . we were born with two patent carotids, although we have a fail-safe mechanism in the form of the circle of Willis and two vertebrals, nevertheless it is important to maintain all arteries patent if at all possible. The British, in best Lockean fashion, favour the empirical approach – we look for a comparative or controlled trial and (as will be argued later) hope, somewhat naively, that the variables in the various groups will in a fortuitous manner balance out, allowing the prime question to be answered. The final form of knowledge, characterized in carotid surgery by our American colleagues is pragmatic. Their argument runs . . . if a carotid endarterectomy can be done at low risk and if it works (i.e. stops TIAs and possibly prevents strokes), then do it. For the benefit of non-vascular specialists reading this chapter, and especially for the benefit of surgical trainees, I admit to this pragmatic approach which therefore colours my views on the operation. However, I hasten to add that reference *will* be made to those who disagree!

In the first section I review the theoretical background to the operation together with some of the difficulties which have to be overcome in successfully proving the operation's efficiency. The next section summarizes the results of some recent series and trials including one from our own Joint Vascular Research Group (JVRG UK). The final section concentrates on the logistics and the technical aspects of the operation.

Theoretical rationale for endarterectomy

Until recently, platelet emboli were thought to be the main source of neurological damage. Thus, the ulcerated plaque in Figure 3.1 could produce the corresponding multi infarct X-ray illustrated in Figure 3.2. This concentration on the classical trilogy of unihemispheric problems, plaque and emboli has blinkered much of the thinking

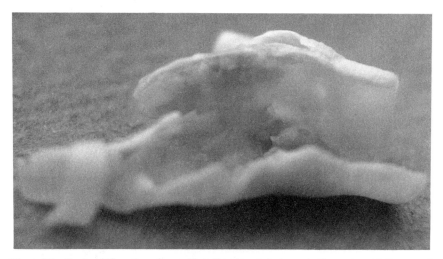

Figure 3.1   Typical bifurcation plaque. Note the ulcerated plaque in the centre and the smooth break-off point obtained in the internal carotid artery. (Picture by D. Gyftocostas)

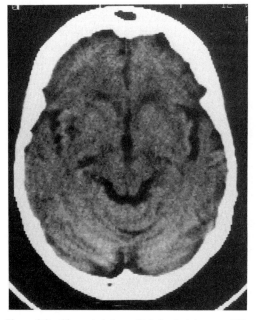

Figure 3.2   Characteristic multi-infarct picture on CT scan often associated with ulcerated plaques. (Courtesy of Dr. P. Cooke)

regarding extracranial vascular disease. Indeed in certain centres, patients with proven bilateral carotid stenosis of >75% suffering with vertigo would *still* be diagnosed as suffering from vertebrobasilar insufficiency and treated with medication.

Evidence has now accumulated to show that the amount of plaque or *degree* of stenosis *per se* is also important. This evidence is reviewed later in the chapter but at this stage it is important to understand that if stenoses >75% *are* high risk lesions then the more hawkish surgeon is likely to want to operate on them *even if* they are asymptomatic. Whereas in the 1960s and 1970s discussions such as those by Wolf *et al.*[2] were based on minimal objective measurements, as our unit has shown[3] a great deal can now be found about individual patients by the use of non-invasive investigations. Thus, Duplex scanning (Figure 3.3) and transcranial mapping (Figure 3.4) are now becoming widely available. With such powerful non-invasive techniques it is now theoretically possible to predict what should and should not be done to individual patients.

The capacity of the cerebral circulation to respond to increased blood flow (so-called cerebral perfusion reserve) can also be assessed non-invasively[4,5]. In severe disease it is now possible to estimate how much each cerebral artery contributes to the total perfusion pattern. Thus in the 30 or so years since the first endarterectomies, which were performed on the basis of clinical acumen and relatively crude arteriography, we now have non-invasive investigations which can provide physiological, pathological and anatomical details to help guide patient selection.

With a complete circle of Willis and an asymptomatic stenosis, little needs to be done. However, with an incomplete circle and a stenosis approaching 70%, there is a theoretical, and as I argue later, probably a real risk of a complete carotid occlusion. Transcranial scanning with cerebral reserve estimations helps to assess this risk. Similarly, even with a complete circle of Willis with one side occluded, significant (>70%) stenosis of the contralateral side puts both sides at risk, for on the already occluded side the possibility of so-called water-shed strokes occurs.

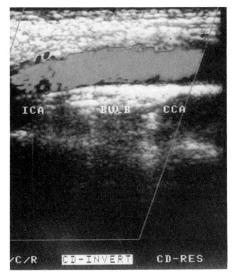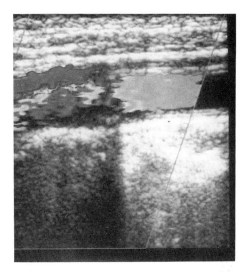

Figure 3.3   Normal (left) and stenosed (right) carotid as shown by Duplex Scanning. (Scans by Dr. S. Powell)

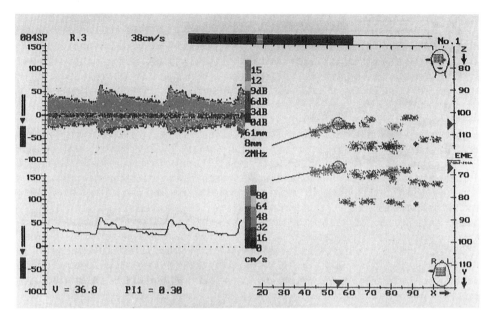

Figure 3.4   Normal transcan demonstrating normal circle of Willis.

The great problem for this theoretical approach is the patient who presents with no symptoms and bilateral occluded carotids. Clearly he or she has been extremely lucky, nevertheless such patients *do* exist and are one of the main props of the therapeutic nihilists who argue fiercely against any intervention.

The contrast between this 'scientific a-priorism' and the Descartian version (represented by opponents to the operation) is marked, for just as Descartes contemplated the theoretical possibility of non-existence, some neurologists contemplate the possibility of no surgical treatment. In the UK this approach is not uncommon despite the fact that, as Sandercock[6] admits, over 90% of strokes are shown to be associated with atheroma or embolism. This might seem an unfair criticism, but a recent conference titled *Stroke: Epidemiological, Therapeutic and Socio-Economic Aspects*, whose report runs to 169 pages, contains virtually no reference to surgery whatsoever[7].

Similarly, review articles[6] can come to the dogmatic conclusion

'Nevertheless, surgery on the carotid artery will only ever be a small part of the management . . .'

on the basis of a literature search which he admits contains no convincing evidence either way!

Kuller and Sutton[8] similarly title their article 'Carotid Artery Bruit: is it safe and effective to auscultate the neck?', and base their argument about neck bruits on the Framingham study[2], when non-invasive studies by Riles *et al.*[9] had already shown that such extrapolations were unsafe. For sound haemodynamic reasons the stenosis shown in Figure 3.3 might well have no bruit over it but nevertheless remains life-threatening. Given such uncertainty therefore, the empiricists clamour for a trial.

The empirical approach

In many clinical situations a well-conducted randomized comparative trial will indicate (if not prove) the answer regarding treatment options. This is the hope of two major studies currently underway; one in Europe, one in North America. What I now say, of course, is hostage to fortune but I suspect just as the North American EC/IC trial reported in 1985[10] attracted, to my mind, fair criticism by Dudley[11], so too will these trials. The controversy centres on patient selection. For a trial to be scientifically sound the population entered into that trial should reflect the population at risk. Secondly it should have clear treatment end-points and comparable treatments. I am not presently convinced that these two conditions apply in the European trial. The North American trial too has certain deficiencies. For both trials, when neurologists and surgeons are involved, patient selection will be difficult.

Starting with the European study; it seeks to examine the benefits of endarterectomy in patients with classical unilateral disease. The protocol presented in 1984[12] allows certain high risk symptomatic patients (for example patients with stenoses > 75%) to be excluded. Similarly asymptomatic patients with severe bilateral stenosis would also be excluded. Right from the start therefore, the trial has limited itself to endarterectomy in a selected group of patients who may or may not reflect the natural history of patients with extracranial disease. The other weakness of this particular trial is that the outcome of carotid endarterectomy not unreasonably includes the influence of coronary artery disease (CAD). However, as CAD and carotid disease are closely related, unless both are equally well documented and treated it will be difficult to sort out quite how much of the outcome is due to surgery, natural history or aspirin. To expect the randomization to separate all of these factors against the background in biased selection is, I believe, somewhat hopeful. The final arbiter for inclusion into this trial (which was conceived in the early 1980s) is four-vessel angiography. According to Sandercock[6] angiography carries a 5–12% risk of complication; on that basis one wonders why the trial was even considered ethical in the first place.

The other major trial currently underway is being run in North America. On the face of it this has a better chance of providing an answer.

Importantly
> 'Surgeons, neurologists and neuroradiologists at the participating centre will have to agree to randomise *all* patients with classical unilateral disease'

These are much tighter criteria than in the European study, where 'grey areas' are allowed. The centres will also be required to 'log all patients who undergo endarterectomy whether or not they are included in the study'. Even so, this same article fails to make clear just how carefully the patients will be scrutinized for other disease. However, stroke or death by stroke will be *the* end point in contradistinction to the more woolly stroke/mortality rate espoused by the European study. Better as this trial potentially is, and despite the early *low* morbidity mortality rate in the initial group undergoing endarterectomy, nevertheless it too could be accused of operating on that group of patients which selects itself with unihemispheric disease. There is a growing body of evidence which suggests that this is not the case. This is exemplified by my own unit's study[3] and reports in the symposium on stroke epidemiology referred to earlier[7]. In other words, the underlying presumption that TIAs/strokes and ipsilateral carotid disease truly represent the majority of extracranial vascular disease prevalent in society is suspect. Such trials therefore, however well conducted, cannot generalize about endarterectomy in *all* cases of cerebrovascular disease.

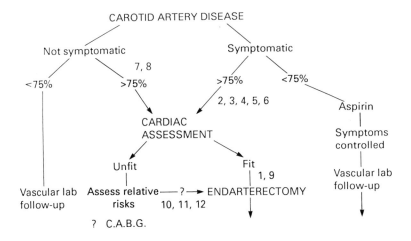

Key	Comment	Reference
1	'Safe Operation', 8535 Patients, 2.5% stroke rate	[13]
2	Endarterectomy better than observation for: stenoses (> 70%), for bilateral stenoses > 50%, and for occlusions plus > 50% stenoses	[14]
3	Natural history study, > 80% stenoses, Stroke/TIA rate seven times greater	[15]
4	> 75% stenoses carry high stroke rate	[16]
5	> 75% stenoses carry high stroke rate	[17]
6	> 75% stenoses carry high stroke rate	[18]
7	> 70% stenoses even if asymptomatic best treated. However, authors admit this may not be the case for women	[19]
8	> 75% or ulcerated lesions dangerous	[20]
9	Despite high risk factors, e.g. hypertension, operative morbidity and mortality in 651 patients only 2%	[21]
10	Combined CAE and CABG safety in doubt	[22]
11	Combined CAE and CABG probably safe	[23]
12	Combined CAE and CABG undergoing randomized trial	[24]

Figure 3.5   (a) Possible decision pathway. The table (b) cites references which support those decisions.

Despite these reservations, the kind of results presently reported from this study, whose perioperative stroke rate is in the order of 1%, is cheeringly different from doubters such as Sandercock who quote figures as high as 11–21%.

Patient selection

For convenience I have attempted to summarize some of the more recent series in some kind of logical order by referencing the kind of decision pathway I use when assessing a patient for surgery (Figure 3.5). A similar review has been presented by Taylor and Porter[25] and this too should help, as these authors suggest, 'the practicing vascular surgeon to make his decision'. Clearly only certain vascular specialists should be performing this operation and they should work hand in glove with a neurologist and, possibly more importantly, a cardiologist. My algorithm for treatment is, by current British Standards, fairly aggressive in stance. Few of my colleagues would operate on asymptomatic stenoses even if they were > 75%, and at this point I would have to admit that such evidence as there is comes for the most part from the large selected retrospective series based on the reasoning outlined in my introduction.

The first, seemingly easy, decision 'is whether or not the patient is symptomatic'. The 'Hawks' on the whole are looking for reasons to operate, the 'Doves' *vice versa*. Thus if a patient presented with a stroke due to the occluded side, I would argue that despite the fact there might be no symptoms attributable to a diseased contralateral carotid, it would not be correct to call the operation a 'prophylactic carotid endarterectomy done for asymptomatic extracranial vascular disease'. This might seem academic but it is at the nub of all the arguments.

The symptomatic patients are most easily dealt with. If one accepts (as I do) that stenosis greater than 75% requires an operation, then lesions below 50% may well not. Thus if aspirin stops further TIAs and the stenosis is < 50% I would opt for conservatism. As Taylor and Porter[25] suggest, the presence of an ulcerated plaque on Duplex scanning or multiple cerebral emboli on CT scanning[20] may well change my mind. The important point of all the decisions is, however, (as in Figure 3.5), cardiac assessment. There really is *very* little point in operating on one part of the cardiovascular system when a potentially more serious lesion lies in another. Deaths from MI postoperatively are a reflection of poor patient selection and a criticism of the doctors rather than of carotid endarterectomy *per se*. Clearly, combined cardiac and carotid operations can be performed[22]. In Southampton we tend to treat whichever lesion appears to be potentially most lethal. However, Hertzer and colleagues are well into a prospective trial of this worrying combination, their initial report suggesting that a rational rather than intuitive approach is possible[24].

Using this rigorous system of screening for coronary disease (which is fairly similar in the four major centres involved in the JVRG UK study) the 215 patients were all recruited within three years and of those, nearly 80% had lesions of > 75% stenosis. Over 90% were alive, well and free of symptoms at 12 months[26]. Like the large North American and Canadian series, the results were achieved with low permanent stroke and mortality (1.5%). Thus pragmatically, these high risk patients *can* be treated reasonably safely and, more importantly, their very worrying symptoms controlled.

Carotid endarterectomy

Investigation

In Southampton[3] and in Bristol[27] the introduction of the kind of non-invasive investigations described above has led to a great reduction in the numbers of arteriograms performed. Following cardiac assessment, on my unit a classical history of unihemispheric problems together with a characteristic bifurcation lesion shown on a Duplex is considered a sufficient preoperative vascular work-up. In instance of diagnostic difficulty, patients also have CT scanning. The development of Magnetic Resonance imaging may have a great simplifying effect on this in that both artery and brain can be assessed simultaneously. In any case I rarely now use arteriography, reserving it for those patients where a complete carotid occlusion is suspected or when proximal disease such as a vertebral steal appears likely.

Hankey and Warlow[28] have shown that observer error in all types of assessment *is* important but those centres (for example Hames *et al.*[29]), whose experience stretched back over the 10 years or so that non-invasive techniques have been available, would see such views as being somewhat over cautious.

The operation

The operation itself should be performed by a consultant vascular surgeon and consultant anaesthetist (Rubin *et al.*[13]); of the two, I suspect the latter is the more important. Figure 3.6 shows our theatre layout. The head end of the table is kept clear for transcranial monitoring. At all stages blood pressure, pulse, etc. are controlled within strict limits. This lesson was learned in the 1960s but still (even on our unit) occasionally gets forgotten. In high risk patients with contralateral occlusions, falls in blood pressure can be disastrous, producing so-called 'paradoxical' or watershed strokes.

The technique

This is well described but there are variants on the technique. I prefer an incision parallel to the line of the sternomastoid.

With high lesions I employ the technique described by Hans *et al.*[30]. Tacking down sutures on the internal carotid often means that the dissection has not been taken high enough: the kind of specimen illustrated in Figure 3.1, with its smooth long posterior tongue, means that it has.

Like Gummerlock and Neveralt[31] I always try to shunt. It makes teaching my vascular trainees easier; I am not convinced it is essential. Whenever I encounter small arteries or have technical difficulties with difficult break-off points in the atheroma, in line with the JVRG trial[26] I always close the arteriotomy with a patch. Before

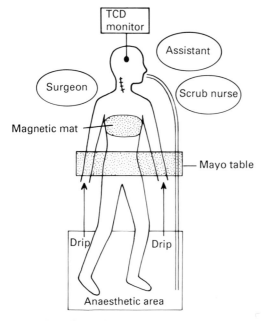

Figure 3.6   Theatre layout during endarterectomy.

closing the wound I like to see a good signal in the middle cerebral artery on transcranial scanning. If I do not, if in the recovery area the signal disappears or if the patient deterioriates neurologically, I immediately re-explore the patient, passing a small embolectomy catheter. The experience of Painter *et al.*[32] confirms the effectiveness of this approach.

Follow up

Having established a vascular laboratory, it is tempting to scan and rescan all patients for 'progression of disease'. For scientific purposes, as for example in our patch/non patch study, this is important; routine follow-up of all patients with extracerebral vascular disease should, however, probably be confined to those patients with bilateral disease or a combination of disease > 50% with other risk factors such as hypertension. Whether or not aspirin (as a prophylactic) is indicated postoperatively is still debatable but such evidence as there is, for example that from Boysen *et al.*[33], is inconclusive.

Conclusion

Clearly our recent series shows that, like many others, our unit is capable of safely performing endarterectomies. Equally clearly there are certain patients, whether symptomatic or otherwise, where non-invasive studies demonstrate that the cerebral circulation is critically impaired. I believe that these patients require an operation, based on our results confirmed by the transcranial studies cited above[4,5]. My grey area, sadly, is the one theoretically amenable to the simple expedient of doing a trial. Regretfully for the reasons stated above, like Relman in his thoughtful review on the EC/IC trial[34] I am not at all sure that such a trial can now be done. In the meantime I continue pragmatically in most instances to do no harm and in the majority to do some good.

References

1. Eascott, H. H. G., Pickering, G. W. and Robb, C. (1954) *Lancet*, **i**, 994–996
2. Wolf, P. A., Kawn, W. B., Sorlie, P. and McNamara, P. (1981) Asymptomatic bruit and the risk of stroke: the Framingham Study. *J. Am. Med. Ass.*, **245**, 1442–1445
3. Chant, A. D. B., Thompson, J. F., Stranks, G. J. *et al.* (1990) Impact of Duplex scanning on carotid artery endarterectomy. *Br. J. Surg.*, **77**, 188–189
4. Bishop, C. C., Powell, S., Insall, M. *et al.* (1986) Effect of internal carotid occlusion on middle cerebral artery blood flow at rest and in response to hypercapria. *Lancet*, **i**, 710–712
5. Ratnatunga, C. and Adiseshiak, M. (1990) Increase in middle cerebral velocity on breath holding. *Eur. J. Vasc. Sur.*, **4**, 519–523
6. Sandercock, P. A. G. (1987) Asymptomatic carotid stenosis spare the knife. *Br. Med J.*, **294**, 1368–1369
7. Royal Society of Medicine *Stroke: Epidemiology, Therapeutic and Socio-Economic Aspects.* Published Royal Society of Medicine Services Symposium No. 99
8. Kuller, L. H. and Sutton, K. C. (1984) Carotid artery bruit: Is it safe and effective to auscultate the neck? *Stroke*, **15**, 944–947
9. Riles, T. S., Lieberman, A., Kopelman, I. *et al.* (1981) Symptoms stenosis and bruit. Inter-relationships in carotid artery disease. *Arch. Surg.*, **116**, 218–220.
10. EC/IC bypass study group (1985) Results of an international randomised study. *New Eng. J. Med.*, **313**, 1191–1200
11. Dudley, H. A. F. (1987) Extracranial–Intracranial bypass one: Clinical Trials nil. *Br. Med. J.*, **294**, 1501–1502

12. Warlow (1984) *European Carotid Surgery Trial* 3rd edition
13. Rubin, J. R., Pitlok, H. C., King, T. A. *et al.* (1986) Surgical versus non-operative treatment of symptomatic carotid stenosis. *Ann. Surg.*, **204**, 154–162
14. Hertzer, N. R., Flanagan, R. A., O'Hara, P. J. and Bevan, E. G. (1986) Surgical versus non-operative treatment of symptomatic carotid stenosis. *Ann. Surg.*, **204**, 154–162
15. Colgan, M. P., Leahy, A. L., Grouden, M. C. *et al.* (1990) The results of an eight-year study in asymptomatic patients. *Br. J. Surg.*, **77**, A344
16. Bogousslavsky, J., Despland, P. A. and Regli, F. (1988) Progress of high risk patients with non-operated symptomatic stenosis. *Stroke*, **19**, 109–110
17. Aldoori, M. I., Benveniste, G. L., Baird, R. N. *et al.* (1987) Asymptomatic murmurs and Duplex scanning. *Br. J. Surg.*, **74**, 496–499
18. Moneta, G. L., Taylor, D. C., Nicholls, S. C. *et al.* (1987) Operative versus (non-operative) management of high grade stenosis. *Stroke*, **18**, 1005–1009
19. Hertzer, N. R., Flanagan, R. A., O'Hara, P. J. and Bevan, E. G. (1986) Surgical versus non-operative treatment of asymptomatic disease. *Ann. Surg.*, **204**, 164–171
20. Sterpetti, A. V., Schultz, R. D. and Feldhaus, R. J. (1988) Asymptomatic carotid artery stenosis on the contralateral side to CAE. *J. Vasc. Surg.*, **8**, 453–459
21. Nunn, D. B. (1988) Carotid artery endarterectomy in patients with territorial TIA's. *J. Vasc. Surg.*, **8**, 447–451
22. Perler, B. A., Burdick, J. F., Minken, S. L. *et al.* (1988) Should we perform CAE and cardiac procedures synchronously. *J. Vasc. Surg.*, **8**, 402–409
23. Cambria, R. P., Ivarrson, B. L., Akins, C. W. *et al.* (1989) Simultaneous carotid and coronary disease. Safety of combined approach. *J. Vasc. Surg.*, **9**, 56–61
24. Cosgrove, D. M., Hertzer, N. R. and Loop, F. D. (1989) Surgical management of synchronous carotid and coronary artery disease *J. Vasc. Surg.*, **3**, 690–692
25. Taylor, L. M. and Porter, J. M. (1986) Basic data related to CAE. *Ann. Vasc. Surg.*, **1**, 264–265
26. Ranaboldo, C., Chant, A. D. B., Bell, P. B. and Barros, D'Sa A. A. B. (1991) Patch angioplasty, a controlled trial for Joint Vascular Research Group UK. *Br. J. Surg.* (in press)
27. Farmilo, R. W., Scott, D. J. A., Cole, S. E. A. *et al.* (1990) Role of Duplex scanning in the selection of patients for CAE. *Br. J. Surg.*, **77**, 388–390
28. Hankey, G. J. and Warlow, C. P. (1990) Symptomatic carotid ischaemic events: safest most cost effective way of selecting patients for angiography before CAE. *Br. Med. J.*, **300**, 1486–1491
29. Hames, T. K., Humphries, R. N., Ratliff, D. A. *et al.* (1985) Validation of Duplex scanning and CW Doppler with angiography. *Ultrasound Med. Biol.*, **11**, 827–834
30. Hans, S. S., Shah, S. and Hans, B. (1989) Carotid Endarterectomy for high plaques. *Am. J. Surg.*, **157**, 431–435
31. Gummerlock, M. K. and Nevarelt, E. A. (1988) Carotid Endarterectomy to shunt or not to shunt. *Stroke*, **19**, 1485–1490
32. Painter, T. A., Hertzer, N. R., O'Hara, P. J. *et al.* (1987) Symptomatic internal carotid thrombosis after CAE. *J. Vasc. Surg.* **3**, 446–451
33. Boysen, G., Sorensen, P. S., Jukler, M. *et al.* (1988) Danish very low dose aspirin study after CAE. *Stroke*, **19**, 1211–1215
34. Relman, A. S. (1987) The extracranial study ... what have we learned? *New Eng J. Med.*, **316**, 809–810

Postscript

My hostage to fortune returned home* unexpectedly early! At the time of printing, after 10 years or so and more than 2000 patients the European Study has confirmed the operation's worth. I am sad for the patients who drew 'no operation' but glad that the issue *seems to have been* resolved.

* *Source:* Anon. (1991) *The Sunday Times*, 24 February

Chapter 4

Carotid body tumours – the premise of the vascular surgeon

Aires A. B. Barros D'Sa

Introduction

The chemodectoma is a tumour of the chemoreceptor system which carries the pathological description of non-chromaffin paraganglioma, differentiating it from the positive chromaffin reaction which characterizes a phaeochromocytoma. Although the chemodectoma occurs rarely, it is most commonly encountered as a carotid body tumour (CBT), that being the sole lesion involving the carotid body.

In recent years progress in vascular surgical skills and techniques and sophisticated preoperative radiodiagnosis have favourably influenced the outcome in the management of carotid body tumours. The high mortality and morbidity once associated with operations on these tumours have both been significantly reduced. These are not grounds for complacency and it is worth emphasizing that the rewards are a product of diligent preoperative preparation, patient surgery and precise operative technique. Undeniably, the vascular surgeon who works in the carotid territory, uses shunts, performs vein graft repairs and has an interest in carotid body tumours, will accumulate the personal experience and confidence required for the proper treatment of this condition. It would be fair to say that this particular repertoire is not to be found in any other surgical specialty and, for this reason, the vascular surgeon has a duty and a responsibility to play the leading role in the management of these tumours.

Anatomy and physiology of the carotid body

Although there is a view that the carotid body originates in the third branchial arch, it is generally conceded that its cells arise from the neural crest and migrate with the autonomic nervous system[1]. On these grounds, the carotid body has been included in the APUD (amine precursor uptake decarboxylase) classification[2], the implication being that its totipotential cells were endocrine in function. Histologically it is composed of cell nests or zellballen of Type 1, or chief cells, containing dense granules which can synthesize catecholamines[1] and Type 2, or sustentaculum cells, which hold these nests together.

Regardless of its embryological origin, the carotid body develops in the adventitia[3], a minute, 0.1–0.5 cm, ovoid structure located on the posterior aspect of the common carotid artery bifurcation, although it may be found on adjacent vessels[4,5]. A tiny channel arising from the external carotid artery close to the bifurcation supplies the carotid body, occasionally assisted by the ascending pharyngeal artery[3,4]. Additional adventitial vessels and others from the superior thyroid, occipital, subclavian, vertebral and thyrocervical arteries may be acquired by an enlarging CBT[6–8]. Afferent branches from the glossopharyngeal and vagus nerves and the cervical sympathetic ganglia innervate the carotid body[9]. The carotid tissue exerts an important but incompletely understood influence on the homeostatic control of arterial blood gases and pH. Similar chemoreceptor tissue is also present in other areas such as the jugular bulb (glomus jugulare), the middle ear (glomus tympanicum), the ganglion nodosum of the vagus nerve (glomus intravagale) and the aortic body.

Pathophysiology of the carotid body

Hyperplasia of carotid bodies and a tenfold increased risk of tumour formation have been observed in populations living at high altitudes[10–12] and in the UK in patients with chronic hypoxaemia due to respiratory disease[13]. In contrast to hyperplastic carotid body tissue, CBTs show proliferation of Type 1 cells with nuclear pleomorphism and vesicular nuclei, maintaining the zellballen architecture but within a field of increased vascularity, while the number of Type 2 cells in the intervening spaces appears unchanged (Figure 4.1). Persistently high arterial $p\text{CO}_2$ and low arterial $p\text{O}_2$ levels accompanying chronic obstructive pulmonary disease appear to be important in the development of bilateral tumours of the carotid body[14]. Not surprisingly, it has been suggested that these pathophysiological stimuli induce simple hyperplasia which may be a precursor to the growth of chemodectomas of carotid bodies and other chemoreceptor structures in genetically predisposed individuals[10,14]. In congenital cyanotic heart disease, chronic hypoxia is again implicated in the aetiology

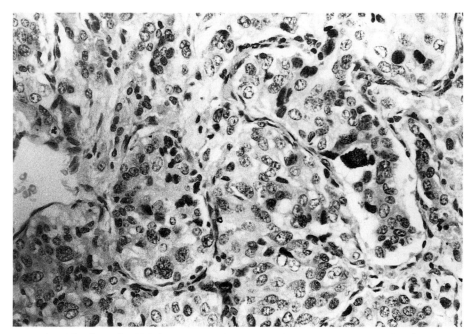

Figure 4.1   Histology of a CBT (H&E stain, original magnification × 500). (From [74] with permission)

of carotid body hyperplasia[15] and CBTs, both solitary[16] and bilateral[17]. Autopsy studies have established a direct correlation between increases in carotid body size and right ventricular weight[18]. For a time, bilateral glomectomy, or the removal of both carotid bodies, was thought to alleviate asthma[19] but once the harmful effects of this operation became known it was soon abandoned[20].

Carotid body tumour (CBT) pathology

The incidence of CBTs is sporadic, occurring in any age group but especially between 50 and 60 years, and slightly more commonly in females[21]. Bilateral CBTs are observed in 5% of cases, which rises to 30% when the condition is familial[21–25]. Hereditary transmission occurs in an autosomal dominant fashion[14,21,26,27], with a varying but unexplained degree of penetration. Although familial tumours tend to appear at an earlier age in subsequent generations[14], this behaviour was not observed in the second generation of a family with bilateral chemodectomas in five siblings[28]. A contralateral second tumour may appear some years after the first has been removed[22]. The rather indolent and symptomless disposition of a CBT may account for the fact that its clinical detection may be delayed until it has achieved considerable maturity.

Bilateral glomus jugulare tumours, which are aggressive and tend to occur in older females, have been discovered in the siblings of patients with familial bilateral CBTs[28,29]. Paragangliomas of other chemoreceptor tissue may coexist with CBTs, particularly in familial cases in the form of a multiple tumour syndrome[21,26,27,30–32]. The categorization of CBT as an apudoma and its allocation to the MEA Type II group remains to be justified[2,33]. Although a hormone unique to the carotid body has yet to be identified, it is suggested that catecholamine-secreting paragangliomas do occur[33–35]. The Type 1, or chief cells, synthesize and store catecholamines, but plasma and urine catecholamine levels are usually normal[7,8,36,37], elevated levels having been observed rarely[1,34,38–47].

Histological criteria alone fail to separate CBTs into the conventionally accepted categories of benign, locally invasive or malignant metastasizing tumour[23,36,48,49]. They are in the main histologically benign but there are reports of local malignancy rates of 3–13.5% and of distant metastases in a further 3%[21,36,37,50,51], although an incidence of metastases in up to 23% has been demonstrated in a long-term follow-up of patients[52]. Invasion by primary or recurrent tumour can be quite destructive locally[8,25,50,53,54]. Preliminary histology cannot always be relied upon to indicate the invasive or malignant potential of a CBT[1,48], the burden of proof of malignancy being dependent on the discovery of a tumour metastatic deposit[1,49]. It must be borne in mind, however, that the chemoreceptor system of a patient may be the seat of multicentric tumours[29,31] and therefore coexisting chemodectomas at other sites must not be mistaken for metastases. A recently reported study[55] attempting to correlate the clinicopathological features of CBTs with their DNA ploidy pattern, as determined by image analysis, showed first that tumour ploidy cannot be used to assess malignant potential, and secondly that there was no relationship between mitotic activity and clinical behaviour, although perineural and vascular invasion was observed only in those with abnormal DNA histograms.

The surgeon dealing with CBTs encounters varying degrees of ease in removing them and is aware that the behaviour of a particular tumour as witnessed at operation is not necessarily reflected in the histological report.

In an effort to grade these tumours according to the progressively increasing difficulties observed in removing them and the corresponding rise in the associated morbidity, the Mayo Clinic series of CBTs was analysed by Shamblin *et al.*[36]. The ensuing classification which bears his name divides CBTs into three groups according to the gross tumour–vessel relationship; group I localized, group II adherent and partially surrounding the vessels, group III intimately surrounding the vessels. On these impressions rest the decisions which must be taken as to the best surgical approach. In most instances the tumour can be excised completely, leaving the carotid arterial system intact, while on the other that can be achieved only by excising a part of the carotid system with the tumour. If the internal carotid artery has to be sacrificed then intraluminal arterial shunting and reconstruction with a vein graft become necessary components of the operative procedure.

Clinical diagnosis

The failure even to consider a possible diagnosis of CBT has, in part, contributed to the notoriety surrounding the complications and mortality of surgery[36,50,56–58]. Certain characteristics of the tumour, namely its rich vascularity, the pressure effects on neighbouring structures further aggravated by its capacity for local invasion, and in some instances the presence of a contralateral tumour, should arouse sufficient suspicion to promote a thorough examination of the head, neck and cranial nerves.

In its classical presentation, a CBT is a painless non-tender mass situated just beneath the upper portion of the sternocleidomastoid muscle (Figure 4.2). While most of these tumours grow steadily, approximately one-fifth of them enlarge rapidly to cause pain, tenderness and increasing pressure on adjacent anatomical structures[2,59]. Up to one-third of all cases will present with cranial nerve palsies

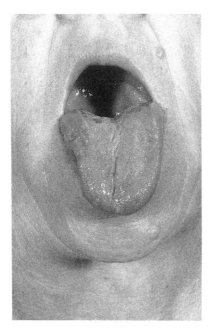

Figure 4.2 A right-sided carotid body tumour associated with some hemiatrophy and deviation of the tongue due to involvement of the hypoglossal nerve

predominantly involving the vagus and hypoglossal, and to a lesser extent the glossopharyngeal and spinal accessory. In a few instances the sympathetic nerve trunk or the pharynx may become involved. The consequent clinical manifestations can be predicted and include hoarseness, irritating pain, deviation and even hemiatrophy of the tongue (Figure 4.2), dysphagia, Horner's syndrome and, rarely, the carotid sinus syndrome[8,36,42,50,52,56–59].

A variety of clinical presentations exist beyond this conventional clinical picture of CBTs. There is some evidence attesting to the occasional secretory potential of CBTs[1,34,38–47]. In such cases, or in the rare instance of a coexisting phaeochromocytoma[32,60–62] the patient may present with episodic flushing, dizziness, palpitations, ventricular tachycardia, hypertension and serious cardiovascular problems which warrant searching enquiry. Tumour pressure on the internal carotid artery can cause transient ischaemic attacks[63], and if the vessel is atheromatous, can conceivably precipitate stroke. External stimuli, including palpation of the tumour, may induce syncope or dyspnoea and one patient was suffocated by massive bilateral tumours[25]. Extension of tumour substance intracranially around the internal carotid artery has proved fatal[25,59].

Located where it is, a CBT is often mistaken for the more commonly observed cervical lymphadenopathy, whether inflammatory, lymphomatous or otherwise neoplastic. Apart from obvious conditions such as carotid aneurysm, branchial cyst or sternomastoid tumour, a differential diagnosis should also take note of rarer possibilities including haemangioma, neurofibroma, Schwannoma, Castleman's disease[64] and, of course, a CBT. On further enquiry, the answer that the swelling has been present for a considerable period of time ought to alert suspicions. In reality, and not infrequently, exploratory biopsy of presumed lymph nodes may be attempted rather precipitously, with dire consequences. Physical signs may be quite non-specific even when a probable diagnosis of CBT is entertained[65]. The classic term 'potato' tumour does convey the correct impression of a mass which is firm and devoid of pulsation, although sustained compression will usually reduce its size. Where the tumour has a softer consistency it may be pulsatile with a continuous audible hum on auscultation. Lateral mobility in the absence of vertical movement is a fairly reliable sign that the mass is a CBT[66].

Investigations

A definitive diagnosis is commonly arrived at by contrast angiography[25,49,67], a potentially hazardous investigation with a low but measurable incidence of morbidity. It certainly ought not to be the first mode of investigation in the atypical cervical gland and the small tumour, or in screening the family of a patient with bilateral CBTs. Doppler ultrasound techniques, including Duplex sonography, are of limited value[68,69] while plain X-rays and tomography[28] have been practically supplanted by computed tomography scanning (CT) and magnetic resonance imaging (MRI). Dynamic scintigraphy or radionuclide perfusion scanning[70,71], using 99-m technetium is an inexpensive, minimally invasive and eminently acceptable technique for demonstrating the vascularity of clinically unsuspected CBTs[28,72,73] (Figure 4.3) and can be safely repeated every few years[74]. It therefore has a special application in the identification of local recurrences or in the location of a contralateral tumour appearing in later years[22,28]. Confronted by a mass in the carotid triangle, this method represents a valuable discriminating tool aimed at either

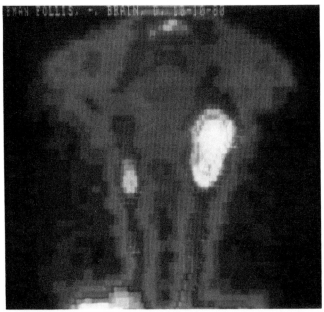

Figure 4.3 Radionuclide scan revealing two clinically undetectable CBTs, one small (right) and one larger (left). (From [28] with permission)

confirming the presence of a CBT or eliminating that possibility, thereby leaving the general surgeon confident to explore the area and to proceed to tissue biopsy if required. Intravenous digital subtraction angiography is rather more invasive than dynamic scintigraphy and provides images poorer in detail and clarity when compared to an intra-arterial study, which, by general acceptance, is unjustifiable as a screening technique.

It is conceivable that extrinsic compression of the internal carotid artery by the tumour, and possibly tumour steal, may compromise cerebral flow to such an extent that the arterial injection of contrast may precipitate stroke[28]. Selectively applied to only those patients with positive radionuclide scans, conventional angiograms display the pathognomonic radiological features of CBTs which have been exhaustively detailed in the literature[8,25,42,52,53,56–59,75–80]. The tumour is highly vascular, producing a 'lyre-like' or goblet-shaped splaying of the carotid bifurcation, pushing and even compressing the internal carotid artery posterolaterally and displacing the external carotid artery anterolaterally (Figure 4.4a). A slightly later phase of the same study outlines a cloud of fine tortuous vessels which may define the key sources of blood supply to the tumour, the dimensions of which are evident from the tumour blush which seems clearly to displace and surround the main arteries (Figure 4.4b). Thus, biplanar angiograms are important and of particular value in planning an operative approach[28,34,78]. This observation is particularly valid in the older patient with coexisting atherosclerotic and ulcerating disease of the internal carotid artery, which is likely to be disturbed during the process of extirpating the tumour causing cerebral thromboembolism[81]. In removing the tumour it may therefore be necessary to resect and reconstruct the relevant segment of artery. Angiographic studies will also expose unsuspected bilateral CBTs[28,37] and metastases to lymph nodes[25]. It has also been argued that contrast angiography may fail to reveal a CBT,

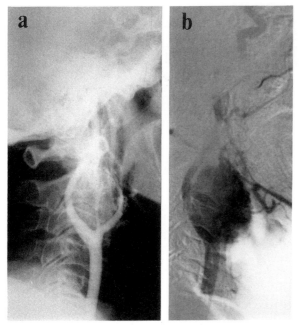

Figure 4.4 (a) Angiography shows a CBT classically splaying the carotid bifurcation; (b) a subtraction film of the arteriolar phase shows a cloud of tumour vessels surrounding the external carotid artery. (From [74] with permission)

too small either to contain a recognizable tumour circulation or, at the other extreme, to distort the configuration of the carotid bifurcation[28]. Exceptions to classic appearances are frequent[59,76,82,83], one being the avascularity of the tumour[10], and it is worth remembering that while the mass may not be a CBT it may still be a variety of chemodectoma such as a glomus intravagale or glomus jugulare tumour.

CT scanning with contrast enhancement of the carotid arteries[28,84] complements angiography by clarifying the dimensions and configuration of the tumour (Figure 4.5) and in advanced cases provides evidence of invasion into the arteries and outwards into adjacent structures[84–86]. Early experience with MRI[87] shows that it has value in defining the anatomy of vascular structures surrounding the tumour and in demonstrating changes in blood flow due to the tumour mass.

Having delineated a CBT anatomically, its occasional endocrine potential[1,34, 38–47,88] must be uncovered by estimating plasma catecholamines, urinary catecholamines and vanillyl-mandelic acid (VMA) and by deducing VMA/creatinine ratios. If these tests are positive, the presence of a coexisting phaeochromocytoma[32,60–62] must be excluded and in either case preoperative preparations with appropriate pharmacological agents will be required.

Fine needle aspiration for cytological diagnosis of a highly vascular tumour, closely related to cranial nerves, major vessels and possibly to atheromatous carotid arteries, is not only partially successful but has resulted in fatality[89] and is therefore contraindicated[90].

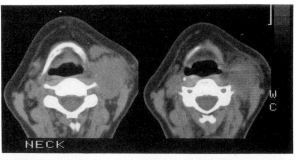

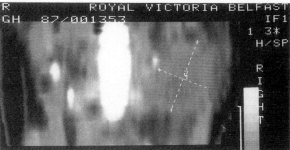

Figure 4.5   CT scan of neck: transverse sections (above) show anatomical boundaries of CBT; coronal section (below) permits assessment of size and extent. (From [74] with permission)

Irradiation treatment

The place of radiotherapy in the management of CBTs has been limited on the one hand by the well-published radioresistance of these tumours[25,36,37,56,66,81,83,91] and on the other by the effects of irradiation injury, resulting in tissue necrosis and other sequelae such as carotid artery stenosis, laryngeal stricture and destruction of the mandible[25,36,50,56,83]. The consequent fibrosis and obliteration of tissue planes compound the inherent difficulties which attend operative removal, thereby rendering surgery doubly hazardous. In practice, the widely held view that CBTs are unresponsive to irradiation therapy is attenuated to some extent by reports of regression and varying degrees of control of the tumour[92–94]. Radiotherapy can also relieve pain caused by bony and other metastatic deposits and, as survival can be prolonged, aggressive palliation is justifiable[65].

Surgical treatment

The effects of growth, local invasiveness and potential malignancy of this tumour, as well as the absence of any evidence to indicate a capacity for spontaneous regression, leave the surgeon with little option but to resort to operation. This line of treatment was first adopted in 1880 and a review of the experience in 27 cases was published in 1906[95]. The entire literature of the past century yields a cohort of just over a thousand case reports, reflecting a rate of diagnosis of approximately ten cases per year, which serves to illustrate the rarity with which a general surgeon will encounter this tumour. In early reports of CBT excision the depressing results of a 30%

mortality rate and a 50% stroke rate are not unexpected when it is realized that a definitive preoperative diagnosis was not available before exploration and that the carotid artery was frequently ligated in the process[66,81,83,96]. A turning point in the management of CBTs followed two observations, first, that the carotid body lies within the adventitia[3] and secondly that a relatively avascular subadventitial plane of dissection, or 'white line', existed allowing excision of the tumour without damaging the carotid vessels[97]. The adoption of a strictly anatomical technique of removal, aided by simultaneous advances in anaesthesia, blood transfusion and vascular surgical techniques, have together contributed to safer surgery and its pre-eminence in the management of this condition[8,25,36,42,50,52].

Any doubts expressed as to the need for early operation[23,25] are dispelled by the relative technical ease of excision of a small tumour with little risk to important neighbouring structures[10,37,49,67,90,91] principally the cranial nerves[51,98–100], thereby keeping morbidity to a minimum. Despite modern vascular surgical techniques the incidence of cranial nerve palsies remains high[52,98,100], approximately half of which are permanent[98], a particular feature of the larger tumour which tends to fall within group II and, especially, group III of Shamblin's classification[36]. Clearly the early diagnosis of this unusual tumour is recommended, but is only likely if there is a general awareness of its existence. If examination of a tumour in the carotid area results in a differential diagnosis which does not include the CBT then exploration or biopsy, oblivious to this possibility, may precipitate a dangerous situation. Explorations for excision or biopsy of a mass in the carotid triangle are not unusual and in as many as one-third of cases have been followed by definitive surgery to remove a CBT[65].

It is interesting to recall that planned open biopsy was recommended at one time as the method of choice in confirming the diagnosis[66]. The deliberate incision into a CBT, the flow rate through which approximates $2 \, l/100 \, g$ per minute[67,101], exceeding that of the brain, must have been an alarming experience for the unprepared surgeon. Life-threatening haemorrhage may demand hurried carotid ligation in a bloody field, inviting the twin dangers of stroke and accidental injury to cranial nerves[25,57,58,91,102,103]. Understandably, this practice of exploratory biopsy is obsolete.

Any general surgeon faced with a mass suspected to be a CBT should refrain from performing a biopsy and, instead, obtain the immediate assistance of a vascular surgeon accustomed to dealing with this condition. To proceed unaided, with neither the experience nor the appropriate surgical instruments, is to invite disaster. All these terrors can be averted by preoperative investigations aimed at eliminating the diagnosis of CBT.

In general, all CBTs should be removed except in the presence of compelling contraindications such as advanced malignant change, prohibitive concurrent cardiac and respiratory risks or senility. In any event, the unoperated patient ought to be kept under review, examining the tumour as it enlarges and perhaps becomes symptomatic. The aim of surgery is to excise the tumour in its entirety while preserving the carotid system and adjacent nerves. In some cases, as with Shamblin's group III tumours[36], excision may not be possible without injury to the common or internal carotid artery. Under such circumstances, these vessels should be sacrificed but they must be replaced by a graft[60,82,104].

Surgical removal of a CBT, especially if it is large and longstanding, should not be undertaken lightly and the patient should be made aware of the nature of the condition before consent is obtained. The information and discussion must contain a sensible assessment of the value of operation but must also identify potential risks and complications such as injury to the cranial nerves and stroke. The occasional patient with elevated plasma catecholamines may be at risk of cardiovascular collapse during induction and surgery[34] and will require the administration of alpha- and beta-receptor blockade, in the form of phenoxybenzamine and propranolol respectively, for a week before surgery, along with fluid expansion of the extracellular space to avert irreversible hypotension following tumour excision[44,62]. Regardless of the technical proficiency of the surgeon, adequate blood and, if available, autotransfusion facilities, must be kept in readiness.

To facilitate removal a large tumour can be subjected to preoperative embolization aimed at reducing its vascularity and size[7,105–108]. This calls for expertise in superselective catheterization of 'feeder' vessels to the tumour arising from all branches of the carotid and subclavian systems. Even if two branches of the external carotid artery can be successfully cannulated, embolization may still be incomplete. In any case, surgery is recommended within a day or two of embolization[107,108]. The potential dangers of inadvertent 'spill' causing necrosis of tissues of the head and face, and of cerebral and ocular infarction, militate against this approach. If, after embolization, some tumour tissue is left behind it has the capacity to acquire a fresh blood supply, leading to recurrence[109]. Surgical excision of a non-embolized CBT may not be as easily accomplished but it offers the best hope of lasting success.

It is an operation which, in the interests of safety and good practice, ought to be undertaken by a vascular surgeon accustomed to operating in this area and experienced in the insertion of intraluminal shunts and vein graft repair. For large tumours which extend distally towards the base of the skull, further exposure may be gained by temporomandibular joint subluxation, if necessary with the help of a maxillofacial surgical colleague[110].

If temporomandibular subluxation is envisaged, nasotracheal intubation is preferable to standard endotracheal anaesthesia. A catecholamine-secreting tumour when compressed may provoke haemodynamic fluctuations in as much as manipulation of the carotid bifurcation can induce bradycardia and hypotension, and in the older patient may cause plaque or thrombus to be dislodged from a diseased carotid artery. Essential to the surveillance of cardiovascular changes are an arterial line and ECG monitoring. The standard 'jack-knife' position with a soft sandbag placed between the scapulae (as used for carotid endarterectomy) will allow sufficient lateral rotation and hyperextension of the neck. Access is maintained to one upper long saphenous vein in case a donor graft is required.

The objectives of operation are the removal of the CBT totally but cosmetically, while at the same time preserving the integrity of the carotid arteries and adjacent nerves, and avoiding excessive loss of blood in the process. The application of clear and established principles of technique will ensure that safe and precise excision are achieved[8,25,28,36,37,49,56–59,79,90,91,103,104,111–114]. These include wide exposure, location of cranial nerves, control of the carotid arterial system, dissection in the correct prescribed plane, preparedness to resort to intraluminal shunting and, if necessary, vein grafting to replace any arterial segment.

An oblique cervical incision anterior to the sternomastoid muscle border gives better access and distal exposure than the curvilinear creaseline approach. The dissection is developed just anterior to the internal jugular vein, exposing the common facial vein, which is ligated after first excluding the (small) possibility of a low-slung hypoglossal nerve. An early tumour tends to be confined largely within the cleft between the internal and external carotid arteries. A large tumour may surround the

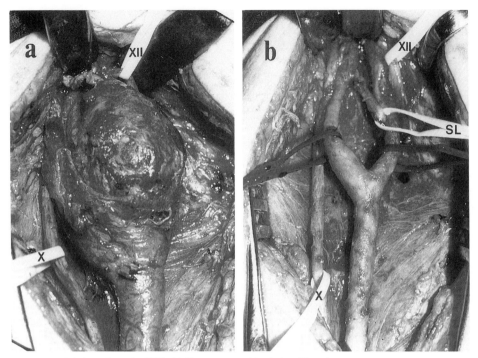

Figure 4.6 Moderately early CBT. (a) Tumour–carotid relationships, the vagus (X) and hypoglossal (XII) nerves within silastic slings; (b) tumour excision leaves the carotid system, vagus (X), its superior laryngeal branch (SL) and hypoglossal (XII) nerves intact

external carotid artery, leaving the internal carotid artery just recognizable (Figure 4.6(a)) but it may grow to a degree where it entirely obscures the distal common carotid and both its main branches (Figure 4.7(a)). Entering the surface of the tumour mass is a plethora of fine tortuous vessels, some of which can be observed coursing proximally down the surface of the common carotid artery. It is this neovascularity which contributes to the bleeding potential of a CBT. Traversing the upper lateral aspect of the tumour in a shallow arc, and sometimes covered by an indistinct capsule, is the hypoglossal nerve. The internal carotid artery when visible, sometimes enveloped by a capsule, appears stretched and flattened posterolaterally but is enclosed by tumour in advanced cases. It may be opportune at this stage to confirm that a CBT can move only from side to side and also that it exhibits fleeting detumescence under sustained compression.

The hypoglossal nerve is carefully freed from the tumour, placed within a silastic sling (Figures 4.6(a), 4.7(a)) and mobilized upwards by dividing the descendens hypoglossi nerve and the occipital branch of the external carotid artery. The common carotid artery is encircled well below the tumour and, if feasible, the distal internal and external carotid arteries are also similarly controlled. Major tumour vessels originating from branches of the external carotid and subclavian arteries are ligated as the boundaries of the tumour are gradually mobilized, to some extent cutting off external blood supply. On anterior rotation of the tumour–carotid mass the vagus nerve is observed (Figures 4.6(a), 4.7(a)), and after placing it within a sling it may just be possible to identify the superior laryngeal nerve. The spinal accessory nerve is

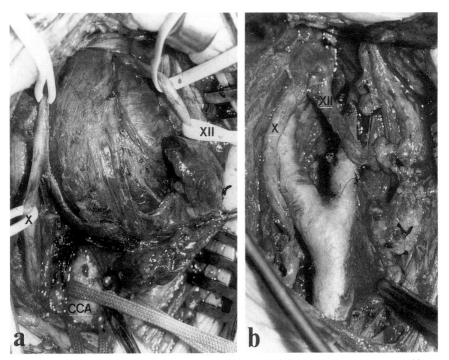

Figure 4.7   Large CBT. (a) Completely surrounding the carotid system; the common carotid artery (CCA) is just visible, the vagus (X) and hypoglossal (XII) nerves are encircled by silastic slings; (b) tumour excision leaves the carotid system, vagus (X) and hypoglossal (XII) nerves intact

rarely involved, except in large and distally invasive tumours. The glossopharyngeal nerve comes to light in the latter stages of dissection at the cranial end of the tumour.

A large tumour severely limits distal access. The division of the digastric muscle, stylohyoid tendon and adjacent veins are helpful measures, taking care not to injure the medially placed hypoglossal nerve. If the tumour has extended into the styloid process or mastoid it must be regarded as virtually inoperable. The ramus of the mandible and the facial nerve, and especially its mandibular branch, can compromise further progress but anterior subluxation of the mandible[110] and lateral mandibulotomy[115,116] will provide ideal access to the distal anatomical structures related to the CBT. The disadvantages of lateral mandibulotomy are that the preferred curvilinear approach provides inadequate exposure and normal nutrition is delayed due to wire fixation of the mandible and intramaxillary fixation with arch bars. Alternatively, an oblique incision extended up to the ear and around it, coupled with resection of the mastoid process, will expose the distal neurovascular structures[117].

Dissection strictly in the subadventitial plane of cleavage, or 'white line'[97] is a precept rewarded by effective extirpation of the tumour while still retaining the integrity of the arteries. Magnification enhances accuracy as sharp dissection is commenced proximally and advanced circumferentially over the common carotid artery, up the internal branch, maintaining haemostasis at each step, and keeping the denuded artery irrigated and moist[74]. Similar dissection is continued up the external carotid artery, alert to the presence of the superior laryngeal nerve (Figure 4.6(b)). At least one large feeding vessel issuing directly from the carotid bifurcation is controlled by a fine prolene stitch. In larger tumours the deep component of the 'collar-stud' configuration which lies parapharyngeally can be surprisingly large.

At this stage formal re-identification of the adjacent anatomy, especially in relation to the ninth cranial nerve, is vital. The tapering tumour tissue along the internal carotid artery converges upwards along with the ninth, tenth, eleventh and twelfth nerves, medial to which lie the upper sympathetic trunk and superior cervical ganglion. Both precision and patience are imperative at this final stage when excision of the tumour must be complete while preserving intact the artery and nerves (Figures 4.6(b), 4.7(b)). The excised tumour usually bears a deep U-shaped imprint of the splayed-out carotid bifurcation[74].

If flow through the internal carotid artery, which may already be compromised by the tumour mass, is further impaired during operation, ischaemia may ensue. Such an outcome could be averted by the use of an intraluminal shunt[30], facilitating a more careful and unhurried approach aimed at preserving the cranial nerves[37,77,91]. In practice, shunting will be infrequently required, as either an emergency step or a planned manoeuvre. For example, an unexpected tear of modest size in the carotid trunk is extended longitudinally away from the undissected tumour and an inlying shunt, perhaps of the Brener type, can be rapidly inserted to maintain cerebral flow[74]. Alternatively, in circumstances either of imminent entry into the artery or the likelihood of prolonged occlusion at an early stage, an outlying shunt of the Pruitt variety may be placed connecting the proximal common to the distal internal carotid artery, while the intervening tumour-bearing arterial segment is isolated within doubly encircled and tightened silastic slings[74].

When the ideal plane represented by the 'white line'[97] is obliterated by an invasive though not necessarily malignant tumour, the carotid trunk should be shunted before excision. If the internal carotid artery is coincidentally atheromatous, requiring endarterectomy, it is preferable to resect the affected segment simply because the combination of subadventitial tumour excision and endarterectomy could leave the arterial wall in a precarious state. On detaching the tumour-bearing segment of carotid artery, the shunt carrying a saphenous vein graft harvested in readiness for this manoeuvre, is inserted to bridge the gap. The interposed vein graft is anastomosed distally and the shunt extracted before completing the proximal anastomosis.

In most instances CBTs can be removed without sacrificing any portion of the carotid system, but in a few the hazards of excision are increased by tumour invasion of the artery, cranial nerves, internal jugular vein and lymph nodes. Despite good preoperative CT scans it may be difficult to differentiate between tumour invasion of the vagus nerve or the jugular vein from a coexisting tumour of the ganglion nodosum or glomus jugulare, respectively. A segment of the external carotid artery can be removed *en bloc* with the tumour after ligating some of its branches. Adjacent lymph nodes infiltrated by tumour should be removed, if necessary by excising a segment of the internal jugular vein, in the knowledge that cranial nerve damage might occur.

Recurrent tumours, some of which probably develop from inadequately removed tissue, can be challenging, not only due to fibrosis and obliteration of planes, but also because the arteries previously denuded of adventitia are more vulnerable to damage during dissection[74]. These are persuasive arguments for a thorough ablation of the tumour at the first operation. A cautious approach is called for, keeping in reserve shunting, arterial excision and vein graft replacement, skills which fall within the domain of the vascular surgeon.

The type of dissection and intimate handling of the carotid vessels may induce spasm which can be abolished by bathing them in warm papaverine solution and any risk of thrombosis countered with an intravenous bolus of heparin. Haemostasis is secured and closed suction drainage is established.

In the early postoperative period, and especially after removal of a large malignant tumour, the airway may be compromised by haematoma, laryngeal oedema or cord paralysis, sufficient to require endotracheal reintubation and even a temporary tracheostomy. Disturbance of baroreceptor function, particularly after previous removal of a contralateral tumour, will be manifested by fluctuations of pulse and blood pressure. Regular monitoring of neurological function will alert the surgeon to the development of cerebrovascular ischaemia, calling into question the possibility of thrombotic occlusion of the internal carotid artery or of the vein graft. Doubts must be resolved by immediate angiography and, if indicated, by expeditious reintervention and corrective repair.

The excised tumour, transferred within an iced container, is submitted to histopathological analysis, electron microscopic search for secretory granules, immunofluorescent, histochemical and radioimmunoassay techniques to identify amines and peptides, while some tissue is deep frozen for future elucidation of its hitherto unknown secretory potential.

Results of surgery

Complications may occur, even during investigation of a CBT; for instance, stroke can follow contrast angiography[28]. The more intimate the tumour–vessel relationship, the greater the technical challenge to the surgeon, and this increasing degree of difficulty is corroborated by Shamblin's classification[36] of CBTs into groups I, II and III. Further, the operative complexity may be reflected in the incidence of both morbidity and mortality[37]. On balance, however, the discovery of a proper plane of dissection[97] allied with the application of modern vascular surgical techniques has meant that the unacceptably high mortality of 30%[66] and rate of hemiplegic stroke of 20%[37], either in the aftermath of *en bloc* resection of the carotid artery and tumour or carotid ligation for haemorrhage, must to a degree be regarded as historical. In a large series, a perioperative mortality rate of 6% and a stroke rate of 2.7% is evidence of improved management[98]. None the less stroke and nerve damage, as well as inadequate excision, give cause for concern, particularly in operations on group III tumours.

The employment of shunts to maintain cerebral perfusion intraoperatively and the preservation or replacement of the internal carotid artery have contributed to a lowering of the incidence of stroke. However, there is no room for complacency as the reduction or arrest of flow by clamping to control bleeding, failure of a shunt, arterial spasm or thrombosis may lead to stroke. This complication will be kept to a minimum as CBTs are increasingly accepted within the repertoire of the vascular surgeon.

During excision of a tumour traction on a cranial nerve usually causes no more than transient neuropraxia. Permanent iatrogenic nerve injury may be a product of surgical inexperience, limited exposure, scanty knowledge of anatomy and failure to identify and protect a nerve within a silastic sling, especially in the final stages of excision. A nerve may have to be sacrificed deliberately when invaded by tumour or in the process of block dissection. Cranial nerve injury, in order of vulnerability, manifests itself in the form of a clumsy tongue or difficulty with chewing (hypoglossal), hoarseness (vagus) and dysphagia or choking (glossopharyngeal and vagus).

Sympathetic trunk injury may not be evident during surgery for large tumour masses until a Horner's syndrome becomes apparent postoperatively[49].

The probability of leaving behind a residue of tumour would seem less likely when it is benign and well circumscribed, but a surgeon who has not previously encountered CBTs will naturally face operation with some trepidation. In good hands, complete excision is possible in the vast majority of cases with a late local recurrence rate of 6%[99], in all cases occurring in the familial variety of CBT. Quite understandably, haemorrhage, cerebral ischaemia and cranial nerve damage are problems which may create anxiety sufficient to discourage complete excision, but a vascular surgeon who regularly operates on the carotid artery and is interested in CBTs can attract enough patients to acquire the confidence to remove these tumours properly and completely, and to review them indefinitely. It is in the surgeon's interest to be thorough, and to avoid having to return to the scene to deal with recurrences which might well be attended by even greater pitfalls. Long-term follow-up is clearly most important to detect local recurrence or metastases, but postoperatively survival has been shown to be equal to that of sex- and age-matched controls[99].

References

1. Glenner, G. G. and Grimley, P. M. (1974) Tumors of the extra-adrenal paraganglion system (including chemoreceptors). *Atlas of Tumour Pathology*, series 2, fascicle 9. Washington: Armed Forces Institute of Pathology
2. Pearse, A. G. E. (1973) Cell migration and the alimentary system: endocrine contribution of the neural crest to the gut and its derivatives. *Digestion*, **8**, 372–385
3. Boyd, J. D. (1937) The development of the human carotid body. *Contrib. Embryol.*, **26** (152), 1–33
4. Adams, W. E. (1958) *The comparative morphology of the carotid body and carotid sinus*. Springfield: Charles C. Thomas, p. 55
5. Smith, P., Jago, R. and Heath, D. (1982) Anatomical variation and quantitative histology of the normal and enlarged carotid body. *J. Pathol.*, **137**, 287–304
6. Hanafee, W. N. and von Leden, H. (1965) Angiography in management of carotid body tumors. *J. Am. Med. Ass.*, **191**, 499–502
7. Borges, L. F., Heros, R. C. and DeBrun, G. (1983) Carotid body tumors managed with preoperative embolization: a report of two cases. *J. Neurosurg.*, **59**, 867–870
8. Davidge-Pitts, K. J. and Pantanowitz, D. (1984) Carotid body tumors. In: *Surgery Annual* (ed. L. M. Nyhus). Norwalk, Conn: Appleton-Century-Crofts, **16**: 203–227
9. Eyzaguirre, C. and Zapata, P. (1984) Perspectives in carotid body research. *J. Appl. Physiol.*, **57**, 931–957
10. Saldana, M. J., Salem, L. E. and Traveean, R. (1973) High altitude hypoxia and chemodectomas. *Hum. Pathol.*, **4**, 251–263
11. Rodriguez-Cuevas, H., Lau, I. and Rodriguez, H. P. (1986) High altitude paragangliomas, diagnostic and therapeutic considerations. *Cancer*, **57**, 672–676
12. Pacheco-Ojeda, L., Durango, E., Rodriguez, C. and Vivar, N. (1988) Carotid body tumors at high altitudes: Quito, Ecuador 1987. *World J. Surg.*, **12**, 856–860
13. Heath, D., Edwards, C. and Harris, P. (1970) Post-mortem size and structure of the human carotid body. *Thorax*, **25**, 129–40
14. Chedid, A. and Jao, W. (1974) Hereditary tumors of the carotid bodies and chronic obstructive pulmonary disease. *Cancer*, **33**, 1635–1641
15. Lack, E. E. (1976) Carotid body hypertrophy in patients with cystic fibrosis and cyanotic congenital heart disease. *Hum. Pathol.*, **8**, 39–47
16. Nissenblatt, M. J. (1978) Cyanotic heart disease: 'low altitude' risk for carotid body tumor? *Johns Hopkins Med. J.*, **142**, 18–21
17. Hirsch, J. H., Killen, F. C. and Troupin, R. H. (1980) Bilateral carotid body tumors and cyanotic heart disease. *Am. J. Radiol.*, **134**, 1073–1075
18. Edwards, C., Heath, D. and Harris, P. (1971) The carotid body in emphysema and left ventricular hypertrophy. *J. Pathol*, **104**, 1–13

19. Nakayama, K. (1961) Surgical removal of the carotid body for bronchial asthma. *Dis. Chest*, **40**, 595–604
20. Wood, J. B., Frankland, A. W. and Eastcott, H. H. G. (1965) Bilateral removal of carotid bodies for asthma. *Thorax*, **20**, 570–573
21. Grufferman, S., Gillman, M. W., Pasternak, L. R., Peterson, C. L. and Young, W. G. (1980) Familial carotid body tumors: case report and epidemiologic review. *Cancer*, **46**, 2116–2122
22. Lund, F. B. (1917) A case of bilateral tumors of the carotid body. *Boston Med. Surg. J.*, **176**, 621–623
23. Wilson, H. (1966) Carotid body tumours. *Surgery*, **59**, 483–493
24. Wilson, H. (1970) Carotid body tumours: familial bilateral. *Ann. Surg.*, **171**, 847–848
25. Dent, T. L., Thompson, N. W. and Fry, W. J. (1976) Carotid body tumours. *Surgery*, **80**, 365–372
26. Kroll, A. J., Alexander, B., Cochios, E. and Pechet, L. (1964) Hereditary deficiencies of clotting factors VII and X associated with carotid body tumor. *New Eng. J. Med.*, **270**, 6–13
27. Parry, D. M., Li, F. P., Strong, L. C., Carney, J. A., Schottenfeld, D. *et al.* (1982) Carotid body tumors in humans: genetics and epidemiology. *JNCI*, **68**, 573–578
28. Hamilton, J. R. L. and Barros D'Sa, A. A. B. (1987) Radionuclide angiography and surgery for familial bilateral chemodectomas. *Eur. J. Vasc. Surg.*, **1**, 97–105
29. Foote, E. L. (1964) Tumors of the glomus jugulare. *Am. J. Clin. Pathol.*, **41**, 72–77
30. Som, M. L., Silver, C. E. and Seidenberg, B. (1966) Excision of carotid body tumors using an internal vascular shunt. *Surg. Gynecol. Obstet.* **122**, 41–44
31. Larraza-Hernandez, Q, Albores Saavedra, J., Benavides, G., Krause, L. G., Perez-Merizaldi, J. C. and Ginzo, A. (1982) Multiple endocrine neoplasia. Pituitary adenoma, multicentric papillary thyroid carcinoma, bilateral carotid body paraganglionoma, parathyroid hyperplasia, gastric leiomyoma, and systemic amyloidosis. *Am. J. Clin. Pathol.*, **78**, 527–532
32. Pritchett, J. W. (1982) Familial concurrences of carotid body tumor and pheochromocytoma. *Cancer*, **49**, 2578–2579
33. Sundaram, M. and Cope, V. (1973) Paraganglioma in the neck. *Br. J. Surg.*, **73**, 182–185
34. Glenner, G. G., Grout, J. R. and Roberts, W. C. (1961) A non-adrenaline secreting carotid body-like tumour. *Lancet*, **2**, 439
35. Levit, S. A., Sheps, S. G., Espinosa, R. E., Remine, W. H. and Harrison, E. G. (1969) Catecholamine secreting paraganglioma of glomus jugulare region resembling phaeochromocytoma. *New Eng. J. Med.*, **281**, 805–811
36. Shamblin, W. R., Remine, W. H., Sheps, S. G. and Harrison, E. G. (1971) Carotid body tumor (chemodectoma): clinicopathologic analysis of ninety cases. *Am. J. Surg.*, **122**, 732–739
37. Lees, G. D., Levine, H. L., Beven, E. G. and Tucker, H. M. (1981) Tumors of carotid body: experience with 41 operative cases. *Am. J. Surg.*, **142**, 362–365
38. Bederal, P., Bratten, M., Cappelen, C., Mylius, E. A. and Walaas, O. (1962) Noradrenaline-adrenaline producing nonchromaffin paraganglioma. *Acta Med. Scand.*, **172**, 249–257
39. Hamberger, C. A., Hamberger, C. B., Wersall, J. and Wagermark, J. (1967) Malignant catecholamine-producing tumor of the carotid body. *Acta Pathol. Microbiol. Scand.*, **69**, 489–492
40. Salyer, K. E., Ketchum, L. D., Robinson, D. W. and Masters, F. W. (1969) Surgical management of cervical paragangliomata. *Arch. Surg.*, **98**, 572–578
41. Clarke, A. D., Matheson, H. and Boddie, H. G. (1976) Removal of catecholamine-secreting chemodectoma. *Anaesthesia*, **31**, 1225–1230
42. Irons, G. B., Weiland, L. H. and Brown, W. L. (1977) Paragangliomas of the neck. Clinical and pathological analysis of 116 cases. *Surg. Clin. N. Am.* **57**, 575–583
43. White, M. C. and Hickson, B. R. (1979) Multiple paragangliomata secreting catecholamines and calcitonin with intermittent hypercalcaemia. *J. R. Soc. Med.*, **72**, 532–538
44. Newland, M. C. and Hurlbert, B. J. (1980) Chemodectoma diagnosed by hypertension and tachycardia during anesthesia. *Anesth. Analg.*, **59**, 388–390
45. Crowell, W. T., Grizzle, W. E. and Siegel, A. L. (1982) Functional carotid paragangliomas: Biochemical, ultrastructural and histochemical correlation with clinical symptoms. *Arch. Pathol. Lab. Med.*, **106**, 599–603
46. Strauss, M., Nicholas, G. G., Abt, A. B., Harrison, T. S. and Seaton, J. F. (1983) Malignant catecholamine-secreting carotid body paraganglioma. *Otolaryngol. Head Neck Surg.*, **91**, 315–321
47. Payne, C. M., Nagle, R. B. and Borduin, V. (1984) An ultrastructural cytochemical stain specific for neuroendocrine neoplasms. *Lab. Invest.*, **51**, 350–365
48. Pryse-Davis, J., Dawson, I. M. and Westbury, G. (1964) Some morphologic, histochemical and chemical observations on chemodectomas and the normal carotid body, including a study on the chromaffin reaction and possible ganglion cell elements. *Cancer*, **17**, 185–202
49. Van Asperen De Boer, F. R. S., Terpstra, J. L. and Vink, M. (1981) Diagnosis, treatment and operation complications of carotid body tumours. *Br. J. Sur.*, **68**, 433–438

50. Lack, E. E., Cubilla, A. L., Woodruff, J. M. and Farr, H. W. (1977) Paragangliomas of the head and neck region. *Cancer*, **39**, 397–409
51. Gaylis, H., Davidge-Pitts, K. and Pantanowitz, D. (1987) Carotid body tumours. A review of 52 cases. *S. A. Med. J.*, **72**, 493–496
52. Krupski, W. C., Effeney, D. J., Ehrenfeld, W. K. and Stoney, R. J. (1982) Cervical chemodectoma: Technical considerations and management options. *Am. J. Surg.*, **144**, 215–220
53. Martin, C. E., Rosenfeld, L. and McSwain, B. (1973) Carotid body tumors: A 16-year follow-up of seven malignant cases. *S. A. Med. J.*, **66**, 1236–1243
54. Occiogrosso, M., DeTommasi, A., Vailati, G. and DeBenedictis, G. (1983) Malignant chemodectoma of the carotid body causing spinal cord compression. *Surg. Neurol.*, **23**, 14–18
55. Barnes, L. and Taylor, S. R. (1990) Carotid body paragangliomas. *Arch. Otol. Head Neck Surg.*, **116**, 447–453
56. Chambers, R. G. and Mahoney, W. D. (1968) Carotid body tumours. *Am. J. Surg.*, **116**, 554–558
57. Chung, W. B. (1979) The carotid body tumor. *Can. J. Sur.*, **23**, 319–322
58. You-Xian, F. and Qun, S. (1982) Surgical treatment of carotid body tumors. *Chin. Med. J.*, **95**, 417–422
59. Javid, H., Dye, W. S., Hunter, J. A., Najafi, H. and Julian, O. C. (1967) Surgical management of carotid body tumour. *Arch. Surg.*, **95**, 771–779
60. Sato, T., Saito, H., Yoshinaga, K., Shibota, Y. and Sasano, N. (1974) Concurrence of carotid body tumor and pheochromocytoma. *Cancer*, **34**, 1787–1795
61. Gibb, M. K., Carney, J. A., Hayles, A. B. and Telander, R. L. (1977) Simultaneous adrenal and cervical pheochromocytomas in childhood. *Ann. Surg.*, **185**, 273–278
62. Glasscock, M. E., Jackson, C. G., Nissen, A. J. and Smith, P. G. (1984) Diagnosis and management of catecholamine-secreting glomus tumors. *Laryngoscope*, **94**, 1008–1015
63. Sanchez, A. C., de Seijas, E. V., Matesanz, J. M. and Trapero, V. L. (1988) Carotid body tumour: Unusual cause of transient ischaemic attacks. *Stroke*, **19**, 102–103
64. Castleman, B., Iverson, L. and Menendex, V. (1956) Localized mediastinal lymph node hyperplasia resembling thymoma. *Cancer*, **9**, 822–830
65. Browse, N. L. (1982) Carotid body tumours. *Br. Med. J.*, **284**, 1507–1508
66. Monro, R. S. (1950) The natural history of carotid body tumours and their diagnosis and treatment. *Br. J. Surg.*, **37**, 445–453
67. Javid, H., Dye, W. S. and Najafi, H. (1976) Carotid body tumour: dissection or reflection. *Arch. Surg.*, **111**, 344–347
68. Lewis, R. R., Beasley, M. G., Coghlan, B. A., Yates, A. K. and Gosling, R. G. (1980) Demonstration of carotid body tumors by ultrasound. *Br. J. Radiol.*, **53**, 368–371
69. Gritzmann, N., Herold, C., Haller, J., Karnel, F. and Schwaighofer, B. (1987) Duplex sonography of tumors of the carotid body. *Cardiovasc. Intervent. Radiol.*, **10**, 280–284
70. Russell, C. D., Jander, H. P. and Dubovsky, E. V. (1975) Demonstration of a chemodectoma by perfusion scanning: case report. *J. Nuc. Med.*, **16**, 472–473
71. Peters, J. L., Ward, M. W. and Fisher, C. (1979) Diagnosis of a carotid body chemodectoma with dynamic radionuclide perfusion scanning. *Am. J. Surg.*, **137**, 661–664
72. Serafini, A. N. and Weinstein, M. B. (1972) Radionuclide investigation of a carotid body tumor. *J. Nuc. Med.*, **13**, 640–643
73. Ruijs, J. H. J., Van Waes, P. F. G. M., De Haas, G., Hoekstra, A., Mulder, P. H. M. and Veldman, J. E. (1978) Screening of a family for chemodectoma. *Radiologia Clin.*, **47**, 114–123
74. Barros D'Sa A. A. B. (1991) Chemodectoma. In *Surgical Management of Vascular Disease*, (eds P. R. F. Bell, C. W. Jamieson and C. W. Ruckley). London: Baillière Tindall (in press)
75. Idbohrn, H. (1951) Angiographical diagnosis of carotid body tumors. *Acta Radiol.*, **35**, 115–123
76. Berrett, A. (1965) Value of angiography in the management of tumors of the head and neck. *Radiology*, **84**, 1052–1058
77. Schechter, M. M. and Chusid, J. G. (1966) Chemodectomas of the carotid bifurcation. *Acta Radiol. (Diagn.) (Stockholm)*, **5**, 488–508
78. Gehweiler, J. A. and Bender, W. R. (1968) Carotid arteriography in the diagnosis and management of tumors of the carotid body. *Am. J. Roentgenol*, **104**, 893–898
79. Westbrook, K. C., Guillamondegui, O. M., Medellin, H. and Jesse, R. H. (1972) Chemodectomas of the neck: Selective management. *Am. J. Surg.* **124**, 760–766
80. Dial, P., Marks, C. and Bolton, J. (1982) Current management of paragangliomas. *Surg. Gynecol. Obstet.*, **155**, 187–192
81. Lahey, F. H. and Warren, K. W. (1951) A long-term appraisal of carotid body tumors with remarks on their removal. *Surg. Gynecol. Obstet.*, **92**, 481–491
82. Conley, J. J. (1963) The management of carotid body tumors. *Surg. Gynecol. Obstet.*, **117**, 722–732

83. Farr, H. W. (1967) Carotid body tumors: A thirty-year experience at Memorial Hospital. *Am. J. Surg.*, **114**, 614–619
84. Ferris, R. A., Kirschner, L. P., Mero, J. H., Fields, R. L. and Fulcher, T. M. (1979) Computed tomography of a carotid body tumor. *J. Comp. Ass. Tom.* **3**, 834–835
85. Chui, M. and Briant, T. D. R. (1982) CT evaluation of carotid sheath lesions. *Br. J. Radiol.*, **55**, 813–816
86. Newmark, H., Mellon, W. S., Bhagwanani, D. G., Bauman, D. H. and Duerksen, R. (1983) Carotid body tumor seen on computed tomography. *CT*, **7**, 155–157
87. Olsen, W. L., Dillon, W. P., Kelly, W. M., Norman, D., Brant-Zawadski, M. and Newton, T.H. (1987) MRI imaging of paragangliomas. *Am. J. Roentgenol.*, **148**, 201–204
88. MacGillivray, D. C., Perry, M. O., Selfe, R. W. and Nydick, I. (1987) Carotid body tumour: atypical angiogram of a functioning tumour. *J. Vasc. Surg.*, **5**, 462–468
89. Engzell, U., Franzen, S. and Zajicek, J. (1971) Aspiration biopsy of tumors of the neck. II. Cytologic findings in 13 cases of carotid body tumour. *Acta Cytologica*, **15**, 25–30
90. Padberg, F. T., Cady, B. and Persson, A. V. (1983) Carotid body tumor – the Lahey Clinic experience. *Am. J. Surg.*, **145**, 526–528
91. Rosen, I. B., Palmer, J. A., Goldberg, M. and Mustard, R. A. (1981) Vascular problems associated with carotid body tumors. *Am. J. Surg.*, **142**, 459–463
92. Lybeert, M. L. M., Van Andel, J. G., Eijkenboom, W. M. A., De Jong, P. C. and Knegt, P. (1984) Radiotherapy of paragangliomas. *Clin. Otolaryngol.*, **9**, 105–109
93. Mitchell, D. C. and Clyne, C. A. C. (1985) Chemodectomas of the neck: the response to radiotherapy. *Br. J. Surg.*, **72**, 903–905
94. Valdagni, R. and Amichetti, M. (1990) Radiation therapy of carotid body tumors. *Am. J. Clin. Oncol.*, **13**, 45–48
95. Keen, W. W. and Funke, J. (1906) Tumors of the carotid gland. *J. Am. Med. Ass.*, **47**, 468–479
96. Pette, J. R., Woolner, L. B. and Judd, E. S. (1953) Carotid body tumors (chemodectomas). *Ann. Surg.*, **137**, 465–477
97. Gordon-Taylor, G. (1940) On carotid tumours. *Br. J. Surg.*, **28**, 163–172
98. Hallet, J. W., Nora, J. D., Hollier, L. H., Cherry, K. J. and Pairolero, P. C. (1988) Trends in neurovascular complications of surgical management for carotid body and cervical paragangliomas: A fifty-year experience with 153 tumors. *J. Vasc. Surg.*, **7**, 284–289
99. Nora, J. D., Hallet, J. W., O'Brien, P. C., Naessens, J. M., Cherry, K. J. and Pairolero, P. C. (1988) Surgical resection of carotid body tumors: Long-term survival, recurrence and metastasis. *Mayo Clin. Proc.*, **63**, 348–352
100. McPherson, G. A. D., Halliday, A. W. and Mansfield, A. O. (1989) Carotid body tumours and other cervical paragangliomas: Diagnosis and management. *Br. J. Surg.* **76**, 33–36
101. Ganong, W. F. (1977) *Medical physiology*, 8th ed, Los Altos, California, Lange Medical Publications p. 504
102. Farr, H. W. (1980) Carotid body tumors: A 40-year study. *CA*, **30**, 260–265
103. Grabowski, E. W., Pilcher, D. B., Schmidek, H. H., Bookwalter, J. R. and Davis, J. H. (1983) Carotid body tumors. *Am. J. Surg.*, **49**, 483–486
104. Anderson, R. and Scarcella, J. V. (1963) Carotid body tumors. *Am. J. Surg.*, **106**, 856–859
105. Schick, P. M., Hieshima, G. B., White, R. A. *et al.* (1980) Arterial catheter embolization followed by surgery for large chemodectoma. *Surgery*, **87**, 459–464
106. Hennessey, Q., Jamieson, C. W. and Allison, D. J. (1984) Pre-operative embolization of a chemodectoma. *Br. J. Radiol.*, **57**, 845–846
107. Ward, P. H., Lin, C., Vinuela, F. and Bentson, J. R. (1988) Embolization: an adjunctive measure for removal of carotid body tumours. *Laryngoscope*, **98**, 1287–1291
108. Robison, J. G., Shagets, F. W., Beckett, W. C. and Spies, J. B. (1989) A multidisciplinary approach to reducing morbidity and operative blood loss during resection of carotid body tumor. *Surg. Gynecol. Obstet.*, **168**, 166–170
109. Martorell, F. (1956) Tumor of the carotid body. *Angiology*, **7**, 228–232
110. Fry, R. E. and Fry, W. J. (1980) Extracranial carotid artery injuries. *Surgery*, **88**, 581–587
111. Farrar, T., Kirklin, J. W., Judd, E. S. and DeVine, K. D. (1956) Resection of carotid body tumors with preservation of the carotid vessels. *Arch. Surg.*, **72**, 595–599
112. Rush, B. F. (1962) Current concepts in the treatment of carotid body tumors. *Surgery*, **52**, 679–684
113. Morris, G. C., Balas, P. E., Cooley, D. A., Crawford, S. E. and DeBakey, M. E. (1963) Surgical treatment of benign and malignant carotid body tumors: Clinical experience with 16 tumors in 12 patients. *Am. J. Surg.*, **29**, 429–437
114. Olcott, C., Fee, W. E., Enzmann, D. R. and Mehigan, J. T. (1981) Planned approach to the management of malignant invasion of the carotid artery. *Am. J. Surg.*, **142**, 123–127

115. Work, W. P. and Hybels, R. L. (1974) A study of tumours of the parapharyngeal space. *Laryngoscope*, **84** (Suppl), 1749–1755
116. Dichtel, W.J., Miller, R. H., Feliciano, D. V. *et al.* (1984) Lateral mandibulotomy: A technique of exposure for penetrating injuries of the internal carotid artery at the base of the skull. *Laryngoscope*, **94**, 1140–1143
117. Purdue, G. F., Pellegrini, R. V. and Arena, S. (1981) Aneurysms of the high internal carotid artery: A new approach. *Surgery*, **89**, 268–270

Chapter 5

Should we operate on thoracoabdominal aneurysms?

John H. N. Wolfe

The repair of a thoracoabdominal aneurysm is a challenge, but enthusiasm must be tempered by the mixed results of this hazardous operation. Since they present a formidable, and relatively uncommon, problem, most vascular surgeons have no, or only limited experience of their treatment. Significant progress has been made in simplifying the procedure, which has encouraged some to undertake this complex operation and there is now sufficient experience to re-evaluate the outcome of these operations and attempt to compare this with a conservative approach.

Are they rare?

Many surgeons maintain that thoracoabdominal aneurysms are so rare that management does not impinge on their own practice. This complacency is probably misplaced, since a study of deaths from aneurysms in the community undertaken in Swansea[1] revealed 78 patients out of 338 (23%) with thoracic and thoracoabdominal aneurysms. Furthermore, with the increased use of abdominal CT scanning and ultrasound patients are more frequently referred with suprarenal aneurysms. Approximately 5% of abdominal aneurysms fall into this category, and these are the ones most likely to present to the general vascular surgeon. However, there are also aneurysms involving the thoracic aorta alone (type I) or the whole of the descending aorta from the left subclavian artery to the iliac bifurcation (type II). Many of these patients are referred to thoracic surgeons; some are treated conservatively and never receive a surgical opinion.

In Stanley Crawford's series of 1193 patients [2] the incidence of thoracoabdominal aneurysms involving the aorta inferior to the pulmonary hilum (types III and IV) was 50%. This is similar to our experience at St Mary's Hospital where 38/65 patients operated upon had a type III or type IV aneurysm. These figures can only give a rough incidence of the types of thoracoabdominal aneurysm and may vary according to referral patterns (Figure 5.1).

How often do they rupture?

There is little conclusive information on the natural history of thoracoabdominal aneurysms. Some surgeons obtain solace from the fact that they have not seen many of them rupture, vindicating their conservative approach. This is not supported by the

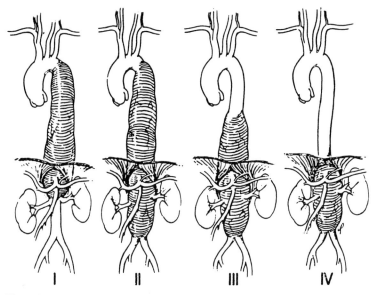

Figure 5.1   Classification of thoracoabdominal aneurysms. (Reproduced from [2] with permission)

information that we have at St Mary's. We accept that the rupture of abdominal aneurysms is a problem of sufficient magnitude for operations to be performed on asymptomatic patients, but in one-quarter of the patients in the Swansea Community study[1] a thoracoabdominal aneurysm was found rather than an infrarenal aneurysm. This supports the hypothesis that the risk of rupture is related to the size rather than the site of the aneurysm. Abdominal aneurysms between 5 cm and 7 cm appear to have an annual incidence of rupture of approximately 12% and those greater than 7 cm a rupture rate of approximately 30% (Szilagyi *et al.*[3]). In an early study by Joyce *et al.*[4] patients with thoracic aneurysms had a five-year survival of approximately 50% if treated conservatively. More recently, Crawford[5] has collated the data on his patients who refused surgery – these had a mortality rate of 76% within two years.

These data must be weighed against the considerable risks associated with surgery.

Progress in surgical intervention

The first successful repair of a thoracoabdominal aneurysm was reported by Etheridge in 1955[6], using homograft. The following year DeBakey reported four similar procedures[7]. Following the death of the first patient from renal failure DeBakey used a shunt. When Dacron became available he modified the technique and sutured the homograft end-to-side proximally and distally to act as a shunt. Side arms of Dacron were sutured to the visceral vessels with a minimum of ischaemic time (Figure 5.2) and the proximal and distal orifices of the aneurysm sac were then sutured off. By 1965 he was able to report 42 of these operations with an operative mortality of 26%[8]; these were outstanding results. Stanley Crawford, working in the same hospital, introduced his simple technique in 1973 (Figure 5.3), which was a major advance and dramatically reduced the mortality rate. His technique greatly

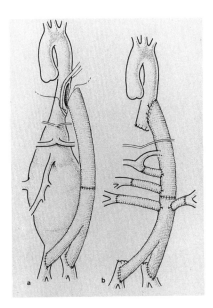

Figure 5.2 DeBakey method of resecting thoracoabdominal aneurysms. (Reproduced from [26] with permission)

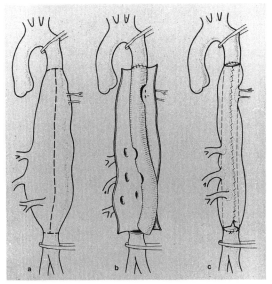

Figure 5.3 Stanley Crawford method of repairing thoracoabdominal aneurysms. (Reproduced from [26] with permission)

reduced the extent of the dissection with a consequent reduction in blood loss; it also avoided the technically demanding anastomoses to each visceral artery. However, it has the disadvantage of a prolonged ischaemia time compared with the deBakey technique.

Various methods have been proposed to reduce this ischaemia. In the 1960s Connelly used a left aortofemoral shunt[9] and Dillon recommended a femorofemoral vein-to-artery shunt using an oxygenator pump[10]. More recently, Korompai and

Hayward have used an external shunt[11]. All these systems, however, require full systemic heparinization which results in increased blood loss. They have been abandoned by most surgeons. Bosher and Brookes have modified Stanley Crawford's technique by advocating total body hypothermia – but this also increases blood loss since clotting is negligible below 27°C[12].

Ischaemia therefore remains the cause of most of the major complications of the operation, which are ischaemia of the spinal cord, renal ischaemia and visceral ischaemia resulting in gut infarction or the systemic manifestations of translocation of the gut flora.

Treatment of spinal cord ischaemia

Mechanical methods

Many methods have been used to prevent paraplegia caused by spinal cord ischaemia. There are theoretical reasons why moderate or profound hypothermia may reduce this problem, but since hypothermia can lead to poor clotting and further blood loss the subsequent hypotension may counterbalance any benefits. Shunting techniques have also been used but the heparinization required carries the same disadvantage as profound hypothermia. Furthermore, it has been shown that the risk of paraplegia is not decreased by the use of shunting in patients operated upon for aneurysms of the descending aorta[13]. There is also experimental evidence (in baboons) to show that spinal cord circulation is not improved by shunting unless the radicular artery is perfused[14].

In the early 1960s experimental evidence was produced which suggested that the removal of cerebrospinal fluid would improve perfusion pressure of the spinal cord and thus reduce the incidence of paraplegia following aortic cross-clamping[15,16]. Stanley Crawford has not found that the drainage of cerebrospinal fluid has reduced his paraplegia rate, but the technique has been advocated by Hollier and colleagues[17]. There is some anecdotal evidence that patients with paresis of the lower extremities may recover if small volumes of cerebrospinal fluid are removed. In this technique a 16-gauge catheter is introduced through the L3/L4 interspace and cerebrospinal fluid (usually approximately 100 ml) removed prior to cross-clamping in order to keep the pressure at approximately zero level.

Modifications of operative technique

Maintenance of blood pressure is an important factor in preventing paraplegia: neural tissue at risk is more likely to infarct if the perfusion pressure is reduced due to a drop in systemic pressure. The duration of ischaemia is also of considerable importance. Although there is no conclusive evidence that the reattachment of intercostal vessels affects rate of paraplegia it seems a logical and important part of the operation. The major anterior spinal artery supplying the lumbar segment of the spinal cord has a variable origin (usually D11/D12) ranging from D6 to L2, and most surgeons arbitrarily reattach one or more pairs of these vessels between these levels[18]. It would be more logical to identify the major source of anterior spinal cord supply by preoperative investigation. Angiography has been used by one group[19] to do this.

Neurophysiological monitoring

This has been used with the idea of selective intercostal artery re-implantation. Somatosensory evoked potentials have been applied[20], they give an indication of the function in the posterior part of the spinal cord and are usually unaffected since ischaemia usually occurs in the anterior part of the cord. Motor evoked potentials have also been used, but Crawford has found these rather unreliable with a relatively high incidence of false negative and false positive recordings[21]. Sandmann[22] has avoided some of these problems by directly recording from the critical segment of the spinal cord. He attributes part of his success in reducing paraplegia rates to this technique.

Pharmacological methods

Papaverine is a powerful topical vasodilator and it has been injected intrathecally, following the drainage of CSF, to reduce ischaemia. Promising results have been obtained in a small series but the method remains relatively untested.

There is some experimental evidence that oxygen free radicals released into the circulation following a period of ischaemia may damage the spinal cord[23] and supra-oxide dismutase has been used to alleviate this. Prostaglandins and calcium channel blockers have also been used, but with the inevitable polypharmacy in these patients it is difficult to ascertain whether they have any significant effect.

Renal ischaemia

Stanley Crawford reported a renal failure rate requiring temporary or permanent haemodialysis of 9%[2]. This was identical to our own figure but in our series no patient has required prolonged haemodialysis since the renal failure was part of multi-system failure[27]. We did have a transient rise in serum creatinine in 17 of the 65 patients, but this returned to normal during their hospital stay. Preoperative renal impairment is the strongest predictor of postoperative problems but it is clearly important to maintain as short a renal ischaemia time as possible. Many surgeons advocate the use of renal perfusion with cold Ringer's lactate solution but we have not employed this method. The use of an occlusion balloon is potentially harmful to these vital arteries: furthermore, the insertion of the balloon and subsequent positioning of the catheters to facilitate the anastomoses may prolong ischaemia time. Stanley Crawford states that there is no significant difference in the incidence of renal failure between the use of the various renal protection techniques and simple aortic cross-clamping[24]. We consider that this supports our current approach of simple aortic cross-clamping which results in a mean ischaemia time to the right kidney of approximately 25 minutes and to the left kidney of approximately 40 minutes.

Visceral ischaemia

The mechanisms of the effects of transient visceral ischaemia are poorly understood, but disruption of the enterocyte barrier probably washes a multitude of unwanted toxic substances into the systemic circulation. We now appreciate that there can be a breakdown of the functional integrity of the gastrointestinal tract without overt ischaemia. This may trigger events which lead to major systemic disturbances and even death. The normal gut teems with pathogenic organisms but the bowel's epithelial lining normally blocks their egress. Even if a few bacteria breach this barrier they are neutralized by the submucosal lymphoid tissue, mesenteric lymph nodes and hepatic kuypffer cells. Breakdown of these various defence mechanisms leads to translocation of the bacteria or their endotoxins with dramatic systemic effects – some of these exogenous and endogenous endotoxins may initiate many of the passive pathophysiological alterations associated with critical illness. Once the enterocyte barrier is breached the gut acts like a large undrained abscess.

A better understanding of the mechanisms and substances involved may lead to development of antibodies that can block or minimize the deleterious effects of partial gut ischaemia.

Bleeding

Perhaps Stanley Crawford's major contribution to the repair of thoracoabdominal aneurysms was the abandonment of cardiopulmonary bypass. The reduced blood loss that resulted from the cessation of heparin use was associated with a dramatic improvement in mortality rates. Some surgeons now advocate cautious heparinization, and the advent of Trasylol (which has been used successfully by cardiac surgeons to reduce bleeding) may also be of value. Meticulous surgical technique is certainly vital and oversewing the aneurysm sac is a useful adjunct to careful haemostasis. We leave the thrombus in the aneurysm sac while performing the proximal anastomosis since this appears to reduce bleeding from the lumbar arteries. Against the current vogue for splenic preservation we have learnt that minor splenic damage should be treated by splenectomy.

Current results

Stanley Crawford's expertise and experience are a benchmark for the rest of us. Mortality rates should be low for type IV aneurysms and the paraplegia rate should also be very low since the major spinal artery is usually above the graft anastomosis. We have not yet had a patient develop paraplegia with a type IV repair.

Type II aneurysms are much more hazardous – Stanley Crawford has a reasonable mortality rate of 10% but the paraplegia rate is 29%.

Our current approach to type IV aneurysms is that of a complex abdominal aneurysm and the indications for surgery are therefore similar; our approach to a type II aneurysm is more circumspect. Elderly asymptomatic patients frequently opt for a conservative approach when faced with the possible complications; these account for most of the 17% of patients treated conservatively in our practice (Figure 5.4). Unfortunately many patients with type II aneurysms have intolerable symptoms such as dysphagia or intractable back pain and request surgery.

Investigation

Thorough investigation is mandatory for these patients and an accurate understanding of the aneurysm's anatomy and associated organ function is essential. A full thoracoabdominal CT scan (Figure 5.5) is an essential first stage in assessing the aneurysm and some patients may be refused surgery on the basis of this alone. The

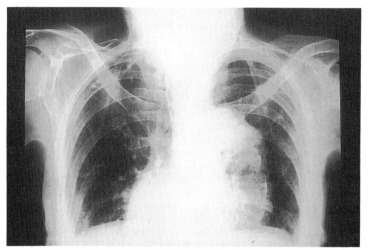

Figure 5.4   Chest radiograph of asymptomatic type II thoracoabdominal aneurysm

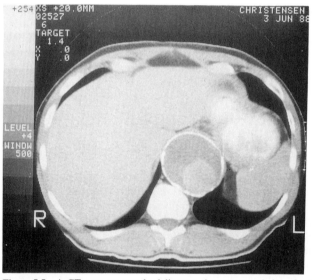

Figure 5.5   A CT scan accurately delineates the extent and size of a thoracoabdominal aneurysm

presence of associated disease of the aorta or aortic branches and the anatomy of these vessels are determined by total aortography (Figure 5.6). With these two investigations it should be possible to plan the technical aspects of surgery.

It is essential to assess the function of the organs that will be affected. Renal function is assessed by serum creatinine levels, and also by a DTPA scan. Poor renal or cardiac function will be associated with greater morbidity and must be carefully assessed preoperatively. If there is significant aortic incompetence the surgery to the aortic valve should precede any attempt to repair the descending aorta (Figure 5.7). Otherwise the massive increase in left ventricular pressure produced by cross-clamping the aorta may be fatal.

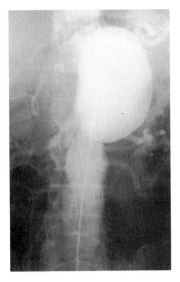

Figure 5.6   Angiogram of type IV thoracoabdominal aneurysm

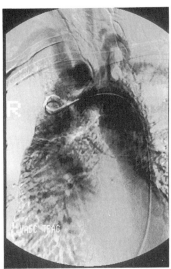

Figure 5.7   Aneurysm in a patient with aortic incompetence and a type II thoracoabdominal aneurysm. The patient was not considered fit for repair of the aortic valve and the thoracoabdominal aneurysm

Most of these aneurysms will be atherosclerotic but the incidence of rarer causes of aneurysm is higher in thoracoabdominal aneurysms. In the younger patient medial degeneration must be considered and patients with true Marfan's syndrome may present major technical problems[25], as will patients with Behçet's disease or Ehlers–Danlos syndrome. Patients with Takayasu's disease or mycotic aneurysms may also present with these aneurysms.

The operation

Each surgeon will have personal nuances of technique but almost all follow the principles of the Stanley Crawford approach. The patient is placed on a bean bag and

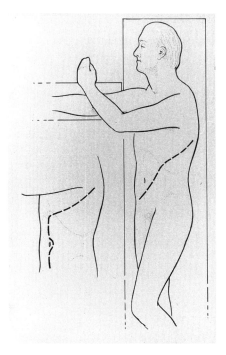

Figure 5.8 Incision for repair of thoracoabdominal aneurysm (inset for types I, II and III) (reproduced from [26] with permission)

rotated 60° to the right with the left arm elevated. The hips are not rotated, thus opening the thoracoabdominal space (Figure 5.8).

For type I, II and III aneurysms we routinely perform the incision through the bed of the 5th or 6th rib. A low thoracic incision can significantly impair access to the proximal part of the descending aorta and embarrass performance at the proximal anastomosis (Figure 5.9).

The retroperitoneal space is approached from behind the descending colon. The left kidney is swung forward with the other viscera and in this way a plane can be manufactured along the inferior aspect of the diaphragm. Great care must be taken to avoid damage to the spleen (which had to be removed in 8% of our patients). The aneurysm then lies exposed in the depths of the wound and the crus of the diaphragm is split in order to obtain access to the lower thoracic aorta. In aneurysms extending into the chest it is *not* necessary to divide the diaphragm. By transecting the anterior aspect of the diaphragm it is possible to open fully the rib cage and expose the intrathoracic aorta. The graft can then be tunnelled through the crura which have been divided and any anastomoses performed above, or below, the diaphragm. By minimizing the disruption of the diaphragm we hope to reduce respiratory morbidity (Figure 5.10).

Once this dissection has been performed there is wide exposure of the aneurysm and there should be little problem with access. The clamps are placed without prior heparinization, and the aneurysm sac opened with diathermy. In order to reduce back bleeding we do not remove the thrombus from the sac until the proximal anastomosis has been performed (using 2/0 or 3/0 Prolene). Before performing the intercostal patches it is essential to ensure that the graft is stretched and oriented correctly so that the orfice in the graft is tailored to the intercostal vessels. Inaccuracies at this juncture can lead to troublesome bleeding.

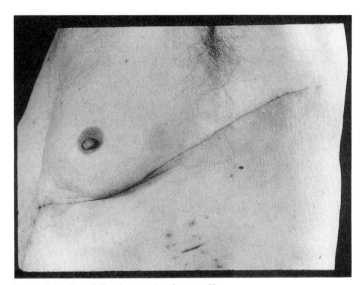

Figure 5.9   Scar following repair of a type II aneurysm

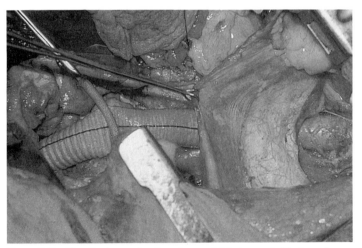

Figure 5.10   The diaphragm has been incompletely transected but good access to both thoracic and abdominal cavities is achieved. The anastomosis has been performed just above the level of the diaphragm

Identification of the visceral orifices is usually straightforward but can on occasion be difficult, particularly in large aneurysms where they can be lost in the folds of the aortic wall. It is essential that all these orifices are carefully identified before the patches are cut. Usually the coeliac artery, superior mesenteric artery and right renal artery can be incorporated in one patch. Back-bleeding from these vessels is minimal and we do *not* use occlusion balloons – we consider that the balloons may damage the vessels and can also get in the way. We have not yet had cause to regret this policy. Having revascularized the right renal artery and gut vessels it is preferable to release the clamp. It is, however, essential to assess the position of the left renal artery anastomosis before the clamps are removed – in some patients the left renal artery is so close to the right that a side biting clamp is difficult to apply to the graft. The surgeon then explains sheepishly to the anaesthetist that the aortic cross-clamp must be re-applied, leading to considerable left ventricular strain and hypertension. A prolonged ischaemia time is better than the unexpected re-application of the aortic cross-clamp. Once these anastomoses have been performed and revascularization of the organs achieved the patient's situation should be more stable.

There are great difficulties in assessing the right kidney and it is therefore essential to ensure that the left kidney is adequately revascularized. Following cross-clamping indigo carmine is injected intravenously so that on release of the clamps the kidneys are perfused with indigo carmine, producing blue urine. This is further reassurance for the surgeon that at least one kidney is functioning.

In most patients the distal anastomosis can be performed to the aortic bifurcation but in a few it will be necessary to perform a bifurcation graft beyond iliac aneurysms. Before completing this anastomosis it is essential to ensure that good back-flow is obtained from the iliac arteries in these non-heparinized patients. It is also essential to ensure that a good flush of blood is obtained from the graft so that any residual clots are removed and are not flushed into the legs.

Following meticulous haemostasis the sac of the aneurysm is closed as a further haemostatic seal. The diaphragm, chest and abdomen are then closed routinely, with a basal chest drain.

Towards the future

In the last 20 years our approach to the infrarenal abdominal aortic aneurysm has changed dramatically. The elective repair of these is now in the standard repertoire of most hospitals. It is unlikely that this will ever be the approach to the thoracoabdominal aneurysm but since Stanley Crawford's historic contribution a large number of patients throughout the world have benefited. We can speculate that improvements in our care of the spinal cord and gut will further improve results, as will the ever-evolving agents available to support heart, lungs and kidneys through the major stresses of this complex procedure.

Acknowledgements

The experience at St Mary's Vascular Unit is the combined experience of Miss A. O. Mansfield and myself together with the anaesthetist Dr P. F. Knight.

References

1. Ingoldby, C. J. H., Wijanto, W. and Mitchell, J. E. (1986) Impact of vascular surgery on community mortality from ruptured aortic aneurysms. *Br. J. Surg.*, **73**, 551–553
2. Crawford, E. S. (1990) Thoraco-abdominal and proximal aortic replacement for extensive aortic aneurysmal disease. In *The Cause and Management of Aneurysms*. (eds R. M. Greenhalgh and J. A. Mannick). W. B. Saunders Co, London, pp. 351–362
3. Szilagyi, D. E., Smith, R. F., DeRusso, F. J., Elliott, F. P. and Sherrin, F. W. (1966) Contribution of abdominal aortic aneurysmectomy to prolongation of life. *Ann. Surg.*, **164**, 153–156
4. Joyce, J. W., Fairbairn, J. F., Kincaid, O. S. and Juergens, J.L. (1964) Aneurysms of the thoracic aorta. A clinical study with special reference to prognosis. *Circulation*, **29**, 176

5. Crawford, E. S. and DeNatale, R. W. (1986) Thoraco-abdominal aortic aneurysms: Observations regarding natural course of disease. *J. Vasc. Surg.*, **3**, 578–582

6. Etheridge, S. N., Yee, J., Smith, J. V., Schonberger, S. and Goldman, M. J. (1955) Successful resection of large aneurysms of the upper abdominal aorta and replacement with homograft. *Surgery*, **38**, 1071

7. DeBakey, M. E., Creech, O. and Morris, G. C. (1956) Aneurysms of the thoraco-abdominal aorta involving the coeliac, superior mesenteric and renal arteries. *Ann. Surg.*, **144**, 459

8. DeBakey, M. E., Crawford, E. S., Garrett, H. E., Beall, A. C. and Howell, J. F. (1965) Surgical considerations in the treatment of aneurysms of the thoraco-abdominal aorta. *Ann. Surg.*, **162**, 650

9. Connolly, J. E., Wakabayashi, A., Serman, J. C. *et al.* (1971) Clinical experience with left ventricular bypass without coagulants for thoracic aneurysms. *J. Thorac. Cardiovasc. Surg.*, **62**, 568

10. Dillon, M. L., Young, W. G. and Sealy, W. C. (1967) Aneurysm of the descending aorta. *Ann. Thorac. Surg.*, **3**, 430

11. Korompai, F. L. and Hayward, R. H. (1975) Preservation of visceral perfusion during resection of thoraco-abdominal aneurysm. *Cardiovascular Diseases: Bull. Texas Heart Inst.*, **2**, 349

12. Bosher, L. H. and Brooks, J. W. (1975) The surgical treatment of thoraco-abdominal aneurysms and aneurysms of the upper abdominal aorta. *Virginia Medical Monthly*, **102**, 116

13. Crawford, E. S. and Rubio, P. A. (1973) Re-appraisal adjuncts to avoid ischaemia in the treatment of aneurysms of the descending aorta. *J. Thorac. Cardiovasc. Surg.*, **66**, 693

14. Svensson, L. G. and Loop, F. D. (1988) Prevention of spinal cord ischaemia in aortic surgery. In *Arterial Surgery, New Diagnostic and Operative Techniques* (eds J. J. Bergan and J. S. T. Yao). Grune & Stratton, London

15. Miyamotok, Uenoa, Wadat, Kimotos (1960) A new and simple method of preventing spinal cord damage following temporary occlusion of the thoracic aorta by drainage of cerebrospinal fluid. *J. Cardiovasc. Surg.*, **1**, 188

16. Blaisdell, F. W. and Cooley, D. A. (1963) The mechanism of paraplegia after temporary thoracic-aortic occlusion and its relationship to spinal fluid pressure. *Surgery*, **51**, 351

17. McCullough, J. L., Hollier, L. H. and Nugent, M. (1988) Paraplegia after thoracic-aortic occlusion; influence of cerebrospinal fluid drainage. Experimental and early clinical results. *J. Vasc. Surg.*, **7**, 153

18. Crawford, E. S., Crawford, J. L., Safi, H. *et al.* (1986) Thoraco-abdominal aortic aneurysms: Pre-operative and intra-operative factors determining immediate and long term results of operations in 605 patients. *J. Vasc. Surg.*, **3**, 389

19. Fereshetian, A., Kadir, S., Caufman, S. *et al.* (1989) Digital subtraction spinal cord angiography in patients undergoing thoracic aneurysm surgery. *Cardiovasc. Intervent. Radiol.*, **12**, 7

20. Cunningham, J. N., Laschinger, J. C., Merkin, H. A. *et al.* (1982) Measurements of spinal cord ischaemia during operations upon the thoracic aorta. *Ann. Surg.*, **169**, 285

21. Crawford, E. S., Mizrahia, M., Hess, K. R., Coselli, J. S., Safi, J. H. and Patel, V. M. (1988) The impact of distal aortic perfusion and somato-sensory evoked potential monitoring on the prevention of paraplegia after aortic aneurysm operation. *J. Thorac. Cardiovasc. Surg.*, **95**, 357

22. Sandmann, W., Grabitz, K., Kniemeyer, H. W., Stuhmeier, K. and Breulmann, M. (1988) Chirurgische Behandlung des Thoraco-Abdominalen und Suprarenalen Aneurysmas. *Zent. bl. Chir.*, **113**, 1305

23. Kirshner, D. L., Kirshner, R. L., Heggeness, L. M. and DeWesse, J. A. (1989) Spinal cord ischaemia and evaluation of pharmacological agents in minimising paraplegia after aortic occlusion. *J. Vasc. Surg.*, **9**, 305

24. Svensson, L. G., Coselli, J. S., Safi, H. J., Hess, K. R. and Crawford, E. S. (1989) Appraisal of adjuncts to prevent acute renal failure after surgery on the thoracic or thoraco-abdominal aorta. *J. Vasc. Surg.* **10**, 230

25. Crawford, E. S. (1983) Marfan's syndrom *Ann. Surg.*, **198**, 487

26. Jamieson, C. W. and Wolfe, J. H. N. (1985) Management of aneurysms involving the visceral arteria. In *Vascular Surgery*. (ed. C. W. Jamieson). Baillière Tindall, London

27. Taylor, P. R., Halliday, A. W., Wolfe, J. H. N. and Manfield, A. O. (1990) Thoraco abdominal aneurysm repair. *Br. J. Surg.*, **77**, A345

Chapter 6

Abdominal aortic aneurysms – a topic of enlarging interest

Roger N. Baird

These lesions are silent and deep and lethal, like the U-boats of old (a U-boat inside the belly), and like them they can be found by reflected sound waves and taken out before they torpedo the patient

Santiago[1]

Increasing incidence

Epidemiological studies in the UK[2] and the US[3] have shown a substantial increase in the incidence of aortic aneurysm from 1950 to the 1980s. The number of deaths in England and Wales attributed to aortic aneurysm in men increased from 202 in 1950 to 4668 in 1984, and in women from 201 to 2591 in the same period. Of course, part of the increase is due to better diagnosis, with the introduction of ultrasound in the 1960s being particularly important in documenting axial diameters and detecting smaller aneurysms. The incidence is also increasing because improved life expectancy has resulted in a greater population of the elderly at risk.

Three recent prevalence studies in the UK have been based on ultrasound screening of general practice populations. Scott *et al.*[4] surveyed 1312 men and women in Chichester aged 65–80 years, of whom 2.6% had abdominal aneurysms greater than 3.5 cm diameter. Collin *et al.*[5] found that 2% of 426 men in Oxfordshire aged 65–74 years had an abdominal aneurysm of greater than 4 cm diameter and O'Kelly and Heather[6] in a similar study in Gloucester found 1.5% with greater frequency amongst hypertensives and smokers.

The cause of most aneurysms is as much an enigma as ever, but the usual explanation is of degeneration of collagen and elastin in the ageing arterial wall. A genetic defect is occasionally responsible for defective collagen production. Quite why the infrarenal aorta is principally affected is unknown; explanations for the initial damage to the arterial wall include hypertension, damage to vasa vasorum, and resonance of standing waves at the aortic bifurcation.

Mortality of rupture

Mealy and Salman[7] collected data for 8 years on ruptured aortic aneurysms from operative and post-mortem registers in Worthing and found an overall mean incidence of 13.9 per 100 000 patient years. The incidence has increased in recent years and with increasing patient age. The overall community mortality rate was 89%, with two-thirds failing to reach hospital alive. A similar figure of 86% was reported by Budd and Finch from Swindon[8]. This appalling mortality has driven demand for population-based screening programmes.

Contained rupture

The accuracy of diagnosis of tender aneurysms has been improved by imaging techniques. Ultrasound will show an aneurysm quickly and easily if abdominal palpation is inconclusive because of guarding or obesity[9]. Better images of the aneurysm are obtained by computed tomography (CT) with arterial enhancement, which may also confirm leakage by the presence of extravasated blood in the retroperitoneal tissues[10]. In one study, a patient with a negative scan was quite fortuitously given a repeat injection of intravenous contrast half an hour later and rescanned, which showed that extensive retroperitoneal haemorrhage had occurred in the interim[11]. Occasionally following a rent in the wall of the aneurysm, the patient's condition stabilizes with an organized haematoma contained by tamponade of surrounding tissues[12]. This *contained rupture* (Figures 6.1 and 6.2) represents an unpredictable state which may at any moment progress to terminal intraperitoneal haemorrhage. The surgeon should not be lulled into a false sense of security, and while there may be time for preoperative assessment, should be prepared to proceed immediately to the operating theatre.

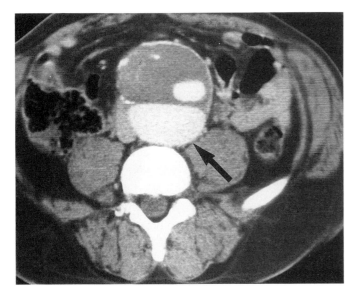

Figure 6.1 CT scan of an abdominal aortic aneurysm with i.v. contrast enhancement, showing a large, thin-walled aneurysm filled by thrombus with a small eccentrically placed lumen. The arrow indicates a posterior contained rupture extending beyond the partly calcified aneurysmal wall

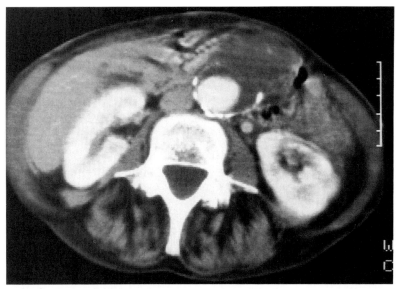

Figure 6.2   Large contained rupture of a small aneurysm shown on CT with contrast enhancement. Note contrast medium in the lumen and in both kidneys, calcium in the wall of a small aneurysm and contained thrombus extending to the abdominal wall, scale in cm

Small aneurysms

The mean infrarenal aortic external diameter increases in men from 1.75 cm at 34 years of age to 2.1 cm at 75 years; comparable values for women are 1.53 cm to 1.75 cm[13]. A localized aortic dilatation to twice the size of arteries on either side is sufficiently abnormal to be called an aneurysm and replacement by a Dacron tube is the orthodox treatment. Unoperated small aneurysms observed by ultrasound or CT increase in size by 0.22–0.33 cm each year[14,15]. Swedenborg's group at the Karolinska Hospital, Stockholm[16] have followed small aneurysms in patients with relative contraindications to surgery by serial CT scans. Their results show a mean growth rate of 0.52 cm/year, and a rapid increase in size or abdominal/back pain presaged rupture[16]. They have withheld surgery in aneurysms of less than 5 cm until repeated estimates approached or exceeded 5 cm[17].

Screening programmes are disclosing asymptomatic small aneurysms, which are a source of anxiety to both patients and vascular surgeons. Repeated scanning is seen by many as procrastination in the face of the inevitable, with a clean surgical strike being preferred. Intervention certainly helps patients with large aneurysms, and *may* confer a survival advantage in those with aneurysms of 4–5 cm external diameter or less. This question raises the daunting prospect of operating on large numbers of small asymptomatic aneurysms detected by screening to prevent unheralded rupture in a few.

Surgeons who are plagued by doubts should consider entering eligible patients into one of the multicentre trials of Dacron replacement vs. surveillance by repeated scans.

Inflammatory aneurysms

Some 7% of aortic aneurysms (Table 6.1) are encased in a pearly white fibrous retroperitoneal tissue to which the duodeno-jejunal flexure is firmly adherent. This causes difficulties in dissecting the aorta above and the iliac arteries below the aneurysm. The neck of an aneurysm is normally approached by scissor dissection to mobilize the duodenum leaving a fringe of posterior peritoneum for later closure. If fibrosis is present, the duodenum is inseparably stuck down, and attempts to dissect it free may result in the lumen of the small bowel being entered and the operative field contaminated with probable abandonment of the operation. To prevent this, the thick wall of peri-aneurysmal fibrosis should be carefully incised, and its outermost layer peeled like an onion skin towards the vena cava, taking the duodenum with it. Further sharp dissection will reveal the uninvolved wall of the neck of the aneurysm which is mobilized sufficiently to be clamped. The potential difficulty in gaining control is highlighted by the occasional need to divide the left renal vein, to clamp the aorta at the diaphragm and to introduce a balloon catheter through the anterior wall of the aneurysm upwards into its neck to occlude it. Rarely the density of fibrosis precludes safe dissection and the aneurysm is deemed inoperable. Provided that the diagnosis is made preoperatively, consideration should be given to a retroperitoneal approach, since less fibrosis is encountered and it is technically easier to gain access to the neck of the aneurysm. Other retroperitonal structures affected include the ureters, vena cava and pancreas, and these appearances are similar to those observed in retroperitoneal fibrosis.

Ureterolysis, once popular, has been replaced by endoscopic insertion of ureteric J-stents, which are removed later once the fibrosis has resolved postoperatively.

In view of these technical difficulties, increases in morbidity and mortality are not unexpected. Sethia and Darke[18] reported one death and one inoperable case from 11 operations; Barr, Cave-Bigley and Harris[19] had one death following 16 operations. Hill and Charlesworth[21] had four deaths amongst 26 elective inflammatory cases.

Patients with inflammatory aneurysms are likely to have symptoms which include backache, malaise and abdominal pain. On examination, there may be a fever, weight loss or swelling of the lower extremities. Raised ESR or viscosity will alert the clinician to review critically preoperative imaging studies. Ultrasound can show a thickened aneurysm wall (Figure 6.3). Nowadays, the diagnosis is usually made by CT. It is likely that as magnetic resonance (Figure 6.4) becomes increasingly available, its usefulness in demonstrating the layers of the fibrotic aneurysm wall will

Table 6.1 Incidence of inflammatory aneurysms

	Inflammatory/total aneurysms	(%)	Reference
Bournemouth	11/157	7	[18]
Liverpool	16/106	15	[19]
Rome	42/695	6	[20]
Manchester	36/780	5	[21]
Bristol	34/279	12	[22]
Total	139/2017	7	

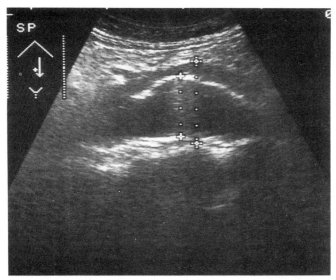

Figure 6.3   Ultrasound scan showing a thickened aneurysmal wall, later confirmed at operation to be an inflammatory aneurysm

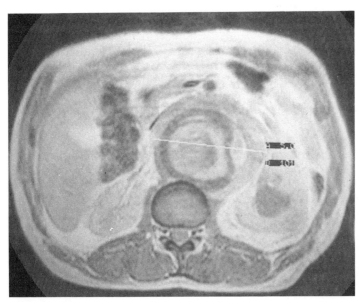

Figure 6.4   Magnetic resonance image of an inflammatory aneurysm showing the layers of the thickened vessel wall

be more widely appreciated. The appearances on short-tau inversion sequence are characteristic, with three or more extra-luminal layers, compared with the two-layered appearance of non-inflammatory aneurysms[22].

Mycotic aortic aneurysms

Mycotic aneurysms were first described by Osler over 100 years ago as caused by weakness of the arterial wall arising from infective emboli from bacterial endocarditis. Septic foci in vasa vasorum of the aortic wall lead to *bacterial aortitis* which is a more accurate description. The clinical features are of fulminant infection, presenting as a painful, pulsatile mass in a pyrexial patient, with a leucocytosis and positive blood cultures. Salmonella is the most common infective organism followed by streptococcus and other gut flora[23,24]. CT scanning with i.v. contrast enhancement will show an uncalcified mass with an irregular lumen[25]. Serial scans may be required, as the aorta may weaken and dilate within a few days, with increasing pain and the risk of rupture. Antibiotic therapy is instituted and the aneurysm is resected. Opinion is divided upon whether the arterial reconstruction should be extra-anatomic or orthotopic. The orthodox approach of an axillo-bifemoral bypass means a protracted operation and the prospect of poor long-term patency[23]. Direct aortic replacement with Dacron is surprisingly free from the risk of cross-infection and is preferred where possible[26]. The time for which antibiotics are needed remains to be determined.

Operative considerations

Anaesthesia

Light general anaesthesia with a thoracic epidural catheter for the infusion of local anaesthetics and opiates is now widely practised. Epidural analgesia by constant infusion pump has transformed the early postoperative days by providing effective pain relief in an alert patient, so that breathing, coughing and mobilization are facilitated.

Incision

Three incisions are used; midline, transverse and retroperitoneal. The midline approach is orthodox and rightly popular, especially in patients with a high narrow costal arch. The incision is quickly made and sewn up and is the only choice for a ruptured case. A transverse incision takes longer, because the rectus abdominis muscles have to be cut, and haemostasis secured. Its advantages include the excellent view of the upper aorta, and the kind healing of the incision. Both transperitoneal approaches give access to co-existent intra-abdominal pathology, and to the right renal and right iliac arteries[27].

The retroperitoneal approach avoids the peritoneal cavity so that the postoperative ileus is shorter by a day or so. It is useful for the few patients where anterior access is difficult, such as inflammatory aneurysms and co-existent horseshoe kidney. For high aneurysms, placement of the aortic clamp is easier, whether at the renal arteries or at the diaphragm[28].

Prosthesis

A woven Dacron tube is quicker, easier and therefore safer to implant than a bifurcation prosthesis. At Bristol Royal Infirmary, a straight tube has been employed in 275 (58%) of 473 aortic aneurysm replacements in the past six years. Bifurcation grafts are needed for aneurysms extending into the iliac arteries. However, moderate iliac artery widening is acceptable, and we have not yet encountered a ruptured iliac aneurysm in patients after tube replacement of an aortic aneurysm. Suprarenal aneurysms can, however, be a late sequel to infrarenal aneurysm repair[29].

Second pathology

Gallstones are not infrequently noted when the abdominal contents are inspected before insertion of a Dacron prosthesis. The incidence of cholelithiasis in aneurysm patients is about 10%, and most are best ignored, especially if the stones are mobile and the gallbladder is thin walled, since acute postoperative biliary disease is rare and often acalculous. An active biliary problem which carries a high incidence of infected bile and the probability that the common bile duct will have to be explored takes operative priority necessitating the postponement of aneurysm repair.

Aneurysm and malignant disease

The decision to repair an aneurysm is a long-term plan to eliminate the threat of rupture. If life expectancy is significantly compromised by co-existent malignant disease, the aneurysm is best left unresected. At Bristol Royal Infirmary, 4 (1.6%) of 247 aortic aneurysm repairs have undergone concomitant excision of intraabdominal malignancy. One, a patient with a small carcinoma of the gallbladder, is tumour-free at more than two years. Three others survived postoperatively but died of malignant disease within six months. These results suggest that the risk of death from metastases is high in coincidental malignant disease and that repair of an aneurysm seldom prolongs life by preventing rupture.

References

1. Santiago, F. (1987) Screening for Abdominal Aortic Aneurysms: the U-boat in the belly. *J. Am. Med. Ass.*, **258**, 1732
2. Fowkes, F. G. R., Macintyre, C. C. A. and Ruckley, C. V. (1989) Increasing Incidence of Aortic Aneurysms in England and Wales. *Br. Med. J.*, **298**, 33–35
3. Bickerstaff, L. K., Hollier, L. H., Van Peenen, H. J. *et al.* (1984) Abdominal Aortic Aneurysms: the changing natural history. *J. Vasc. Surg.*, **1**, 6
4. Scott, R. A. P., Ashton, H. A. and Kay, D. N. (1988) Ultrasound screening of a general practitioner population for aortic aneurysm. *Br. Med. J.*, **296**, 1709–1710
5. Collin, J., Araujo, L., Walton, J. and Lindsell, D. (1988) Oxford screening programme for abdominal aortic aneurysm in men aged 65 to 74 years. *Lancet*, **ii**, 613–615
6. O'Kelly, T. J. and Heather, B. P. (1989) General practice-based population screening for abdominal aortic aneurysms: a pilot study. *Br. J. Surg.*, **76**, 479–480
7. Mealy, K. and Salman, A. (1988) The true incidence of ruptured abdominal aortic aneurysms. *Eur. J. Vasc. Surg.*, **2**, 405–408
8. Budd, J. S. and Finch, D. R. (1988) Management of abdominal aortic aneurysm. *Br. Med. J.*, **297**, 484
9. Shuman, W. P., Hastrup, W. Jr., Kohler, T. R. *et al.* (1988) Suspected leaking abdominal aortic aneurysm: use of sonography in the emergency room. *Radiology*, **168**, 117–119
10. Zarke, M. D., Gould, H. R. and Goldman, M. H. (1988) Computed tomography in the evaluation of the patient with symptomatic abdominal aortic aneurysm. *Surgery*, **103**, 638–642

11. Greatorex, R. A., Dixon, A. K., Flower, C. D. R. and Pulvertaft, R. W. (1988) Limitations of computed tomography in leaking abdominal aortic aneurysms. *Br. Med. J.*, **297**, 284–285

12. Jones, C. S., Reilly, K., Dalsing, M. C. and Glover, J. L. (1986) Chronic contained rupture of abdominal aortic aneurysms. *Arch. Surg.*, **121**, 542–546

13. Horejs, D., Gilbert, P. M., Burstein, S. and Vogelzang, R. L. (1988). Normal aorto-iliac diameters by CT. *J. Com. Ass. Tom.*, **12**, 602–603

14. Collin, J., Araujo, L. and Walton, J. (1989) How fast do very small aneurysms grow? *Eur. J. Vasc. Surg.*, **3**, 15–17

15. Walsh, A. K. M., Briffa, N., Nash, J. R. and Callum, K. G. (1990) The natural history of small abdominal aortic aneurysms: an ultrasound study. *Eur. J. Vasc. Surg.*, **4**, 459–461

16. Delin, A., Ohlsen, H. and Swedenborg, J. (1985) Growth rate of abdominal aortic aneurysms as measured by computed tomography. *Br. J. Surg.*, **72**, 530–532

17. Johansson, G., Nydahl, S., Olofsson, P. and Swedenborg, J. (1990) Survival in patients with abdominal aortic aneurysms. Comparison between operative and non-operative management. *Eur. J. Vasc. Surg.*, **4**, 497–502

18. Sethia, B. and Darke, S. G. (1983) Abdominal aortic aneurysm with retroperitoneal fibrosis and ureteric entrapment. *Br. J. Surg.*, **70**, 434–436

19. Barr, H., Cave-Bigley, D. J. and Harris, P. L. (1985) The management of inflammatory abdominal aortic aneurysms. *J. R. Coll. Surg. Ed.*, **30**, 217–220

20. Fiorani, P., Lauri, D., Faraglia, V. *et al.* (1990) The Recognition and Management of the Non-Specific European Inflammatory Aortic Aneurysm. In *The Cause and Management of Aneurysms* (eds R. M. Greenhalgh and J. A. Mannick). Saunders, London, pp. 189–202

21. Hill, J. and Charlesworth, D. (1988) Inflammatory Aortic Aneurysms; a report of thirty-seven cases. *Ann. Vasc. Surg.*, **2**, 352–357

22. Tennant, W. G., Hartnell, G. G., Wyatt, M. G., Baird, R. N. and Horrocks, M. (1990) Inflammatory aortic aneurysms. Characteristics and specific features on magnetic resonance imaging. *J Cardiovasc. Surg.*, **31**, 105

23. Reddy, D. J. and Ernst, C. B. (1989) Infected Aneurysms. In *Vascular Surgery* 3rd Edition (ed. R. B. Rutherford). Saunders, Philadelphia, pp. 983–996

24. Baird, R. N. (1989) Mycotic Aortic Aneurysms. *Eur. J. Vasc. Surg.*, **3**, 95–96

25. Gonda, R. L., Gutierrez, O. H. and Azodo, M. V. U. (1988) Mycotic aneurysms of the aorta; radiologic features. *Radiology*, **168**, 343–346

26. Chan, F. Y., Crawford, E. S., Coselli, J. S., Safi, H. J. and Williams, T. W. (1989) In situ prosthetic graft replacement for mycotic aneurysm of the aorta. *Ann. Thorac. Surg.*, **47**, 193–203

27. Mannick, J. A., Whittemore, A. D. and Donaldson, M. C. (1990) Elective abdominal aortic aneurysm surgery by the transperitoneal route. In *The Cause and Management of Aneurysms* (eds R. M. Greenhalgh and J. A. Mannick). Saunders, London, pp. 293–302

28. Taylor, P. R. and Wolfe, J. H. N. (1990) When is the retroperitoneal route preferred for elective intra-abdominal aneurysms? In *The Cause and Management of Aneurysms* (eds R. M. Greenhalgh and J. A. Mannick). Saunders, London pp. 311–319.

29. Griffiths, D., Scott, D. J. A. and Horrocks, M. (1990) Spontaneous rupture of suprarenal aneurysms: a late sequel to infrarenal aortic aneurysm repair. *Eur. J. Vasc. Surg.*, **4**, 431–433

Chapter 7

How can we prevent complications from elective aortic surgery?

W. Bruce Campbell

Introduction

We can now offer the patient with an aortic aneurysm or aortoiliac occlusive disease relatively safe operative treatment. Postoperative death is mostly from cardiac causes in the elective setting, and although very low figures are often quoted mortality rates overall remain around 5% or higher[1–4] and clearly there is room for improvement. Some of the later complications of aortic grafting, such as graft sepsis and aortoenteric fistula may also prove fatal, and there are measures that the surgeon can take to minimize the chance of these. Other complications, such as limb ischaemia and sexual dysfunction, may cause long-term morbidity which can be avoided by careful operative technique.

This chapter considers the measures we can take to reduce complications after elective aortic surgery. Areas of controversy are described, and distinctions drawn between those techniques for which there is documented evidence of benefit and those used on a hypothetical basis. Finally, there are some complications, such as spinal cord ischaemia, which we are largely powerless to prevent, and these are also described.

Early complications

Cardiac complications

Cardiac events are by far the most common cause of death after elective aortic surgery and non-fatal myocardial infarction is not infrequent. Reviewing the causes of death in 134 patients out of 3138 having elective grafting for aortic aneurysm, 56% died from cardiac events alone, and cardiac problems contributed to the deaths of many others[5–11]. Recognizing patients with ischaemic heart disease is the first step towards reducing morbidity and mortality. This recognition depends initially on a good history which will detect those at highest risk, who can then be referred for further assessment by a cardiologist and/or an experienced anaesthetist before planning surgery.

The best test for determining cardiac status remains controversial. An ECG is essential, but opinions differ on the relative merits of Goldman risk factor analysis (Goldman et al. [12]), exercise testing, echocardiography, measurement of ejection fraction, and dipyrimadole–thallium scanning in quantifying cardiac risk. Dipyrimadole–thallium scanning has recently been advocated as especially helpful in predicting perioperative cardiac morbidity[13]. Some patients with severe ischaemic heart disease may benefit from coronary angiography and bypass grafting before abdominal aortic surgery. Hertzer's group have advocated an aggressive approach to coronary reconstruction before aortic grafting and have claimed improved survival thereby[7] but the experience of others has not supported this claim[2].

Many patients have subclinical ischaemic heart disease and high levels of monitoring and care should therefore be routine, with the aim of optimizing cardiac function in all patients[14]. Monitoring should include pulmonary wedge pressure measurement in obviously high risk cases which helps to maintain cardiac function at ideal levels during operation[15]. However, even this does not eliminate the possibility of serious cardiac problems[16].

Especial care is required to maintain haemodynamic stability during clamping and unclamping of the aorta[17] and this demands good communication between the surgeon and the anaesthetist. Before unclamping the surgeon should give several minutes' warning so that the patient is well volume-loaded. For an aortic bifurcation graft one limb should be released at a time (this is usually convenient, since each leg can be revascularized as soon as the anastomosis is completed). If serious hypotension occurs then a clamp should be reapplied, but this can usually be left fractionally open to allow a small volume of blood flow which avoids the possibility of clotting within the graft.

Appropriate use of vasodilators, inotropic agents and vasopressors is frequently necessary to maintain optimal cardiac function[18]. Hollier *et al.*[18] have described the use of aortic balloon counter-pulsation during grafting with uniformly good results in a few patients with severely compromised cardiac performance.

Monitoring and care of the highest order is also important in the early postoperative period and an intensive care setting is ideal[19]. Some units achieve this in their own high-dependency area on a ward, but the most important aspect is readily available attention from a doctor experienced in the management of cardiopulmonary physiology.

Clearly patient selection will influence the incidence of cardiac morbidity and mortality, and decisions may be difficult. For high-risk patients with aortoiliac occlusive disease extra-anatomic grafting (e.g. axillo-bifemoral) is always an alternative. For patients with aneurysms and severe ischaemic heart disease the risk of serious cardiac problems must be balanced against the chance of aneurysm rupture (related to aortic diameter), and the life expectancy of the patient from cardiac and other medical problems. Finally, the wishes of the informed patient may be an important influence for or against operation.

Pulmonary complications

Pulmonary complications are common after aortic surgery[7,20] and it is important to identify patients at high risk by preoperative pulmonary function testing of those with a history of chest problems. For practical purposes simple measurement of vital capacity and FEV_1 give a good indication of the patient's ventilatory reserve, but mean forced expiratory flow during the middle half of the forced vital capacity (FEV_{25-75}) has been claimed to be the single most reliable test for predicting pulmonary complications[21]. Apart from expert ventilatory management, good postoperative physiotherapy is the cornerstone to avoiding pulmonary problems, but two additional measures deserve mention.

First, there may be a relationship between the type of incision used and pulmonary complications, although this is controversial. There are suggestions that a transverse incision is preferable to a vertical incision for the anterior approach to aortic reconstruction, being associated with less postoperative pulmonary problems[22]. The retroperitoneal approach, too, has been claimed to reduce pulmonary complications[23,24], but Sicard *et al.*[25] and Cambria *et al.*[26] have failed to show any significant difference. These approaches may have other advantages and disadvantages but the case for reducing pulmonary complications is not proven.

The second measure aimed at reducing postoperative chest problems in these patients is the use of epidural analgesia and, although good objective evidence of its value is difficult to find it transforms postoperative pain relief and allows much easier respiration, coughing and physiotherapy.

Renal failure and ureteric injuries

Renal failure is an important contributor to mortality after surgery for ruptured aneurysms, but can also complicate elective aortic reconstruction. Preoperative raised creatinine is well documented as a risk factor for mortality after aortic surgery[7,27,28]. In most cases, recognizing this risk, and taking meticulous care with haemodynamic stability and fluid balance are the key factors to preserving renal function. Mannitol has been shown to help if the patient is transiently hypovolaemic[29].

There has been considerable discussion on the importance of ligating the left renal vein during aortic surgery. Some surgeons suggest repairing this vein if it needs to be divided, while others simply take care to divide the vein as close as possible to the vena cava in order to preserve collateral venous drainage from the left kidney. Renal failure is more common after left renal vein ligation[2] but is nevertheless an infrequent consequence. Awad and colleagues[30] have reported a small decrease in glomerular filtration rate in a substantial proportion of patients after infrarenal aortic reconstruction, which still affects some patients after six months. All six of their patients whose left renal veins were ligated showed some compromise of renal function, but none developed renal failure. In summary, the left renal vein should only be ligated when really necessary, and then close to the vena cava. Repair is probably necessary only when right-sided renal function is absent or poor.

Occlusion or embolization of the renal arteries at operation are causes of immediate postoperative anuria[27]. Emboli are a special risk when the aorta is filled with loose thrombus and instruments are passed proximally for thrombectomy. Suprarenal aortic grafting requires particular attention to renal perfusion, and good preoperative arteriograms are essential to delineate all arteries to the kidneys. The kidneys can tolerate a warm ischaemia time up to about 45 min[31] but for longer periods renal perfusion should certainly be used. I perfuse the left kidney during reconstruction for suprarenal aneurysm because it remains ischaemic longer than the right; the perfusion system does not interfere with the aortic anastomosis. It is essential to check that good pulsatile flow has been restored to reconstructed renal arteries and that the kidney looks well perfused.

Ureteric injuries are another risk of aortic surgery[32] particularly during reoperations[33]. The ureters are particularly difficult to identify and may be damaged when dealing with inflammatory aneurysms[34]. In difficult reoperative procedures McCarthy *et al.*[35] recommend the use of ureteric stents which can be palpated during dissection. If ureteric injury is suspected at the time of surgery it can be confirmed by intravenous injection of indigo carmine dye[36]. Early recognition allows repair, stenting, and nephrostomy when indicated, all of which reduce the chance of later nephrectomy.

Gastrointestinal complications

Gastrointestinal complications caused the death of 2.7% patients in a series of 476 elective aortic aneurysm grafts reported by Crowson and colleagues[37]. The most common problem was ischaemic bowel. Subclinical colonic ischaemia occurs in about 5% of patients after elective aortic grafting[38,39] but only a few develop obvious clinical signs, and transmural ischaemia is rare[40]. When this does occur the outlook is very bleak and few patients survive. Attention to the gut blood supply is therefore important. Schroeder et al.[40] advocated careful assessment of the gut vasculature by preoperative aortiography. Others advocate measurement of inferior mesenteric artery stump pressure[41] or the use of Doppler measurements[42], but these techniques are not commonly used.

The gut artery most involved in infrarenal aortic reconstruction is the inferior mesenteric artery (IMA). Bast and colleagues[39] failed to show any association between ligation of a patent IMA and development of ischaemia on colonoscopy. Few surgeons preserve this vessel as a matter of routine, and it is, in any event, often occluded in patients with aneurysms.

Bast et al.[39] did confirm an increased incidence of colonic ischaemia if both internal iliac arteries were occluded or ligated, and this supports the common practice of ensuring that at least one of the IMA and two internal iliac arteries are patent, even if this means reimplantation or grafting. In patients whose marginal artery is discontinuous or who lack a middle colonic artery, bowel ischaemia remains a small risk. Hypotension increases the chance of colonic infarction and is one reason for the much higher incidence of this complication after operation for ruptured aneurysm.

Small bowel ischaemia is rare and is related to pre-existing atheroma of the coeliac axis and superior mesenteric artery, which may then be compounded by ligation of the inferior mesenteric artery[43]. This is more common after surgery for occlusive disease than that for aortic aneurysm[44].

Prolonged paralytic ileus or mechanical obstruction complicate aortic surgery infrequently[37] but are difficult to prevent, other than by taking the normal precautions to return the bowel properly to the peritoneal cavity and to avoid catching bowel loops with sutures. Peptic ulceration is another complication and we routinely use H_2-receptor blockers in the postoperative period as prophylaxis against acute ulcers.

Bleeding

The most troublesome sites for potential bleeding at the time of operation are veins adjacent to the aorta and iliac arteries, and there are some special areas where attention to technique avoids this complication. In the juxtarenal area tributaries of the renal vein must not be torn during mobilization. Absence of a renal vein anterior to the aorta should raise suspicion of a retro-aortic vein which can be damaged, resulting in profuse haemorrhage.

Some surgeons advocate using a vertical clamp on the aorta to avoid tearing lumbar veins, but the preference for a 'spoon-shaped' horizontal clamp gives an absolute guarantee of controlling aortic bleeding, makes the anastomosis easier, and avoids clamp handles getting in the surgeon's way. Encircling the aorta with the finger to place this clamp rarely causes bleeding problems. By contrast, there is nothing to be gained by dissecting circumferentially around the common iliac arteries, unless there is a need to ligate these vessels. The iliac veins are often adherent to the arteries, and are easily damaged. Vertical clamps should be applied carefully to avoid damaging the iliac veins with their tips, and clamps with blunt ends (e.g. Fogarty Hydragrip) are ideal. If serious venous bleeding does occur behind an iliac artery, early transection of the artery allows good visualization and rapid control.

Tunnelling from groin to abdomen for placement of a bifurcation graft can cause venous bleeding deep in the pelvis which is difficult to control, and which is a special risk in re-do procedures. A finger, rather than any instrument, should always be used, introducing it lateral to the external iliac artery in the groin.

Postoperatively, arterial bleeding is the most common reason for re-exploration. Bergqvist and Ljungström[45] reported a 1.3% incidence of postoperative haemorrhage among 864 patients having aortic reconstruction, but the overall incidence of this complication is probably greater, since another Scandinavian series documented a 10% incidence of re-laparotomy for bleeding after elective aortic surgery, three of the twelve patients who bled dying as a result[28].

Vessels which open into the sac of an aneurysm (the inferior mesenteric and lumbar arteries) are important sites for re-bleeding since their orifices are open, often calcified, and cannot contract. They must be effectively oversewn and checked meticulously at the end of aneurysm grafting. Small bleeders on the sac edge also need haemostasis by diathermy or suturing. These, and any ligated or oversewn major vessel (such as a distal aortic stump) must be checked at the end of the operation, after the graft has been opened and they have been subjected to the full force of arterial backflow. Checking anastomoses is self-evident.

If re-exploration for bleeding is required after an aortic reconstruction it is not uncommon for the source of the haemorrhage to be obscure, even when a large amount of blood has been lost into the abdominal cavity. This situation demands checking and rechecking of all possible sites, but the surgeon may be left with the unsatisfactory conclusion of failing to identify a major bleeding source.

In prevention and control of all bleeding complications after aortic surgery it is important to be sure that blood clotting is normal, and clotting abnormalities should be corrected as a first step unless bleeding is profuse and demands urgent surgery.

Acute limb ischaemia

Lower limb ischaemia after aortic grafting may be due to embolism, thrombosis or technical errors (which in most instances can be avoided by careful technique).

Embolism was the most common cause reported by Strom, Bernhard and Towne in their series of 262 aortic reconstructions, of whom 10.3% had some kind of ischaemic complication[45a]. Embolic material is most commonly dislodged from within the sac of an aneurysm, and fragments enter the small vessels of the foot resulting in the classic 'trash foot' (Figure 7.1) which is usually irrecoverable. The problem is doubly disastrous because material can only pass to the foot down the patent arteries of a 'good' leg, whereas occlusive disease stops its distal passage. Debris can rarely pass to other vessels, such as the internal iliac arteries ('trash buttock').

Attention to technique should virtually eliminate the occurence of embolism during aortic reconstruction. Gentle initial dissection, with minimal handling of an aneurysm is fundamental. Distal clamps should be applied early[46] and certainly before final

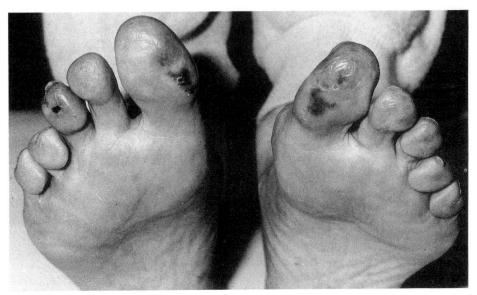

Figure 7.1 Trash foot. During operation for aortic aneurysm embolic material has been dislodged and has entered branches of the digital arteries, causing small areas of infarction in the toes

mobilization and clamping of the proximal aorta which is a manoeuvre especially likely to dislodge thrombus. Later in the operation a number of points are important. These consist of 'external flushing' to allow any debris from the proximal aorta or graft to be evacuated during momentary release of the graft clamp before completion of distal anastomoses. Following this a back bleed should be allowed from the distal vessels, and the lumen should then be sucked out by gentle use of a fine sucker. If back bleeding is absent or poor Fogarty catheters should be passed distally (this may be difficult down tortuous or diseased iliac arteries, and in these cases transfemoral embolectomy should be undertaken later). In addition wherever possible 'internal flushing' is done whereby blood flow is allowed into the 'least important' arteries first. For groin anastomoses this means the serial releasing of clamps on the proximal common femoral artery, the profunda femoris artery and finally the patent, femoral artery.

It is important to recognize acute ischaemia immediately by inspecting the feet, feeling pulses, and measuring Doppler systolic pressures. Sometimes, however, it can be difficult to be certain whether poorly perfused toes are the site of microemboli or whether they will simply warm up in the early postoperative period. If pulses or pressures are inadequate the vessels in the groin should be explored by the passage of embolectomy catheters, and on-table arteriography should be performed if the situation remains unsatisfactory.

Technical errors are an uncommon reason for ischaemia in most reports of aortic reconstruction[47,48], although intimal flaps have been the most common cause in another series[49]. Twisting or kinking of a graft limb, graft compression in the 'tunnel' to the groin, a technically faulty anastomosis or an intimal flap are all avoidable. The risk of clamp damage to the common iliac arteries, which are often calcific or aneurysmal, has been stressed and a strong case made for clamping the external and internal iliac arteries instead[50]. Others have not found this to be a common problem, and I clamp the common iliacs routinely (using atraumatic Fogarty Hydragrip clamps).

In patients with occluded superficial femoral arteries care to revascularize the profunda femoris properly is another important factor in preventing both early and later graft occlusion[47]. This is achieved by extending the distal anastomosis onto the profunda femoris to a point at which that vessel is healthy.

Coagulopathy is sometimes the cause of early graft or distal vessel thrombosis[48]. Underlying causes include thrombocythaemia, antithrombin deficiency or heparin-induced platelet aggregation. A preoperative platelet count and clotting profile is important in prevention.

Any patient is at risk of thrombosis during prolonged clamping, and the use of intravenous heparin (e.g. 5000 units) is standard practice for most surgeons during elective aortic work. The traditional belief that heparin is beneficial has never been proven, nor is there unity of opinion on the optimum dose[51,52]. The Joint Vascular Research Group UK is currently conducting a study of heparin versus no heparin in elective aortic aneurysm surgery.

Hypotension is another cause of ischaemia, either by simple reduction of peripheral perfusion or by causing thrombosis.

Finally, in some cases the exact cause of early graft thrombosis or distal ischaemia remains obscure. 'Poor outflow' may account for a few, but many of these cases have been attributed to inadequate flushing of clot from the proximal graft[47] (avoided by external flushing – see above).

Spinal cord ischaemia

This is a very rare complication of infrarenal aortic surgery and is both unpredictable and unpreventable[53]. The artery of Ademkiewicz usually arises between T8 and L1, but this origin is variable. The spinal cord is more at risk during suprarenal or thoracoabdominal aneurysm surgery. Reimplantation of larger intercostal vessels may help to guard against paraplegia, but neither this precaution nor other measures such as cerebrospinal fluid drainage give a guarantee of avoiding permanent injury to the spinal cord. The management of this condition has been the subject of succinct review by Gewertz[54].

Wound complication

Local wound complications, such as haematoma, lymph fistula and necrosis of the skin edges are quantitatively the most common reasons for prolonged hospital stay after vascular surgical procedures[20] (Figures 7.2 and 7.3). Prevention of haematomata demands good attention to haemostasis. Lymph leaks are said to be reduced by ligating transected lymphatics. In practice it is difficult to do more than ligate obviously divided lymph nodes, and in any event these are hardly ever the source of a lymph leak when re-exploration is necessary. Care to perform an adequate wound closure not only guards against dehiscence, but also contributes to the prevention of haematoma and lymph leaks. Two subcutaneous layers are a minimum, and although an absorbable suture is desirable, it should be of a type which is reasonably durable (I use 0 catgut, or No 1 catgut in obese patients or re-do procedures). The use of suction drains seems to have no influence on the incidence of wound complications[55,56]. Necrosis of wound edges can occur despite careful suturing techniques (Figure 7.2). It may sometimes be related to infection, especially in the deep groin crease of the obese patient.

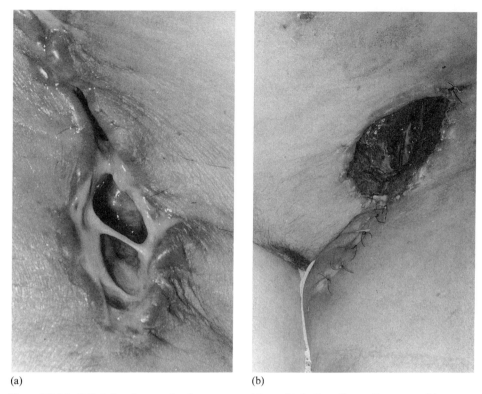

(a)   (b)

Figure 7.2 (a)   Infected groin wound – the commonest type of infection after aortic surgery; (b) infection in this deep groin crease has tracked down to expose the graft

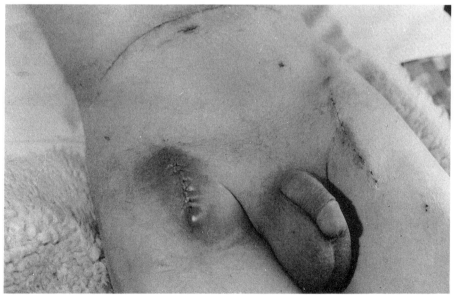

Figure 7.3 Lymphatic collection. A tense collection of sterile lymph has accumulated in the right groin wound. These collections may resolve, but sometimes revision of the wound with placement of a large suction drain is required

Late complications

Graft infection

Aortic graft infection is a serious threat to both life and limb and affects 1–2% of patients[56a–58]. This complication usually presents months or even years after operation, although some cases arise early from infected groin wounds[57] (Figure 7.2). A few late infections may be caused by haematogenous spread of bacteria to parts of the graft devoid of pseudointima, but in most instances contamination at the time of implantation is the likely cause. This means that steps to ensure the strictest asepsis and freedom of the tissues from bacteria are vital, although it is difficult to prove the specific efficacy of most preventive measures because the incidence of graft infection is so low.

Preoperatively it is important to control obvious sites of infection anywhere in the body. Infected lesions at or near incision sites are unacceptable. Looking further from the operative site, Earnshaw *et al.*[59] have shown that patients with rest pain and skin necrosis have a greatly increased risk of wound infection compared with claudicants. Over half of their wound infections were caused by organisms isolated preoperatively from the foot, although no relationship has been proven between bacteria from lesions on the foot before operation and those actually causing aortic graft infections[57]. Nevertheless, every effort should be made to treat distal infection before operation, using good local care and aggressive antibiotic therapy.

General medical problems such as anaemia, uraemia, or malnutrition should be corrected preoperatively, as these may delay wound healing and so encourage infection. It is worth noting however that prolonged preoperative hospital stay increases wound infection rate[60]. Another point to note is that transfemoral aortography predisposes to groin infection on the corresponding side[61]. If possible, surgery involving that groin should be delayed until the puncture site has healed, and perhaps transfemoral aortography should routinely be covered with antibiotics. Some surgeons recommend the use of bactericidal soap for a couple of days preoperatively to reduce numbers of bacteria on the skin[62].

Operative technique is clearly important in preventing graft infection. In his classic paper on graft infection Bunt[63] observes that 'Vascular surgery demands technical expertise, judgement, a certain sense of aesthetics, and most particularly a sufficiently obsessive–compulsive complex as regards attention to operative detail'. But he continues 'most (techniques for preventing graft infection) are anecdotal and although theoretically sound, they are unproven'. General principles include meticulous attention to asepsis, careful handling of tissues, good haemostasis and sound wound closure. The incidence of sepsis is lower if groin anastomoses are avoided[56,57], and indeed most graft infections start in the groin (Figure 7.2). This makes a strong case for anastomosing to the iliac arteries whenever reasonable in aneurysm surgery, although this should not be at the expense of an excellent haemodynamic result.

Bowel surgery at the same time as aortic grafting should generally be avoided whenever possible, although cholecystectomy seems relatively safe[64]. Aortoenteric fistulae and colonic ischaemia are both causes of graft infection and technical measures to avoid these are considered elsewhere.

Some surgeons take special precautions to prevent contact of the graft with the wound edges by using swabs soaked in bactericidal agents[62]. The value of this manoeuvre is certainly unproven, and may be superfluous in view of the well-documented occurrence of bacteria both within aortic aneurysms[65] and in arterial walls and adjacent adipose tissue[66]. In view of the frequent finding of bacteria within the tissues near sites of grafting, prophylactic antibiotics are mandatory, and a review of the evidence for this is almost superfluous[67]. Pitt *et al*.[68] demonstrated a reduction in wound infection among vascular surgical patients using topical, systemic, or combined antibiotic prophylaxis but they showed no differences between the three groups. Systemic prophylaxis is now the accepted method and cephalosporins are popular[69,70] but do not provide guaranteed efficacy against all the organisms commonly recognized as causing graft infection[71]. I use amoxycillin/clavulanic acid (Augmentin) as a routine.

The duration of antibiotic prophylaxis varies. Evidence from other fields of surgery suggests that single dose prophylaxis works well, although some surgeons recommend administration for 5–7 days after arterial grafting[72]. Certainly, one dose is required shortly before operation, and another during or shortly after surgery if there is any amount of blood loss. Thereafter 24 hours of antibiotic therapy is documented as sufficient[67,68] unless there are special indications to continue for a longer period. Work has been reported on pretreatment of vascular prostheses with antibiotics[73] but such techniques are still experimental.

Aortoenteric fistulae

Aortoenteric fistula is the most common cause of gastrointestinal bleeding after an aortic graft[74]. Bunt[75] has defined a true graft enteric fistula as one involving the suture line, which differs in its implications from the more common involvement of the graft wall alone by the gut (graft–enteric erosion). Infection may be important in the development of a graft–enteric fistula and measures to prevent infection at the time of surgery have already been considered. Damage to the duodenal wall must be avoided and Elliot, Smith and Szilagyi[76] advise minimal mobilization of the duodenum with this in mind. Separating the duodenum from the upper anastomosis and the graft is desirable, but surgeons probably delude themselves in their ability to achieve this in all cases. Simple closure of the retroperitoneum generally brings the duodenum back into normal anatomical proximity with the aorta, while closing the body of an aneurysm sac over a graft patently does not always separate the duodenum from the graft. The use of a cuff of graft over the upper anastomosis is recommended by some surgeons[77] but this is difficult to place if the back wall of an aneurysm neck is left intact. Others advocate plication of the retroperitoneum over the graft, or interposition of omentum between duodenum and graft.

Modern synthetic suture materials lower the risk of aortoenteric fistula (compared with silk) and there have been suggestions that end-to-end aortic anastomoses have a lower risk of this complication than end-to-side anastomoses.

It is not surprising that most of the literature on aortoenteric fistula deals with diagnosis and treatment, because the success of most specific measures in prevention is largely hypothetical.

Anastomotic aneurysms

False aneurysms at the site of anastomoses of aortobifemoral Dacron grafts to the femoral arteries are the type of anastomotic aneurysm most frequently seen after vascular reconstruction[78] although iliac and rarely aortic anastomotic aneurysms also occur[79].

Degeneration of the arterial wall is the most common cause of aneurysm and there is a controversial suggestion of an association with hypertension[78,80,81], not substantiated in recent reports[82,83]. Apart from these most of the factors predisposing to false aneurysms are preventable by the surgeon. Endarterectomy at the site of anastomoses has been associated with subsequent false aneurysm formation[80,81]. Excessive anastomotic tension is a contributing factor[78] but failure of the graft or suture materials themselves is now an uncommon cause[83] although Wandschneider, Bull and Deck[82] found suture disruption in 10% of their cases. Wound complications including infection, haematoma, lymph leak and skin necrosis are associated with an increased incidence of false aneurysm formation[78,83,84].

In prevention, femoral endarterectomy should be avoided prior to anastomosis of aortobifemoral grafts whenever possible, adequate sutures should be used, and excess anastomotic tension should be avoided. Operative technique and antibiotic therapy should aim to avoid wound complications and infections.

Anastomotic aneurysms usually present some years after the original operation and identifying a precise cause in each case may be difficult.

Sexual dysfunction

The incidence of impotence or reduced sexual function is higher in patients with aortoiliac vascular disease than in the general population, but some patients suffer deterioration after aortic grafting[85]. The reasons for this are damage to autonomic nerves or disturbances of the blood supply to the pelvis.

The para-aortic autonomic plexus is located primarily on the left side of the infrarenal aorta, and crosses the left common iliac artery to become the superior hypogastric plexus. If these nerves are damaged many patients lose the ability to ejaculate and a few become impotent[86]. Use of the inlay technique of grafting (rather than excising aortic aneurysms) is now standard, and is important in avoiding extensive damage to these nerves[87]. Dissection should not involve the left side of the aorta. Clamping and proximal anastomoses should be kept above the level of the inferior mesenteric artery; and dissection of that vessel should be avoided. The tissues over the left common iliac artery should not be disturbed, and left iliac aneurysms should preferably not be opened, but the graft tunnelled through them. All these measures help to avoid nerve damage[88].

Maintaining blood flow to the pelvis through the internal iliacs is important. The one absolute indication for an end-to-side proximal anastomosis of graft to aorta is bilateral occlusion of the external iliac arteries, which would prevent retrograde perfusion of these vessels after an end-to-end aortic anastomosis.

The incidence of serious disturbance in sexual function after aortic surgery may be lower than has sometimes been claimed, and we must also bear in mind that a proportion of patients are improved[89].

Miscellaneous complications

Minor nerve complications are common in the early weeks after aortofemoral grafting, and consist of dysaesthesia on the thigh due to traction injury of the cutaneous nerves in the femoral incision. These usually resolve. Care to avoid retractor damage to the femoral nerve or to divide its branches (especially during re-do surgery) will avoid more serious or permanent neurological deficits, which should be rare. *Algodystrophy* describes a group of painful conditions including causalgia, reflex sympathetic dystrophy and Sudeck's atrophy, which may occur after aortic bifurcation surgery[90]. It is possible that the measures taken to avoid sexual dysfunction (avoiding the autonomic plexuses) may also guard against this problem.

Perigraft seromas are rare. These are non-infected collections of fluid around grafts, and they may represent an inflammatory response to Dacron[91] (Figure 7.3). Seromas cannot be anticipated and nothing can be done to avoid them.

Finally, we should consider complications which can affect the surgeon rather than the patient. The most important of these is now HIV infection, and all vascular surgeons need to be aware of this risk when assessing patients and when operating. The use of eye protection should now be routine, but the extent of other precautions remains a difficult compromise between what is ideal and what is practical.

References

1. Hertzer, N. R., Avellone, J. C., Farrell, C. J., Plecha, F. R., Rhodes, R. S. *et al.* (1984) The risk of vascular surgery in a metropolitan community. *J. Vasc. Surg.*, **1**, 13–21.
2. Johnston, K. W. and Scobie, T. K. (1988) Multicenter prospective study of nonruptured abdominal aortic aneurysms. I. Population and operative management. *J. Vasc. Surg.*, **7**, 69–81
3. Guy, A. J., Lambert, D., Jones, N. A. G. and Chamberlain, J. (1990) After the confidential enquiry into perioperative deaths – aortic aneurysm surgery in the Northern Region. *Br. J. Surg.*, **77**, A344
4. Campbell, W. B. (1991) Morality statistics for elective aortic aneurysms. *Eur. J. Vasc. Surg.*, (in press)
5. Crawford, E. S., Saleh, S. A., Babb, J. W., Glaeser, D. H., Vaccaro, P. S. and Silvers, A. (1981) Infrarenal abdominal aortic aneurysm. Factors influencing survival after operation performed over a 25-year period. *Ann. Surg.*, **193**, 699–709
6. Soreide, O., Grimsgaard, C. H. R., Myhre, H. O., Solheim, K. and Trippestad, A. (1982) Time and cause of death for 301 patients operated on for abdominal aortic aneurysms. *Age and Ageing*, **11**, 256–260
7. Diehl, J. T., Cali, R. F., Hertzer, N. R. and Beven, E. G. (1983) Complications of abdominal aortic reconstruction. *Ann. Surg.*, **197**, 49–56
8. Bickerstaff, L. K., Hollier, L. H., Van Peenen, H. J., Melton, L. J., Pairolero, P. C. and Cherry, K. J. (1984) Abdominal aortic aneurysms: The changing natural history. *J. Vasc. Surg.*, **1**, 6–12
9. Campbell, W. B., Collin, J. and Morris, P. J. (1986) The mortality of abdominal aortic aneurysm. *Ann. R. Coll. Surg.*, **68**, 275–278
10. Reigel, M. M., Hollier, L. H., Kazmier, F. J., O'Brien, P. C., Pairolero, P. C. *et al.* (1987) Late survival in abdominal aortic aneurysm patients: The role of selective myocardial revascularization on the basis of clinical symptoms. *J. Vasc. Surg.*, **5**, 222–227
11. Johnston, K. W. (1989) Multicenter prospective study of nonruptured abdominal aortic aneurysm. Part II. Variables predicting morbidity and mortality. *J. Vasc. Surg.*, **9**, 437–447
12. Goldman, L., Caldera, D. L., Nussbaum, S. R., Southwick, F. S., Krogstad, D. *et al.* (1977) Multifactorial index of cardiac risk in noncardiac surgical procedures. *New Eng. J Med.* **297**, 845–850
13. McEnroe, C. S., O'Donnell, T. F., Yeager, A., Konstam, M. and Mackey, W. C. (1990) Comparison of ejection fraction and Goldman risk factor analysis to dipyridamole-thallium 201 studies in the evaluation of cardiac morbidity after aortic aneurysm surgery. *J. Vasc. Surg.*, **11**, 497–504
14. Perry, M. O. and Calcagno, D. (1988) Abdominal aortic aneurysm surgery: the basic evaluation of cardiac risk. *Ann. Surg.*, **208**, 738–742
15. Whittemore, A. D., Clowes, A. W., Hechtman, H. B. and Mannick, J. A. (1980) Aortic aneurysm repair. Reduced operative mortality associated with maintenance of optimal cardiac performance. *Ann. Surg.*, **192**, 414–421
16. Kalman, P. G., Wellwood, M. R., Weisel, R. D., Morley-Forster, P. K., Teasdale, S. J. *et al.* (1986) Cardiac dysfunction during abdominal aortic operation: The limitations of pulmonary wedge pressures. *J. Vasc. Surg.* **3**, 773–781
17. Harpole, D. H., Clements, F. M., Quill, T., Wolfe, W. G., Jones, R. H. and McCann, R. L. (1989) Right and left ventricular performance during and after abdominal aortic aneurysm repair. *Ann. Surg.* **209**, 356–362

18. Hollier, L. H., Reigel, M. M., Kazmier, F. J., Pairolero, P. C., Cherry, K. J. and Hallett, J. W. (1986) Conventional repair of abdominal aortic aneurysm in the high-risk patient: A plea for abandonment of nonresective treatment. *J. Vasc. Surg.*, 3, 712–717

19. Campbell, W. B., Goodman, D. A. and Ballard, P. K. (1990) Postoperative care in abdominal aortic surgery – the first 48 hours. *Br. J. Surg.*, 77, A350

20. Lausten, G. S. and Engell, H. C. (1984) Postoperative complications in abdominal vascular surgery. *Acta Chir Scand.*, 150, 457–461

21. Gracey, D. R., Divertie, M. B. and Didier, E. P. (1979) Preoperative pulmonary preparation of patients with chronic obstructive pulmonary disease. A prospective study. *Chest*, 76, 123–129

22. Becquemin, J. P., *et al.* (1985) Pulmonary function after transverse or midline incision in patients with obstructive pulmonary disease. *Int. Care Med.*, 11, 247–251

23. Shepard, A. D., Scott, G. R., Mackey, W. C., O'Donnell, T. F., Bush, H. L. and Callow, A. D. (1986) Retroperitoneal approach to high-risk abdominal aortic aneurysms. *Arch. Surg.* 121, 444–449

24. Nevelsteen, A., Smet, G., Weymans, M., Depre, H. and Suy, R. (1988) Transabdominal or retroperitoneal approach to the aorto-iliac tract: a pulmonary function study. *Eur. J. Vasc. Surg.*, 2, 229–232

25. Sicard, G. A., Freeman, M. B., Vander-Woude, J. C. and Anderson, C. B. (1987) Comparison between the transabdominal and retro-peritoneal approach for reconstruction of the infrarenal abdominal aorta. *J. Vasc. Surg.*, 5, 19–27

26. Cambria, R. P., Brewster, D. C., Abbott, W. M., Freehan, M., Megerman, J. *et al.* (1990) Transperitoneal versus retroperitoneal approach for aortic reconstruction: A randomized prospective study. *J. Vasc. Surg.*, 11, 314–325

27. Bergqvist, D., Olsson, P.-O., Takolander, R., Almen, T., Cederholm, C. and Jonsson, K. (1983) Renal failure as a complication to aortoiliac and iliac reconstructive surgery. *Acta Chir Scand.*, 149, 37–41

28. Bjerkelund, C. E., Smith-Erichsen, N. and Solheim, K. (1986) Abdominal aortic reconstruction: Prognostic importance of coexistent diseases. *Acta Chir Scand.*, 152, 111–115

29. Barry, K. G., Mazze, R. I. and Schwartz, F. D. (1964) Prevention of surgical oliguria and renal-hemodynamic suppression by sustained hydration. *New Eng. J. Med.* 270, 1371–1377

30. Awad, R. W., Barham, W. J., Taylor, D. N., Woodward, D. A. K. and Bullen, B. R. (1990) Technical and operative factors in infrarenal aortic reconstruction and their effect on the glomerular filtration rate in the immediate postoperative period and 6 months later. *Eur. J. Vasc. Surg.*, 4, 239–245

31. Stoney, R. J. and Rabahie, G. N. (1989) Management of juxtarenal and pararenal aortic atherosclerosis. In *Aortic Surgery* (eds J. J. Bergan and J. S. T. Yao). Philadelphia, W. B. Saunders, pp. 161–174

32. Schapira, H. E., Li, R., Gribetz, M., Wulfsohn, M. A. and Brendler, H. (1981) Ureteral injuries during vascular surgery. *J. Urol.*, 125, 293–297

33. Dowling, R. A., Corriere, J. N. and Sandler, C. M. (1986) Iatrogenic ureteral injury. *J. Urol.*, 135, 912–915

34. Henry, L. G. and Bernhard, V. M. (1978) Ureteral pathology associated with aortic surgery: A report of three unusual cases. *Surgery*, 83, 464–469

35. McCarthy, W. J., Flinn, W. R., Carter, M. F. and Yao, J. S. T. (1989) Prevention and management of urologic injuries during aortic surgery. In *Aortic Surgery* (eds J. J. Bergan and J. S. T. Yao). Philadelphia, W. B. Saunders, pp. 539–546

36. Fry, D. E., Milholen, L. and Harbrecht, P. J. (1983) Iatrogenic ureteral injury: Options in Management. *Arch. Surg.*, 118, 454–457

37. Crowson, M., Fielding, J. W. L., Black, J., Ashton, F. and Slaney, G. (1984) Acute gastrointestinal complications of infrarenal aortic aneurysm repair. *Br. J. Surg.*, 71, 825–828

38. Ernst, C. B., Hagihara, P. F., Daugherty, M. E., Sachatello, C. R. and Griffen, W. O. (1976) Ischemic colitis incidence following abdominal aortic reconstruction: A prospective study. *Surgery*, 80, 417–421

39. Bast, T. J., van der Biezen, J. J., Scherpenisse, J. and Eikelboom, B. C. (1990) Ischaemic disease of the colon and rectum after surgery for abdominal aortic aneurysm: A prospective study of the incidence and risk factors. *Eur. J. Vasc. Surg.*, 4, 253–257

40. Schroeder, T., Christoffersen, J. K., Andersen, J., Bille, S., Gravgaard, E. *et al.* (1985) Ischemic colitis complicating reconstruction of the abdominal aorta. *Surg. Gynecol. Obst.* 160, 299–303

41. Ernst, C. B. (1983) Prevention of intestinal ischaemia following abdominal aortic reconstruction. *Surgery*, 93, 102–106

42. Hobson, R. W., Wright, C. B., Rich, N. M. and Collins, G. J. (1976) Assessment of colonic ischaemia during aortic surgery by Doppler ultrasound. *J. Surg. Res.*, 20, 231–235

43. Williams, L. F., Kim, R. M., Tompkins, W. and Byrne, J. J. (1968) Aortoiliac Steal – a cause of intestinal ischaemia. *New Eng. J. Med.*, 278, 777–778

44. Johnson, W. C. and Nabseth, D. C. (1974) Visceral infarction following aortic surgery. *Ann. Surg.*, **180**, 312–318

45. Bergqvist, D. and Ljungstrom, K-G. (1987) Hemorrhagic complications resulting in reoperation after peripheral vascular surgery. A fourteen-year experience. *J. Vasc. Surg.*, **6**, 134–138

45a. Strom, J. A., Bernhard, V. M. and Towne, J. B. (1984) Acute limb ischaemia following aortic reconstruction: A preventable cause of increased mortality. *Arch. Surg.*, **119**, 470–473

46. Starr, D. S., Lawrie, G. M. and Morris, G. C. (1979) Prevention of distal embolism during arterial reconstruction. *Am. J. Surg.*, **138**, 764–769

47. Brewster, D. C., Meier, G. H., Darling, R. C., Moncure, A. C., LaMuraglia, G. M. and Abbott, W. M. (1987) Reoperation for aortofemoral graft limb occlusion: Optimal methods and long-term results. *J. Vasc. Surg.*, **5**, 363–374

48. Towne, J. B. (1989) Acute limb ischaemia following aortic surgery. In *Aortic Surgery* (eds J. J. Bergan, and J. S. T. Yao). Philadelphia, W. B. Saunders, pp. 511–518.

49. Ameli, F. M., Provan, J. L., Williamson, C. and Keachler, P. M. (1987) Etiology and management of aortofemoral bypass graft failure. *J. Cardiovasc. Surg.* **2**, 695–700

50. Imperato, A. M. (1983) Abdominal aortic surgery: Prevention of lower limb ischaemia. *Surgery*, **93**, 112–116

51. Mashiah, A., Thomson, J. M., Poller, L. and Charlesworth, D. (1989) Changes in the coagulation of blood during resection of the abdominal aorta. *Surg. Gynecol. Obs.*, **149**, 214–216

52. Quigley, F. G., Jamieson, G. G., Lloyd, J. V. and Faris, I. B. (1988) Monitoring of heparin in vascular surgery. *J. Vasc. Surg.*, **8**, 125–127

53. Crawford, E. S. (1983) Symposium: Prevention of complications of abdominal aortic reconstruction. Introduction. *Surgery*, **93**, 91–96

54. Gewertz, B. L. (1989) Monitoring spinal cord function. In *Aortic Surgery*, (eds J. J. Bergan and J. S. T. Yao). Philadelphia, W. B. Saunders, pp. 78–83

55. Healy, D. A., Keyser, J., Holcomb, G. W., Dean, R. H. and Smith, B. M. (1989) Prophylactic closed suction drainage of femoral wounds in patients undergoing vascular reconstruction. *J. Vasc. Surg.*, **10**, 166–168

56. Dunlop, M. G., Fox, J. N., Stonebridge, P. A., Clason, A. E. and Ruckley, C. V. (1990) Vacuum drainage of groin wounds after vascular surgery: A control trial. *Br. J. Surg.*, **77**, 562–563

56a. Szilagyi, D. E., Smith, R. F., Elliott, J. P. and Vrandecic, M. P. (1972). Infection in arterial reconstruction with synthetic grafts. *Ann. Surg.*, **176**, 321–323

57. Lorentzen, J. E., Nielsen, O. M., Arendrup, H., Kimose, H. H., Bille, S. *et al.* (1985) Vascular graft infection: An analysis of sixty-two graft infections in 2411 consecutively implanted synthetic vascular grafts. *Surgery*, **98**, 81–86

58. O'Hara, P. J., Hertzer, N. R., Beven, E. G. and Krajewski, L. P. (1986) Surgical management of infected abdominal aortic grafts: Review of a 25-year experience. *J. Vasc. Surg.*, **3**, 725–731

59. Earnshaw, J. J., Hopkinson, B. R., Makin, G. S. and Slack, R. C. B. (1988) Risk factors in vascular surgical sepsis. *Ann. R. Coll. Surg.*, **70**, 139–143

60. Cruse, P. J. E. and Foord, R. (1973) A five-year prospective study of 23,649 surgical wounds. *Arch. Surg.*, **107**, 206–210

61. Landreneau, M. D. and Raju, S. (1981) Infections after elective bypass surgery for lower limb ischaemia: The influence of preoperative transcutaneous arteriography. *Surgery*, **90**, 956–961

62. Goldstone, J. and Effeney, D. J. (1985) Prevention of Arterial Graft Infections. In *Complications in Vascular Surgery* (eds V. M. Bernhard and J. B. Towne). Grune and Stratton, New York, pp. 487–498

63. Bunt, T. J. (1983) Synthetic vascular graft infections. I. Graft infections. *Surgery*, **93**, 733–746

64. Bickerstaff, L. K., Hollier, L. H., Van Peenen, H. J., Melton, L. J., Pairolero, P. C. and Cherry, K. J. (1984) Abdominal aortic aneurysm repair combined with a second surgical procedure – Morbidity and mortality. *Surgery*, **95**, 487–491

65. Buckels, J. A. C., Fielding, J. W. L., Black, J., Ashton, F. and Slaney, G. (1985) Significance of positive bacterial cultures from aortic aneurysm contents. *Br. J. Surg.*, **72**, 440–442

66. Wakefield, T. W., Pierson, C. L., Schaberg, D. R., Messina, L. M., Lindenauer, S. M. *et al.* (1990) Artery, periarterial adipose tissue, and blood microbiology during vascular reconstructive surgery: Perioperative and early postoperative observations. *J. Vasc. Surg.*, **11**, 624–628

67. Kaiser, A. B., Clayson, K. R., Mulherin, J. L., Roach, A. C., Allen, T. R. *et al.* (1978) Antibiotic prophylaxis in vascular surgery. *Ann. Surg.*, **188**, 283–289

68. Pitt, H. A., Postier, R. G., MacGowan, W. A. L., Frank, L. W., Surmak, A. J. *et al.* (1980) Prophylactic antibodies in vascular surgery. Topical, systemic, or both? *Ann. Surg.*, **192**, 356–364

69. Fradet, G., Brister, S., Richards, G. K., Prentis, J., Brown, R. A. *et al.* (1986) Antibiotic prophylaxis in vascular surgery: Pharmacokinetic study of four commonly used cephalosporins. *J. Vasc. Surg.*, **3**, 535–539

70. Sunderland, G. T. and McKay, A. J. (1987) Survey of antibiotic use by members of the Vascular Society. *Br. J. Surg.*, **74**, 331–332
71. Bandyk, D. F., Berni, G. A., Thiele, B. L. and Towne, J. B. (1984) Aortofemoral graft infection due to staphylococcus epidermidis. *Arch. Surg.*, **119**, 102–108
72. Rutherford, R. B. (1989) In *Vascular Surgery*, (ed. R. B. Rutherford) Philadelphia, W. B. Saunders
73. Webb, L. X., Myers, R. T., Cordell, R. *et al.* (1986) Inhibition of bacterial adhesion by antibacterial surface pretreatment of vascular prosthesis. *J. Vasc. Surg.*, **4**, 16–21
74. Yeager, R. A., Sasaki, T. M., McConnell, D. B. and Vetto, R. M. (1987) Clinical spectrum of patients with infrarenal aortic grafts and gastrointestinal bleeding. *Am J Surg.*, **153**, 459–461
75. Bunt, T. J. (1983) Synthetic vascular graft infections. II. Graft-enteric erosions and graft-enteric fistulas. *Surgery*, **94**, 1–9
76. Elliott, J. P., Smith, R. F. and Szilagyi, D. E. (1974) Aortoenteric and paraprosthetic enteric fistulas. *Arch. Surg.*, **108**, 479–490
77. Umpleby, H. C. and Turnbull, A. R. (1988) Arterioenteric fistulas. *Br. J. Hosp. Med.*, **39**, 488–496
78. Szilagyi, D. E., Smith, R. F., Elliott, J. P., Hageman, J. H. and Dall'Olmo, C. A. (1975) Anastomotic aneurysms after vascular reconstruction: Problems of incidence, etiology, and treatment. *Surgery*, **78**, 800–816
79. Sieswerda, C., Skotnicki, S. H., Barentsz, J. O. and Heystraten, F. M. J. (1989) Anastomotic aneurysms – an underdiagnosed complication after aorto-iliac reconstructions. *Eur. J. Vasc. Surg.*, **3**, 233–238
80. Youkey, J. R., Clagett, G. P., Rich, N. M., Brigham, R. A., Orecchia, P. M. and Salander, J. M. (1984) Femoral anastomotic false aneurysms. An 11-year experience analysed with a case control study. *Ann. Surg.*, **199**, 703–709
81. Di Marzo, L., Strandness, E. L., Schultz, R. D. and Feldhaus, R. J. (1987) Reoperation for femoral false aneurysm. *Ann. Surg.*, **206**, 168–172
82. Wandschneider, W., Bull, P. and Denck, H. (1988) Anastomotic aneurysms – an unsolvable problem. *Eur. J. Vasc.*, **2**, 115–119
83. Clarke, A. M., Poskitt, K. R., Baird, R. N. and Horrocks, M. (1989) Anastomotic aneurysms of the femoral artery: aetiology and treatment. *Br. J. Surg.*, **76**, 1014–1016
84. Hollier, L. H., Batson, R. C. and Cohn, I. (1980) Femoral anastomotic aneurysms. *Ann. Surg.*, **191**, 715–720
85. Miles, J. R., Miles, D. G. and Johnson, G. (1982) Aortoiliac operations and sexual dysfunction. *Arch. Surg.*, **117**, 1177–1181
86. Sabri, S. and Cotton, L. T. (1971) Sexual function following aortoiliac reconstruction. *Lancet*, **2**, 1218–1219
87. Depalma, R. G. (1982). Impotence in vascular disease: relationship to vascular surgery. *Br. J. Surg.*, **69**, (suppl.), s14–s16.
88. Flanigan, D. P. and Schuler, J. J. (1989) Sexual function and aortic surgery. In *Aortic Surgery*, (eds J. J. Bergan and J. S. T. Yao). Philadelphia, W. B. Saunders, pp. 547–560.
89. Nevelsteen, A., Beyens, G., Duchateau, J. and Suy, R. (1990) Aorto-femoral reconstruction and sexual function: A prospective study. *Eur. J. Vasc. Surg.*, **4**, 247–251
90. Churcher, M. D. (1984) Algodystrophy after aortic bifurcation Surgery. *Lancet*, **2**, 131–132
91. Blumenberg, R. M., Gelfand, M. L. and Dale, W. A. (1985) Perigraft seromas complicating arterial grafts. *Surgery*, **97**, 194–203

Chapter 8

Mesenteric ischaemia – recognition reaps rewards

Paul Lieberman

All surgeons must have had the unforgettable experience of operating on a patient with extensive infarction of the bowel. Not many, however, will have had to manage a patient with chronic intestinal ischaemia and even they will have seen fewer patients with intestinal ischaemia than they have read articles about it.

Over 50 years ago Dunphy established at post mortem[1] the link between intestinal infarction and a previous history of ischaemic abdominal pain, thus providing a logical and attractive foundation for the possibility of relieving pain and preventing fatal infarction by reversing intestinal ischaemia.

This chapter attempts to present a brief review of the problems of acute and chronic intestinal ischaemia and to indicate possibly helpful directions in practical diagnosis and management. The more familiar we become with the practicalities of revascularization of ischaemic intestine the more likely is it that patients with intestinal angina, as Mikkelson termed the symptoms of pain from chronic intestinal ischaemia[2], will be treated and infarction avoided. It is to be hoped also that as more experience is gained in operations for revascularization the procedures will be applied to more patients who have reached the point of intestinal infarction and may therefore have an improved chance of survival.

Pathophysiology

Most cases of chronic intestinal ischaemia are due to atheromatous plaques at the origins of the coeliac axis (CA), superior mesenteric artery (SMA) and inferior mesenteric artery (IMA). If the arteries are sufficiently narrowed or occluded the splanchnic blood supply is derived from a rich collateral circulation which, while allowing adequate flow for resting demands, in rare instances may be inadequate for peak post-prandial requirements and may therefore give rise to intestinal angina[3]. If the collateral blood supply becomes inadequate for resting metabolic demands, mesenteric infarction results.

Infarction

When ischaemia progresses to the point of bowel infarction, whether the initiating cause is chronic or acute, the final outcome is the same. In the face of falling perfusion pressure there is a homeostatic increase in collateral flow, dilatation of intestinal vessels, redistribution of flow from muscularis to mucosa and increase in oxygen extraction

As anoxia becomes more profound AMP accumulates and breakdown products of hypoxanthine, a derivative of AMP, give rise to the free radicals which are so damaging in the 'reperfusion injury'. In experimental situations the use of free radical scavengers such as SOD and allopurinol reduce the amount of damage after limited periods of ischaemia[4,5], but if ischaemia is prolonged cell death is inevitable.

Following infarction, visible histological changes occur within an hour but subcellular changes can be demonstrated within 10 minutes of occlusion[6]. The later gross changes of haemorrhagic necrosis of the gut, toxaemia and massive intralumi-nal fluid loss become manifested by increasingly severe symptoms of peritonitis and systemic illness leading to death from multiorgan failure within hours or days.

Infarcted bowel induces many systemic consequences with increased leucocyto-sis[7], haematocrit, and marked acidosis[8]; in some patients serum amylase is raised. The liver enzymes ALT and AST, together with LDH and CPK all may be elevated in the serum, but it is disappointing that none of these measurable systemic effects occurs sufficiently early in the course of the disease to make them useful as a diagnostic marker. The earliest rise is seen in the isoenzyme CPK-BB derived from smooth muscle, which reaches a peak value six hours following experimental infarction[9].

Acute ischaemia

Causes

Acute infarction of the small bowel is not uncommon, with an incidence of presentation in Glasgow of perhaps ten cases per year for a population of 200 000[7]. The majority of cases (33%) were the result of embolic occlusion of the SMA, thrombosis of an atherosclerotic vessel (26%) or a failure of intestinal perfusion without major vessel occlusion (24%). Just as peripheral emboli to the limbs are becoming less common in clinical practice, so cardiac emboli as a cause of acute ischaemia are less frequently seen and thrombotic occlusion is more frequent[10].

Acute non-occlusive mesenteric ischaemia can follow any period of profound hypotension from heart failure, bleeding or sepsis but can also be precipitated by other stimuli such as drugs[11,12,13] which can initiate a vicious circle of vasocon-striction, hypoxia, sepsis and progression to bowel necrosis. The symptoms are similar to those of occlusive ischaemia but are easy to overlook in a patient who is usually desperately ill from another cause. If a case is diagnosed either by timely angiography before laparotomy or at operation it should be treated by specific vasodilators such as intra-arterial papaverine[14] as well as general supportive measures.

Recognition

Revascularization for acute ischaemia can only be of value early in the course of the disease and it is this that makes it so necessary to be alert for possible cases. The vast majority of emboli occur in patients with a history of cardiac disease, and a minority have a past history of a previous embolic event. Of course, as Dunphy showed[1], many patients whose infarction is due to thrombosis have a prior history of mesenteric angina and are very likely to have had claudication or angina pectoris as well. On examination such patients will very frequently have evidence of atheroma at other peripheral sites such as the femoral or carotid vessels.

The initial symptoms, which may be insidious or of sudden onset, are of severe abdominal pain with gut emptying by vomiting or diarrhoea. The pain, which may initially be central and colicky and later becomes continuous and diffuse, is often more severe than seems to be accounted for by the signs which are, initially, few.

The most persuasive sign is the appearance of a patient who appears ill and in obvious pain but has perhaps only a little tenderness in the RIF. The bowel sounds may be enhanced initially in the course of the illness and disappear later when ileus and peritonitis supervene producing increasing abdominal tenderness.

Diagnosis

Unfortunately, there are no simple investigations which can reliably help to substantiate a clinical suspicion of early intestinal ischaemia. Raised transaminases and LDH are not specific and in many cases the amylase is normal[7]. A leucocytosis above 15 000 and acidosis with base excess below − 10 may be helpful later in the condition, and a plain abdominal X-ray is useful to exclude other major causes of severe abdominal pain. The film may show gas in the wall of the infarcted bowel or in the portal system, but this is a very late sign.

As soon as the condition is suspected, if the patient's signs do not warrant an immediate laparotomy, an aortogram should be obtained. This may be a counsel of perfection for most units in the UK which do not have a 24 hour angiographic service available, but if available it must be done immediately to avoid any delay to laparotomy. Ideally, preoperative resuscitation and angiography should proceed together. Views should be taken with a flush aortogram, AP and lateral. Selective angiography may be very helpful in those with non-occlusive ischaemia as the angiography catheter can be used subsequently for intra-arterial infusion[15,16].

Management

The general preoperative management and resuscitation should be the same as for any other severely ill patient. Depleted circulating volume is replaced using serum electrolytes, the CVP, Swan Ganz catheter and PCV as a guide while urine output is measured with a bladder catheter and blood pressure with a radial line. Blood is cross-matched, antibiotics are given and a nasogastric tube passed.

Non-operative management
When prior angiography has shown non-occlusive ischaemia or minimal distal emboli the selective angiogram catheter offers the possibility of infusing the SMA with papaverine solution (30–60 ml/h) or other arterial vasodilator.

The use of low dose intra-arterial thrombolysis has occasionally been described for embolic lesions of the SMA[17,18] but opportunities for treatment are rare and this is a slow and uncertain therapy during which it is impossible to determine the condition of the bowel. It could be considered if there are very powerful reasons to avoid laparotomy or if the emboli are seen to be peripheral on angiography.

Operative management
A midline exploratory laparotomy will allow the diagnosis of ischaemia to be confirmed, an assessment of the condition of the gut to be made and the cause to be

determined. Bergan[19] has described how, by inspection of the root of the mesentery and proximal jejunum, it is usually possible to distinguish easily between cases caused by emboli and those caused by thrombosis. Emboli tend to lodge distally about 5 cm from the origin of the SMA at the middle colic branch, thus allowing a palpable pulse to be felt at the very root of the SMA as well as giving good perfusion of the proximal jejunum. This is in contrast to cases caused by thrombosis when the SMA is occluded from its origin and signs of ischaemia are present even in the proximal loop of the jejunum at the duodeno-jejunal flexure.

The early case may look deceptively normal with only pallor and pulseless vessels evident but it is only too often the case that massive necrosis is found with dilated loops of greenish black malodorous bowel. If the whole small bowel is frankly gangrenous no remedial operation may be possible, while in fortunate cases a limited ischaemic segment with well perfused margins requires only a limited resection.

When an extensive resection seems necessary, or when there seems to be a prospect of avoiding resection, a revascularization procedure should be considered first, as such a procedure may well improve perfusion sufficiently to modify the decision about the need for resection or the length of gut to be resected.

Embolectomy   If an embolus is suspected, embolectomy should be attempted. The operation is in principle no different from embolectomy at other sites, and as at other sites careful technique, gentle manipulation of the balloon catheter and precise suture closure are necessary.

The transverse mesocolon is lifted and the small gut mesentery drawn downwards and to the right. It may be necessary to divide the ligament of Trietz and mobilize the proximal jejunum and 4th part of the duodenum. If the origin of the SMA is pulsatile it is reasonably simple to expose the artery using careful dissection through a longitudinal incision in the overlying peritoneum.

Once exposed, the artery and its branches are secured and controlled with silastic rubber loops and appropriate clamps. The artery is incised through a transverse incision and gently swept proximally and distally with 4 fr and 3 fr Fogarty catheters. It is usually simple to achieve good proximal clearance of clot with brisk blood flow, but clearance of distal arcades can be a problem.

It has been suggested[20] that by using a temporary intraluminal vascular shunt, such as a Javid carotid shunt, to allow perfusion of the distal gut before closing the arteriotomy it is possible to identify those bowel loops which are not well perfused and which might therefore require further distal passage of a fine Fogarty catheter.

Another manoeuvre borrowed from peripheral arterial practice[20] is the suggested use of 100 000 units of urokinase or similar thrombolytic agent for instillation into the distal arterial bed. Closure of the arteriotomy requires the usual precise arterial suture technique and if the vessel is too narrow or if there is coexisting atheroma it may be wise to use a vein patch[21].

Grafting   If the acute ischaemia is a result of thrombosis an arterial graft is needed for revascularization. There are nowadays no enthusiasts for the early technique of retrograde TEA of the origin of the SMA[22].

Because of the risk of graft infection, with or without bowel resection, a vein graft should be the first choice and in desperately ill patients an infrarenal aortic origin for the graft is the best site. The precise technique can be similar to that suggested for the chronic ischaemic patient, but may have to be adjusted to allow for the length of graft available. Again, the interesting suggestion has been made[20] that a temporary intraluminal Javid shunt is sufficiently stiff to allow it to be introduced through the proximal SMA stenosis enabling perfusion of the bowel preparation for the grafting procedure.

Resection   With the revascularization completed, the need for resection must be assessed after a period of 30 minutes or so during which the bowel is covered by warm packs. Bowel which is obviously necrotic must be resected but it can be difficult to be sure about intestinal viability on clinical grounds. Following revascularization there is sometimes only patchy reperfusion apparent at first and there is frequently doubt about the viability of bowel at the margins of infarcted segments. Various tests for bowel viability have been described using Doppler ultrasound, infrared photoplethys-mography (PPG), fluorescein, laser doppler flowmetry, surface oximetry and pulse oximetry[23–28]. In experienced hands these may contribute to the operative decision about resection but all require experience and specialized equipment which may not always be available.

If a resection is performed it is best to avoid primary anastomosis and to bring out the divided ends of bowel to the skin surface. This allows subsequent inspection of the bowel mucosa and avoids the disaster of a dehisced or leaking anastomosis.

There is a good case to be made for planning a second look laparotomy within 24 h in cases where revascularization has been performed without bowel resection and viability is in question[29–31]. In these cases arrangements for re-operation should be established in advance and the patient maintained on artificial ventilation in an intensive care unit.

Postoperative care

Fluid losses into the gut are likely to be large and fluid balance must be closely monitored and regulated. The patient is maintained on parenteral nutrition and may require this for some weeks depending on the length and degree of adaptation of the remaining gut. Unless there is a specific contraindication the patient who has had an embolus should be maintained on lifelong anticoagulation (S1,40).

Clinical experience

Our local experience of acute infarction[7] with an overall mortality of 92% is as dismal as many other reports which have shown how little results have changed in 30 years. All authors agree that early awareness and recognition of the condition are vital and have a significant effect on outcome. The place of early angiography is universally recommended by both those who have failed to use it extensively and those who have found it useful in practice.

The most impressive demonstration of what can be achieved comes from New York. Boley's study used a simple clinical protocol in which all patients with a high-risk history and abdominal pain of longer than two hours were given an aortogram unless a plain abdominal X-ray showed another lesion. With early angiographic diagnosis, aggressive embolectomy for major clots and the use of intra-arterial papaverine mortality was reduced to less than 50%. These results have never been bettered.

Chronic ischaemia

Causes

The vast majority of cases of chronic intestinal ischaemia are caused by atheromatous plaques at the origins of the visceral vessels, but on occasion miscellaneous other conditions are responsible. These include systemic lupus erythematosus, rheumatoid arthritis, radiation vasculitis, methysergide, fibromuscular hyperplasia, arteritis, Takayasu's disease, neurofibromatosis and Buergers syndrome[33–40].

It has long been recognized that very severe disease can exist in the mesenteric vessels without giving rise to symptoms. Indeed, in 1869 a case was reported in which a woman who had died from an unrelated cause showed at post-mortem complete occlusion of all the vessels supplying the intestine[42]. A recent British post-mortem investigation[43] in an unselected population revealed the widespread nature of atherosclerotic mesenteric lesions and showed that stenoses were critical in about 10% of IMAs, 5% of SMAs and 3% of CAs.

Presentation

The patient with mesenteric angina may well have a long history of vague abdominal pain which is usually related to meal times and may be affected by the size of the meal. He or she will probably have had many investigations for the pain with negative or non-specific results and very frequently has a history of, or shows signs of, atherosclerosis at other peripheral sites.

The precise cause of the pain is not understood, but it is thought to be related to muscular spasm or anaerobic metabolism in the wall of the gut which occurs when it is unable to achieve the normal post-prandial flow increase[44] which accompanies an increased oxygen uptake. To explain the observation that the pain of intestinal angina starts before food arrives in the small gut it has been suggested that the pain is due to shunting of blood to the stomach from the intestine[45].

In addition to pain, patients with intestinal angina present with weight loss. Indeed, the combination of abdominal pain and a cachectic appearance often prompts multiple investigations for malignancy[46]. Many investigations have failed consistently to show evidence of malabsorption in mesenteric angina[47] but there have been some reports[48,49] which document reversal of poor absorption following revascularization. Most would accept that most patients do not suffer weight loss from malabsorption but do have an inadequate food intake because conditioning links eating with pain – the 'food fear'

An abdominal bruit is frequently present, but extensive aortic and visceral atheroma is common in these patients and a bruit is not a specific sign for intestinal ischaemia.

Diagnosis

The mainstay of the diagnosis of chronic intestinal ischaemia (CII) is angiography. A lateral subtraction angiogram of the aorta and splanchnic vessel origins is adequate to show localized stenoses or occlusions but a Seldinger aortogram with AP and lateral films is also required to identify other lesions which may require correction, to assess collateral and to plan surgery.

Apart from the demonstration of the blocked arterial origins, the most striking feature in many aortograms is the marked collateral flow either through the pancreatico-duodenal anastomoses or, where the SMA is occluded and the small intestine derives flow from the IMA, through the 'meandering mesenteric artery'[50] (Figure 8.1). It is widely held that it is necessary to demonstrate occlusion of two out of the three splanchnic vessels, of which one must be the SMA, in order to entertain a diagnosis of symptomatic CII[51] (Figure 8.2) but there are a few patients in most reported series who have had symptoms of intestinal angina with only SMA occlusion[52]. The angiogram demonstrates only the anatomy of the atherosclerotic disease – it cannot indicate its functional significance.

There are no clinically useful tests of intestinal function which can help and it has to be emphasized that the best available guide to function is the history of pain and weight loss. It is still true that 'To distinguish the life-threatening from the insignificant mesenteric block remains very difficult'[53].

It has been possible for about ten years to image the origin of the visceral vessels using ultrasound. As the machines have become more sophisticated and the operators more accomplished, particularly with the advent of colour Duplex systems, there is increasing enthusiasm for ultrasound examination of these vessels[54] but unfortunately only about 85% of arteries can be insonated[55] and the significance of the flow measurements which can be made is still being assessed. It is tempting to consider that a stress test of SMA flow with a meal or flow stimulant such as glucagon[56] should be sensitive for mesenteric arterial insufficiency but since the flow may be enhanced quite adequately through collateral circulation which is not measured by the examination, definite conclusions about impaired intestinal function cannot be drawn. None the less, Duplex ultrasound is, and will increasingly become, very valuable as a screening test for exclusion of non-ischaemic patients because demonstration of a normal peak

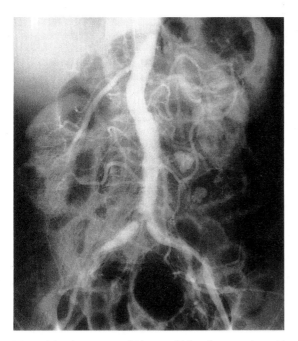

Figure 8.1 Aortogram of 74-year-old female presenting with post-prandial pain and intermittent claudication, showing meandering mesenteric artery

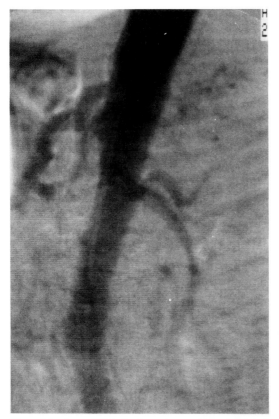

Figure 8.2 Lateral digital subtraction angiography showing stenosis of coeliac axis and occlusion of the superior mesenteric artery. At operation the blood pressure in the distal arcades of the mesenteric artery was 40 mm Hg

systolic flow velocity in the SMA virtually rules out the presence of significant SMA stenosis[55,57].

Treatment

Percutaneous angioplasty
There have been a number of case reports[58–60] of splanchnic arterial stenoses treated by percutaneous angioplasty (PTA), the attraction being the minimally invasive nature of the technique.

Unfortunately, most mesenteric atheroma lies at the ostia of the vessels in the aortic wall and it is now recognized that these ostial lesions are not best managed by PTA[61]. In addition, thrombosis following failed angioplasty might result in disastrous infarction and PTA should therefore only be performed where immediate revascularization is available. However, for the rare cases with a distal lesion or with fibromuscular hyperplasia PTA should certainly be considered.

In the future these difficult ostial lesions may be amenable to dilatation with endoluminal stent to maintain patency, but at present surgery is the treatment of choice.

Operation for chronic ischaemia
Operation for revascularizing the SMA or CA should only be considered when a patient has the diagnosis of symptomatic chronic visceral ischaemia firmly established by a typical history, exclusion of other possible causes and an angiogram which confirms the presence of severe mesenteric arterial disease. However, operations on the infrarenal aorta may well compromise intestinal blood supply from either the IMA or the internal iliac arteries and not uncommonly the IMA has to be revascularized to be certain about colonic perfusion. When there is severe disease of the SMA and CA, concomitant revascularization of these vessels can avoid the risk of intestinal infarction[62–64].

Prophylactic surgery of this nature tends to be self-justifying and without a trial cannot truly be shown to be necessary. Nevertheless, when the risk of postoperative intestinal infarction exists it is worth considering the place of concomitant mesenteric grafting since it causes little extra disturbance to the patient for great potential benefit.

The number of vessels which require reconstruction will depend on the extent of disease. Most authors take the view that restoration of flow to both SMA and CA is advantageous when both are blocked as it gives some degree of protection to the gut in the event that one of the grafts should fail[65]. One functioning graft, however, is sufficient to ensure viability and pain relief[66].

Technique   The first operation performed for mesenteric revascularization was a retrograde endarterectomy (reported in 1958[67]) and since then many operative procedures have been described[65,68–73].

There have been two main approaches to the practical problems of grafting to the mesenteric vessels. One well-supported view advocates direct revascularization of the SMA by prograde grafting from the supracoeliac aorta[68], by reimplantation of the transected SMA[70] or by transaortic disobliteration of the SMA and coeliac axis via a thoracoabdominal retroperitoneal approach[65]. While the prograde approach may be necessary on occasion because of infrarenal problems, there is no doubt that the supracoeliac approach is more demanding both for the patient, whose supracoeliac aorta must be clamped, and the surgeon, who may have to work in unfamiliar territory.

The other view recommends an indirect approach to the mesenteric vessels. This is usually easier because it involves a familiar dissection of the infrarenal aorta or iliacs and avoids a supracoeliac aortic clamp. Perhaps the most widely accepted technique is that described in a standard text in which a short vein graft is taken from the aorta to the root of the SMA[74]. A practical problem is that there is a great disparity between the relative positions of the SMA and the aorta when the SMA is displayed for anastomosis and in its resting position with the abdomen closed. With a short graft there is the possibility of kinking and there seems to be great merit in the method used by a group from Portland which uses a longer prosthetic graft.

The lazy loop   This is the name given in our hospital to the technique described by Porter's group in Portland[71,75] which we have found to be very useful (Figures 8.3 and 8.4). In this technique, a prosthetic graft of 6–8 mm diameter is anastomosed at its proximal end to the aorta, the iliac artery or an aortic graft. A retroperitoneal pocket is made by blunt dissection to the left of the midline in front of the kidney and this space allows the graft to pass upwards in a gentle curve, concave to the right, sitting comfortably in the retroperitoneum. The graft then skirts the lower border of

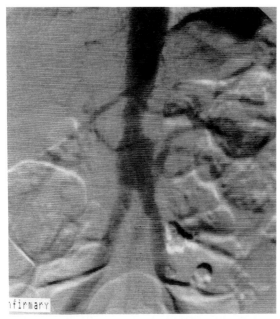

Figure 8.3   Postoperative intravenous digital subtraction angiography showing position of 'lazy loop' in front of the left kidney and the anterograde entry of graft into the superior mesenteric artery. Note the origin of the graft from the body of a Dacron trouser graft. The flow in this 6 mm graft was 450 ml/min

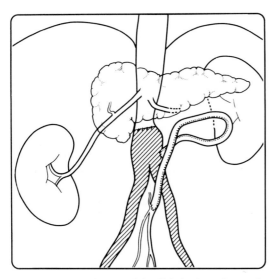

Figure 8.4   Line diagram of the digital subtraction angiography in figure 2 to emphasize the anatomical relationship of the graft

the pancreas continuing its curve and finally is anastomosed obliquely to a good quality segment of the proximal SMA to allow antegrade blood flow.

The anastomosis is constructed conventionally, the mobility of the graft allowing easy completion. Because of the length of the graft, any torsion or movement induced by the mesentery lying flat against the aorta after operation is easily taken up by the graft without inducing kinks. If the coeliac axis also requires attention, another long graft, which can be the second limb of a 12 × 7 bifurcation graft, is taken from the same origin through a retropancreatic tunnel and anastomosed, again in a prograde fashion, to the common hepatic artery. The technique is very suitable for those patients who require an aortic graft in addition to mesenteric repair since in these cases the mesenteric limb, taken from the anterolateral aspect of the body of the aortic graft, achieves inflow (Figures 8.3 and 8.4). Because of the retroperitoneal course of the graft, made by creating the pocket in front of the left kidney, good graft coverage is easily achieved.

Although there is an understandable surgical instinct to keep grafts short, in the mesenteric circulation where there are high graft flow rates to maintain patency, the length of the graft confers a practical advantage. Porter[75] recommends the use of intraoperative flowmetry for monitoring the graft flow and, using a 7 mm woven Dacron graft, describes flow rates from 500–800 ml/min.

Postoperative care

After operation, the patient may suffer a period of intestinal ileus, distension and fluid loss and so should be managed with nasogastric suction and close control of fluid and electrolyte balance as well as TPN. If graft occlusion occurs, massive infarction could result although this has only rarely been reported. More often graft occlusion seems only to be marked by a failure of the patient to progress smoothly. Because of this, an angiogram is performed before the patient is discharged to check graft patency. If found to be occluded the graft should be revised as resumption of a full diet may precipitate infarction.

Clinical experience

Since adopting the lazy loop in 1986 we have used it in six patients with intestinal angina: five with atheroma and one with Takayasu's arteritis. In all patients only the SMA was revascularized. No patients died at the time of operation but two grafts were found to be occluded at a week on routine postoperative angiography. While one is functioning well at 18 months following thrombectomy, consent for re-operation on the other was refused because the patient was symptom-free on a hospital diet. Sadly he was readmitted and died a month later with intestinal infarction. There have been two late deaths at one year and at seventeen months from renal failure and a CVA respectively. All other patients are pain-free and have gained weight.

The patient numbers are small but the frequency of presentation is in keeping with the experience from other centres. A leading British referral centre reported 37 symptomatic cases in a 25-year period, of which 31 underwent mesenteric anterior reconstruction[53]. If 30% of the ten or so patients who die annually with intestinal infarct in our hospital did so from mesenteric thrombosis, then it may be calculated that only three patients per annum are available to be saved by elective operation, and only one or two of these will have had prodromal symptoms of intestinal angina.

Encouragingly good results of mesenteric grafting have been widely reported from many centres, regardless of the operative technique used[76–84]. In all these studies, about 90% of survivors achieve relief of symptoms, and operative mortality is in single figures. Late deaths from mesenteric infarction also seem to be infrequent.

From the perspective of the clinical surgeon, the satisfaction of the patient who can again enjoy eating is persuasive evidence for continuing to treat patients with symptoms of chronic ischaemia by revascularization.

Summary

The outlook for patients with established intestinal infarction is still bleak: with the most aggressive approach to active management the best results in embolic cases show no more than about 50% surviving and most of us cannot hope to emulate even this degree of success. Every author writing on this subject makes a plea for early recognition but this is unlikely to come about until current diagnostic procedures change.

Perhaps in the future every admitting surgeon will have, in addition to a sound management protocol, the ability to use a colour Duplex ultrasound in the way that a stethoscope or abdominal X-ray is now used. If these or some other advances come about then early recognition and mesenteric artery revascularization might just allow us to improve on the results of our colleagues of 40 years ago.

Although a rare condition, chronic intestinal ischaemia is a rewarding one to treat. Because the need for this type of surgery is infrequent, the simplicity of the lazy loop reconstruction has encouraged us in a more confident approach to operation than was the case when we used a retroaortic supracoeliac dissection. One consequence is that symptomatic patients are more actively sought and, with colour Duplex mesenteric arterial investigation now available, in practice it is quite simple to assess patients as candidates for angiography and possible surgical revascularization.

References

1. Dunphy, J. E. (1936) Abdominal pain of vascular origin. *Am. J. Med. Sci.*, **192**, 109–113
2. Mikkelson, W. P. (1957) Intestinal angina: its surgical significance. *Am. J. Surg.*, **94**, 262–269
3. Hansen, H. J., Engell, H. C., Ring-Larsen, H. and Ranek, L. (1977) Splanchnic blood flow in patients with abdominal angina before and after arterial reconstruction. A proposal for a diagnostic test. *Ann. Surg.*, **186** (2), 216–220
4. Parks, D. A., Bulkley, G. B. and Granger, D. N. (1983) Role of oxygen-derived free radicals in digestive tract diseases. *Surgery*, **94**, 415
5. S. Parks, D. A., Bulkley, G. B., Granger, D. N. *et al.* (1982) Ischaemic injury in the small intestine: role of superoxide radicals. *Gastroenterology*, **82**, 9
6. Brown, R. A., Chiv, C., Scott, J. H. *et al.* (1970) Ultrastructural changes in the canine mucosal cell after mesenteric arterial occlusion. *Arch Surg.*, **101**, 290
7. Wilson, C., Gupta, R., Gilmour, D. G. and Imrie, C. W. (1987). Acute superior mesenteric ischaemia. *Br. J. Surg.*, **74**, 279–281
8. Brooks, D. H. and Carey, L. C. (1973) Base deficit in superior mesenteric artery occlusion: an aid to early diagnosis. *Ann Surg.*, **177**, 352–353
9. Graeber, G. M., Wolf, R. E. and Harmon, J. E. (1984) Serum creatine kinase and alkaline phosphatase in experimental small bowel infarction. *J. Surg. Res.*, **37**, 25–32
10. Mosley, J. G. and Marston, A. (1989) Acute intestinal ischaemia. In *Splanchnic ischaemia and multiple organ failure* (eds A. Marston, G. B. Bulkley, R. G. Fiddian Green and Ulf Haglund) pp. 279–289
11. Nalbaudiau, H., Sheth, M. and Dietrich, R. (1985) Intestinal ischaemia caused by cocaine ingestion: report of two cases. *Surgery*, **97**, 374–376

12. Roberts, C. and Maddison, F. E. (1976) Partial mesenteric arterial occlusion with subsequent ischemic bowel damage due to pitressin infusion. *Am. J. Roentgenol.*, **126** (4), 829–831

13. Holt, P. M. and Hollanders, D. (1980) Massive arterial thrombosis and oral contraception. *Br. Med. J.*, **280**, 19–20

14. Aldrete, J. S., Han, S. Y., Laws, H. L. and Kirklin, J. W. (1977) Intestinal infarction complicating low cardiac output states. *Surg. Gynecol. Obstet.*, **144** (3), 371–375

15. Carrasco, D., Gordo, R., Olaso, V., Baguena, J. and Berenguer, J. (1978) The value of emergency angiography in the diagnosis and prognosis of acute mesenteric arterial insufficiency. *Am. J. Gastroenterol.*, **69** (3, 1), 295–301

16. Clark, R. A. and Gallant, T. E. (1984) Acute mesenteric ischemia: angiographic spectrum. *Am. J. Roentgenol.*, **142** (3), 555–562

17. Jamieson, A. C., Thomas, R. J. and Cade, J. F. (1979) Lysis of a superior mesenteric artery embolus following local infusion of streptokinase and heparin. *Aust. NZ. J. Surg.*, **49** (3), 355–356

18. Hillers, T. K., Ginsberg, J. S., Panju, A., Gately, J., Gill, G. and Waterfall, W. E. (1990) Intra-arterial low-dose streptokinase infusion for superior mesenteric artery embolus. *Can. Med. Assoc. J.*, **142** (10), 1087–1088

19. Bergan, J. J. (1967) Recognition and treatment of intestinal ischaemia. *Surg. Clin. N. Am.*, **47**, 109–206

20. Whitehill, T. A. and Rutherford, R. (1990) Acute intestinal ischaemia caused by arterial occlusions: optimal management to improve survival. *Sem. Vasc. Surg.*, **3**, 149–156

21. Pearce, W. H. and Bergan, J. J. (1989) The management of visceral ischaemic syndromes. In *Vascular Surgery* vol. 11 (ed. R. B. Rutherford) W. B. Saunders, pp. 1086–1096

22. Brittain, R. S. and Early, T. K. (1963) Emergency thromboendarterectomy of the superior mesenteric artery. Report of four cases. *Ann. Surg.*, **158**, 138–143

23. Wright, C. B. and Hobson, R. W. (1975) Prediction of intestinal viability using doppler ultrasound technique. *Am. J. Surg.*, **129**, 642–645

24. Denobile, J., Guzzetta, P. and Patterson, K. (1990) Pulse oximetry as a means of assessing bowel viability. *J. Surg. Res.*, **48**, 21–23

25. Bulkley, G. B., Zuidema, G. D., O'Mara, C. S. *et al.* (1981) Intraoperative determination of viability following ischaemic injury: a prospective, controlled trial of adjuvant methods (Doppler and fluorescin) compared to clinical judgement. *Ann. Surg.*, **193**, 628

26. Locke, R., Hauser, C. J. and Shoemaker, W. C. (1984) The use of surface oximetry to assess bowel viability. *Arch. Surg.*, **119**, 1252

27. Pearch, W. H., Jones, D. N., Warren, G. H. *et al.* (1987) The use of infrared plethysmography in identifying early intestinal ischaemia. *Arch. Surg.*, **122**, 308

28. Johansson, K., Ahn, H. and Lindhagen, J. (1989) Intraoperative assessment of blood flow and tissue viability in small-bowel ischaemia by laser Doppler flowmetry. *Acta Chir. Scand.*, **155** (6–7), 341–346

29. Van Weel, M. W. (1956) Acute mesenteric arterial occlusion successful treatment by embolectomy and limited intestinal resection. *Acta Chir. Neerl.*, **8**, 147

30. Smith, X. Y. and Bloggs, A. B. (1957) Superior mesenteric artery embolectomy in the treatment of massive mesenteric infarction. *New Eng. J. Med.*, **252**, 595

31. Lindblad, B. and Hakansson, H. (1987) The rationale for second look operation in mesenteric vessel occlusion with uncertain viability at primary surgery. *Acta Chir. Scand.*, **153**, 53–534

32. Elliott, J. P., Hageman, J. H. and Szilyagi, D. E. (1980) Arterial embolization: problems of source, multiplicity, recurrence and delayed treatment. *Surgery*, **88**, 833–840

31. Lindblad, B. and Hakansson, H. (1987) The rationale for second look operation in mesenteric vessel occlusion with uncertain viability at primary surgery. *Acta Chir. Scand.*, **153**, 530–534

32. Elliott, J. P., Hageman, J. H. and Szilyagi, D. E. (1980) Arterial embolization: problems of source, multiplicity, recurrence and delayed treatment. *Surgery*, **88**, 833–840

33. Ripley, H. R. and Levin, S. R. (1966) Abdominal angina associated with fibromuscular hyperplasia of the coeliac and superior mesenteric arteries. *Angiology*, **17**, 297–310

34. Wolf, E. A., Summer, D. S. and Strandness, D. E. (1972) Disease of the mesenteric circulation in patients with thromboangiitis obliterans. *Vasc. Surg.*, **6**, 218–223

35. Mosley, J. G., Desai, A. and Gupta, I. (1990) Mesenteric arteritis. *Gut*, **31** (8), 956–957

36. Nussaume, O, Bouttier, S., Duchatelle, J. P., Valere, P.E. and Andreassian, B. (1990) Mesenteric infarction in Takayasu's disease. *Ann. Vasc. Surg.*, **4** (2), 117–121

37. Brunner, H., Stacher, G., Bankl, H. and Grabner, G. (1974) Chronic mesenteric arterial insufficiency caused by vascular neurofibromatosis. A case report. *Am. J. Gastroenterol.*, **65** (5), 442–447

38. Arnold, G. L., Fawaz, K. A., Callow, A. D. and Kaplan, M. M. (1982) Chronic intestinal ischaemia associated with oral contraceptive use. *Am. J. Gastroenterol.*, **77** (1), 32–34

39. Rybka, S. J. and Novick, A. C. (1983) Concomitant carotid, mesenteric and renal artery stenosis due to primary intimal fibroplasia. *J. Urol.*, **129** (4), 798–800

40. Rosen, N., Sommer, I. and Knobel, B. (1985) Intestinal Buerger's disease. *Arch. Path. Lab. Med.*, **109** (10), 962–963
41. Meacham, P. W. and Brantley, B. (1987) Familial fibromuscular dysplasia of the mesenteric arteries. *South. Med. J.*, **80** (10), 1311–1316
42. Chiene, J. (1869) Complete obliteration of the coeliac and mesenteric arteries. *J. Anat. Physiol.*, **3**, 65–72
43. Croft, R. J., Menon, G. P. and Marston, A. (1981) Does intestinal angina exist? A critical study of obstructed visceral arteries. *Br. J. Surg.*, **68**, 316–318
44. Quamar, M. I., Read, A. E. and Skidmore, R. (1986). Transcutaneous doppler ultrasound measurement of superior mesenteric artery blood flow in man. *Gut*, **27**, 100–105
45. Poole, J. W., Sammartano, R. J. and Boley, S. J. (1987) Haemodynamic basis of the pain in chronic mesenteric ischaemia.*Am. J. Surg.*, **153**, 171–176
46. Glueklich, B., Deterling, R. A. Jr., Matsumoto, G. H. and Callow, A. D. (1979) Chronic mesenteric ischemia masquerading as cancer. *Surg. Gynecol. Obstet.*, **148** (1), 49–56
47. Marston, A., Clarke, J. M. F. Garcia, J. and Miller, A. L. (1985) Intestinal function and intestinal blood supply. *Gut*, **26**, 656–666
48. Watt, J. K., Watson, W. C. and Haase, S. (1967) Chronic intestinal ischaemia. *Br. Med. J.*, (3), 199
49. Tilson, M. D. and Stansel, H. C. (1976). Abdominal angina. Intestinal absorption eight years after successful mesenteric revascularization. *Am. J. Surg.*, **131** (3), 366–368
50. Fisher, D. F. and Fry, W. J. (1987) The collateral mesenteric circulation. *Surg. Gynecol. Obstet.*, **164**, 487–491
51. Hansen, H. J. B. (1976) Abdominal angina. *Acta Chir. Scand.*, **142**, 319–325
52. Hollier, L. H., Bernatz, P. E. and Pairolero, P. C. (1981). Surgical management of chronic visceral ischaemia: A reappraisal. *Surgery*, **90**, 940–946
53. Marston, A. (1989) Chronic intestinal ischaemia. In *Splanchnic Ischaemia and Multiple Organ Failure* (eds A. Marston, G. B. Bulkley, R. G. Fiddian Green and Ulf Haglund) pp. 323–336
54. Strandness, D. E. Jr. (1986) Ultrasound in the study of atherosclerosis. *Ultrasound Med. Biol.*, **12** (6), 453–464
55. Moneta, G. L. (1990) Diagnosis of chronic intestinal ischaemia. *Sem. Vasc. Surg.*, **3**, 176–185
56. Lilly, M. P., Harward, T. R., Flinn, W. R., Blackburn, D. R., Astleford, P. M. and Yao, J. S. (1989) Duplex ultrasound measurement of changes in mesenteric flow velocity with pharmacologic and physiologic alteration of intestinal blood flow in man. *J. Vasc. Surg.*, **9** (1), 18–25
57. Nicholls, S. C., Kohler, T. R. and Martin, R. L. (1986). Use of haemodynamic parameters in the diagnosis of mesenteric insufficiency. *J. Vasc. Surg.*, **3**, 507–510
58. Furrer, J., Gruntzig, A., Kugelmeier, J. and Goebel, N. (1980) Treatment of abdominal angina with percutaneous dilatation of an arteria mesenterica superior stenosis. Preliminary communication. *Cardiovasc. Intervent. Radiol.* **3** (1), 43–44
59. Golden, D. A., Ring, E. J., McLean, G. K. and Freiman, D. B. (1982) Percutaneous transluminal angioplasty in the treatment of abdominal angina. *Am. J. Roentgenol.*, **139** (2), 247–249
60. Roberts, L. Jr., Wertman, D. A. Jr., Mills, S. R., Moore, A. V. Jr. and Heaston, D. K. (1983) Transluminal angioplasty of the superior mesenteric artery: an alternative to surgical revascularization. *Am. J. Roentgenol.*, **141** (5), 1039–1042
61. Cicuto, K. P., McLean, G. K and Oleaga, J. A. (1981) Renal artery stenosis – anatomic classification for percutaneous transluminal angioplasty. *Am. J. Roentgenol.*, **137**, 599–601
62. Johnson, W. C. and Nasbeth, D. C. (1974) Visceral infarction following aortic surgery. *Ann Surg*, **180**, 312
63. Connolly, J. E. and Kwaan, J. H. (1982) Management of chronic visceral ischemia. *Surg. Clin. North Am.*, **62** (3), 345–356
64. Jaxheimer, E. C., Jewell, E. R. and Persson, A. V. (1985) Chronic intestinal ischemia. The Lahey Clinic approach to management. *Surg. Clin. North Am.*, **65** (1), 123–130
65. Stoney, R. J., Ehrenfeld, W. K. and Wylie, E. J. (1977) Revascularisation methods in chronic visceral ischaemia. *Ann. Surg.*, **121**, 736
66. Jaffe, M. S. (1971) Status of abdominal visceral circulation via superior mesenteric prosthesis. *Am. J. Surg.*, **121**, 736
67. Shaw, R. S. and Maynard, E. P. (1958) Acute and chronic thrombosis of the mesenteric arteries associated with malabsorption: A report of two cases successfully treated by thromboendarterectomy. *New Eng. J. Med.*, **258**, 874–878
68. Beebe, H. G., MacFarlane, S. and Raker, E. J. (1987) Supraceliac aortomesenteric bypass for intestinal ischemia. *J. Vasc. Surg.*, **5** (5), 749–754
69. Hollier, L. H. (1982) Revascularization of the visceral artery using the pantaloon vein graft. *Surg. Gynecol. Obstet.*, **155** (3), 415–416

70. Kieny, R., Batellier, J. and Kretz, J. G. (1990) Aortic reimplantation of the superior mesenteric artery for atherosclerotic lesions of the visceral arteries: sixty cases. *Ann. Vasc. Surg.*, **4** (2), 122–125

71. Baur, G. M., Millay, D. J., Taylor, L. M. Jr. and Porter, J. M. (1984) Treatment of chronic visceral ischemia. *Am. J. Surg.*, **148** (1), 138–144

72. Crawford, E. S., Morris, G. C. Jr., Myhre, H. O. and Roehm, J. O. Jr. (1977) Celiac axis, superior mesenteric artery, and inferior mesenteric artery occlusion: surgical considerations. *Surgery*, **82** (6), 856–866

73. Adashek, K. and Wittenstein, G. (1979) Mesenteric revascularization: an operative approach. *Am. J. Surg.*, **137** (6), 821–823

74. Bergan, J. J. and Yao, J. S. T. (1989) Chronic intestinal ischaemia. In *Vascular Surgery* vol. 11 (ed. R. B. Rutherford) W. B. Saunders, pp. 1097–1103

75. Taylor, L. M. and Porter, J. M. (1990) Treatment of chronic intestinal ischaemia. *Sem. Vasc. Surg.*, **3**, 186–199

76. Kwaan, J. H., Connolly, J. E. and Coutsoftides, T. (1980) Concomitant revascularization of intestines during aortoiliac reconstruction: deterrent to catastrophic bowel infarction. *Can. J. Surg.*, **23** (6), 534–536

77. Rogers, D. M., Thompson, J. E., Garrett, W. V., Talkington, C. M. and Patman, R. D. (1982) Mesenteric vascular problems. A 26-year experience. *Ann. Surg.*, **195** (5), 554–565

78. Pokrowsky, A. V., Kasantchjan, P. O. and Spiridonov, A. A. (1980) A new method of one-stage revascularization of the visceral arteries. Experience with 25 operations. *J. Cardiovasc. Surg. (Torino)*, **21** (6), 659–664

79. Reul, G. J. Jr., Wukash, D. C., Sandiford, F. M., Chiarillo, L., Hallman, G. L. and Cooley, D. A. (1974) Surgical treatment of abdominal angina: review of 25 patients. *Surgery*, **75** (5), 682–689

80. Stanton, P. E., Jr., Hollier, P. A., Seidel, T. W., Rosenthal, D., Clark, M. and Lamis, P. A. (1986) Chronic intestinal ischemia: diagnosis and therapy. *J. Vasc. Surg.*, **4** (4), 338–344

81. van Lanschot, J. J. and van Urk, H. (1984) Vascular reconstruction in intestinal angina. *Netherland J. Surg.*, **36** (6), 151–155

82. Povrovsky, A. V. and Kasantchjan, P. O. (1980) Surgical treatment of chronic occlusive disease of the enteric visceral branches of the abdominal aorta. Experience with 119 operations. *Ann. Surg.*, **191** (1), 51–56

83. Hertzer, N. R., Beven, E. G. and Humphries, A. W. (1977) Chronic intestinal ischemia. *Surg. Gynecol. Obstet.*, **145** (3), 321–328

84. McCollum, C. H., Graham, J. M. and DeBakey, M. E. (1976) Chronic mesenteric arterial insufficiency: results of revascularization in 33 cases. *South. Med. J.*, **69** (10), 1266–1268

Chapter 9

Renal artery disease – when should it be treated surgically?

John A. Murie

Surgical reconstruction of a renal artery is performed infrequently in most centres in the UK, the total number of such operations annually is currently unlikely to exceed a few hundred. Despite their small number, the operations are of great interest because the indications for this type of surgery are often controversial and almost always worthy of debate. The reason for this lies in the 'difficult' nature of the criteria to be met if renal artery disease is to be appropriately dealt with by operation:

1. The disease causes a physiological problem which operation is likely to benefit.
2. Other non-invasive or less invasive techniques are unlikely to achieve comparable results.

Why these criteria are 'difficult' provides the reason for this chapter. They have been contrived not only to get away from the usual worthy classification of renal artery disease and its treatment, but also to allow the current questions which surround the management of renal artery disease to be highlighted. Each criterion will be approached in turn and only those pathologies, investigations and treatments which are topics of current debate will be discussed at length. As disease affecting the artery of a renal allograft provides a not uncommon reason for renovascular surgery, this type of lesion is described concurrently with those of the native vessel when appropriate.

What are the diseases and physiological problems which operation may benefit?

Diseases

Renal artery disease may be broadly classified into two types, stenosing and dilating. The pathologies causing stenosis and eventually occlusion in the native renal artery are mainly atheroma (78%), fibromuscular dysplasia (17%) and trauma (5%)[1,2]. The true incidence of renal artery stenosis (RAS) is unknown and is, in any event, dependent on definition. The principal lesion affecting transplant arteries is less well characterized; atheroma plays a part but fibrosis, perhaps due to the general allograft immune reaction, also occurs and tends to affect the vessel about 1 cm distal to the anastomosis as shown in Figure 9.1[3]. Significant transplant RAS affects at least 1.3% of patients with renal allografts[4].

The dilating disease responsible for renal artery aneurysm (RAA) is ill-understood.

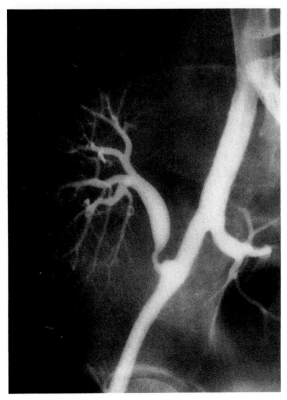

Figure 9.1   Angiogram showing transplant renal artery stenosis. Note the lesion lies about 1 cm distal to the end-to-side anastomosis between the renal artery and the recipient external iliac artery

Macroaneurysm is often associated with atheroma but may be a secondary rather than a primary feature. Microaneurysm and dissection are quite different entities and are not considered here. In a population undergoing aortography, and therefore highly selected, the incidence of RAA has been shown to be about 0.1%. Two-thirds of those affected have solitary lesions; over 90% of RAAs are saccular in nature[5].

Physiological problems

Hypertension
A low blood pressure distal to an RAS (and sometimes distal to an RAA or combination of RAA with RAS) causes increased renin secretion from the juxtaglomerular cells. Renin is a protease which interacts with angiotensinogen to produce angiotensin I. Through the action of a converting enzyme this becomes the octapeptide angiotensin II, a potent vasopressor, making *part* of the chain from RAS to hypertension complete[6]. In truth, however, the relationship of hypoperfusion to hypertension is far more complex than suggested by the original experiment of Goldblatt *et al.*[7] and involves impaired renal production of systemic vasodilators such as prostaglandins, kinins and renomedullary lipids[8].

Nevertheless, it is not the incomplete understanding of the mechanism that causes clinical difficulty; the problem is twofold. First, 'essential' hypertension affects at least 20% of the adult population[8] in Western societies and frequently coexists with RAS. Treatment for RAS may not, therefore, uniformly relieve hypertension. Secondly, even if RAS *is* the primary cause, hypertension may persist after its resolution if the opposite kidney has been sufficiently damaged in the meantime by blood pressure elevation, or if irreversible structural changes in resistance vessels have occurred.

The diagnosis of renovascular hypertension (RH), as opposed to renovascular disease, is difficult to establish as it is *retrospective* in character, i.e. RH is hypertension which is cured by treating renovascular disease. This clinical dilemma is not insignificant as the prevalence of RH in the general hypertensive population is said to be about 1%[9,10], but estimates of up to 5%[11] have been made. The most recent literature review accepts 3% as a reasonable current figure[12].

Renal failure
This problem generally results from the progression of atherosclerosis. Severe atheromatous narrowing of the renal arteries is a bilateral phenomenon in over one-third of patients with RH[11] and RAS may be responsible for the elevation of blood pressure in almost half of those with renal insufficiency in addition to refractory hypertension[13]. The risk of an arteriosclerotic RAS progressing to occlusion is quite high compared with that caused by fibromuscular dysplasia. Several authors have reported that 10–17% of atherosclerotic stenoses occlude within 2–3 years of diagnosis[14–16]. It has also been reported that about 40% of patients with unilateral stenoses develop contralateral stenosis within 52 months[16].

It is not yet possible to predict early which individuals will exhibit such progressive disease[4] but some general remarks can be made from studies comparing patients who have occluded their stenoses during preoperative assessment or during conservative treatment of RAS[17] with those who have not. Patients who occlude tend to be older (median age 64 compared with 55 years); they have narrower stenoses (1.0 mm versus 1.5 mm); they have more contralateral renal artery disease (50% versus 9%), and more ischaemic heart disease (90% against 70%)[18]. These patients represent a high-risk group for surgery.

It is interesting that the diagnosis of renal artery occlusion is not always easy if the opposite kidney is functioning adequately. This is especially so in the chronic case in which RAS progresses gradually to occlusion. Such patients usually have only vague symptoms at the time of occlusion, which are easy to overlook[19]; only about 20% have any flank pain and this is not usually severe. The most useful feature for the clinician is the slight but significant rise in creatinine level, which is seen in over 90% of patients, indicating coexisting impairment of the opposite kidney[17,18].

Haemorrhage
The true incidence of RAA (Figure 9.2) is unknown and so the risk of aneurysm rupture is uncertain. Nevertheless, it is possible to say that among a population recognized as having RAA – by abdominal radiograph, intravenous urogram or angiogram – the risk of an external rupture is about 3%. The magnitude of risk of a covert rupture into the adjacent renal vein is similar[5]. Over 80% of aneurysms are asymptomatic; some produce flank discomfort.

While the physiological problem may not appear great, it should be remembered that RAA may occur at almost any age, even in childhood. Although rupture rarely results in death (loss of the kidney being the usual outcome) pregnant women who harbour an RAA are especially vulnerable – the mortality rate on rupture is 56% for the mother and 82% for the fetus[20]. The transplant renal artery is not immune from the problem which, again, is a specific hazard in pregnancy[21].

Surgery: benefits (and problems)

It should be appreciated that all the pathophysiologies (and diseases) so far described may coexist sometimes within a single kidney.

The aim here is to describe the potential benefit which may be derived from *operation*; competing forms of management for renovascular disease are discussed later. There is no doubt that the renal artery affected by stenosis or aneurysm can generally be reconstructed or bypassed; this is also true to a lesser degree for occlusion. The nature of the surgery is well described in technical manuals[22] and there is little controversy about operative details. A variety of procedures exist which can be tailored to individual circumstances. These include:

Commonly used
- Aortorenal bypass[4,23]
- Renal endarterectomy[24]
- Renal artery implantation

Less common
- Autotransplantation which allows easy access for the extracorporeal repair of renal artery branch lesions[25–27]

Relatively unusual
- Renal revascularization using arterial autografts[28] or a variety of visceral vessels, such as the hepatic[29], splenic[30,31], gastroduodenal[31] or mesenteric arteries[33].

While simultaneous aortic and renal artery reconstruction is recognized as carrying a higher morbidity and mortality rate than renal artery surgery alone (20% versus 4.6% in one recent series)[34] it may nevertheless be worthwhile in carefully selected patients[35].

Recognition of renal artery disease
Before any form of operation can be contemplated the disease must first be recognized. The question of how best to recognize RAS has been around for many years, the answer changing subtly as medical technology advances. *Radioisotope studies* were suggested in the 1950s and a recent review of nine angiographically controlled trials of isotope renography, involving 934 patients with RAS and 951 without, has suggested an overall sensitivity of 74% and a specificity of 77%[36].

Intravenous urography has been around even longer than radioisotope studies. Recent reports on its efficacy are conflicting. Some describe a sensitivity of less than 60%[37], while others report a value of nearly 80%[38]. All the angiographically controlled trials of urography taken together contain 2040 patients with proven RAS and 2133 with normal angiograms and essential hypertension – intravenous urography achieved a sensitivity of 75% and a specificity of 86%[36].

Despite recent enthusiastic reports of screening tests such as the *captopril-enhanced diethylenetriamine penta-acetic acid scan*, the reported sensitivity of 78% and specificity of 52% are unimpressive[39]. Nevertheless, it has been claimed that this test not only identifies RAS but also may predict the outcome of surgery for putative renovascular hypertension[40].

Duplex ultrasonography has been very successful in many areas of vascular assessment and in experienced hands it is said to have an accuracy of 93% in differentiating RAS of less than 60% from that of 60–99% and from occlusion[41]. It is easily repeatable and so it is ideal for serial or follow-up studies[42]. While few centres have as yet the necessary experience to use the technique with confidence for assessing the renal vessels, duplex ultrasonography is likely to become a widespread and useful tool in the future.

One of the newest methods of assessing renovascular disease which has already been integrated into most surgeons' current practice is *digital subtraction angiography* (DSA); this has rendered the isotope renogram and the intravenous urogram obsolete in many centres[43–45]. DSA has considerable attractions, especially if the contrast agent is injected intravenously (IVDSA), either via a central catheter in the superior vena cava[46] or via a peripheral vein[47]. Compared with conventional angiography, IVDSA involves the patient in less risk and less discomfort; it also requires less time, is cheaper and can be performed on an outpatient basis. Nevertheless, IVDSA has some inherent problems, especially when compared with conventional angiography. It requires more patient co-operation to exclude motion artefacts, and even bowel gas moving in the gut may prevent adequate imaging of the renal arteries[48]. It also has a decreased spatial resolution which limits its ability to identify lesions in the branches of the main renal artery and in the distal aspect of the main artery itself. Unlike selective arterial injection studies IVDSA may show mesenteric vessels overlapping the renal arteries, making interpretation difficult without the use of additional injections of contrast medium, which prolongs the procedure and increases the risk of contrast agent-induced renal dysfunction. Perhaps the main disadvantage of IVDSA, however, is that it regularly produces a proportion of non diagnostic images, especially in patients suffering from obesity or reduced renal or cardiac function[36]. A review of 13 papers on the accuracy of IVDSA compared with conventional angiograms, which analysed the outcome for 406 hypertensives who underwent both investigations, demonstrated that the sensitivity of IVDSA ranges from 75%[49] to 100%[50] and the specificity from 76%[47] to 100%[51]. These data can be used to calculate an overall sensitivity and specificity of 88% and 90% respectively. One word of caution: a literature review of the results of 965 renal IVDAs has shown 7.4% to be uninterpretable, which suggests that the above calculations are likely to overestimate the actual performance of IVDSA[36].

IVDSA as a screening test outshines the older isotope studies and intravenous urography, but it is not perfect and some authors advocate conventional angiography. An important retrospective analysis of patients with renovascular disease undergoing conventional renal angiography and other studies has suggested that intravenous urography and isotope renography are so inaccurate that many affected patients are missed, that conventional angiography is relatively safe, that it allows simultaneous angioplasty and that, if there are no contraindications to the test, conventional angiography is the only investigation that should be done to demonstrate RAS[52].

A test which allows not only diagnosis but also intervention by balloon angioplasty, or at least provides a definitive image for the surgeon, is very appealing. It is worthy of note, however, that digital subtraction technology can be used to advantage in conventional intra-arterial studies. Intra-arterial DSA (IADSA) allows smaller diameter catheters and smaller, less concentrated, volumes of contrast agent to be used. IADSA should be regarded as a safer form of conventional angiography rather than a new technique in its own right; it is quietly making the standard conventional method obsolete.

It is widely recognized that the suspicion of renal artery aneurysm is appropriately confirmed by angiography (Figure 9.2); computer tomography or duplex ultrasonography may yield further useful information, but are second-line investigations. Now, too, one may say that the suspicion of stenosis is appropriately confirmed by proceeding directly to angiography and that IADSA is particularly attractive in many respects. Transplant renal artery disease, generally stenosis, is likewise best confirmed or refuted by IADSA.

Functional tests
These are required for patients with RAS and hypertension because of the inevitable doubt as to whether or not the RAS is causal. Several types of test are in current use:

- those which rely on angtiotensin-converting enzyme inhibition
- those which rely on parenchymal transit time.

The measurement of supine[53] or stimulated[54] plasma renin levels has not proved useful as a functional test of RH because peripheral plasma renin levels are influenced by factors other than the renal ischaemia[54]. Of all the proposed renin-based tests to date only *divided renal vein renin studies* have been used extensively as a predictor of the outcome of intervention for putative RH. This rather invasive test, requiring catheterization of the vena cava and renal veins, has been available for

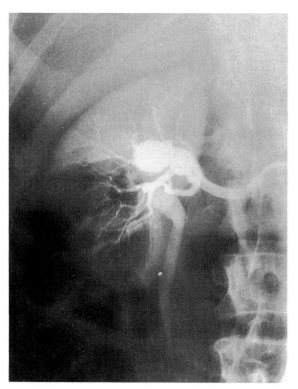

Figure 9.2 Angiogram showing a renal artery aneurysm. This type of lesion is best diagnosed using angiography

many years, although the results obtained are not universally considered worthwhile[55–57]. A ratio of renin activity of more than 1.5 between a stenosed and a non-stenosed side has been said to indicate a functional stenosis, but such a ratio occurs in less than one half of the patients affected by RAS and in no less than a quarter of those with normal angiograms[52]; also in some series patients with a negative ratio have done just as well after intervention as those with a positive ratio[52], and improvement or cure may be expected in over half of patients with non-lateralizing ratios[58]. It has been suggested that the ratio might be useful in lateralizing the functional disorder in bilateral RAS, but inconclusive ratios occur in over one-third of patients[59]. In the author's experience renal vein renin assays can only be relied on if a high output of renin from the side of a unilateral stenosis is associated with complete suppression of renin secretion from the contralateral side. Their poor predictive ability should remind us that factors other than the renin–angiotensin system cause or contribute to the hypertension of RAS[59,60].

Deterioration in renal function related to antihypertensive drug therapy is now well recognized in patients with RAS; the *angiotensin-converting enzyme inhibitors* captopril and enalapril have, in particular, been shown to cause reversible renal failure in patients with bilateral RAS, with RAS in a solitary kidney[61] or in a transplanted organ[62]. The effect may occur because angiotensin II mediates efferent arteriolar tone, maintaining the glomerular filtration rate at low perfusion pressures[63]. The long-term response to captopril may be a useful predictor of response to surgery[64] but prolonged exposure to captopril is likely to impair renal function permanently[65]. Captopril renal scintigraphy is more practical[66,67]. This uses $^{99}Tc^m$-diethylenetriamine-penta-acetic acid (DTPA) scintigraphy before and after the injection of captopril. An increase in time to maximum activity in the affected kidney combined with a reduction in glomerular filtration rate is suggestive of RH due to RAS on that side. Initial results are promising but test numbers so far are small[40].

Some workers contend that the use of the isotope renogram may make a comeback, not as a screening test for RAS but as a predictor of outcome of intervention for hypertension. The proposed discriminator is the '*parenchymal transit time*' and while such quantitative renography may hold some hope for the future, so far the number of patients reported to have been investigated by this method is small[68].

Summary

1. Operations which are technically successful are available to reconstruct or bypass diseased renal arteries.
2. Surgery would appear a reasonable choice for RAA and renal failure due to renal artery disease.
3. A major problem in diagnosing renovascular *hypertension* as opposed to renovascular *disease* exists which makes surgery for hypertension alone less attractive.

What other non-invasive or less invasive techniques are available and do they achieve results comparable with those of surgery?

To assess the place of other techniques in renovascular disease we must first know the results obtained by operation. This section is devoted to the results of surgery for RH, renal failure and RAA, and compares these results with those which might be achieved using other forms of management.

Hypertension

Renovascular reconstruction improves blood pressure in 59–95% of patients, depending on a variety of circumstances[4,69–72]. In general, improvement in blood pressure is less likely when aortoiliac reconstruction is required in addition to renal artery surgery (59–67%) than when operation is carried out for isolated RAS (79%)[70,73]. It has also been suggested that a less favourable result is likely when the underlying pathology is atheroma than when fibromuscular dysplasia is present; a recent series from Oxford bears this out, showing 77% with atheroma 'cured' or 'improved' compared with 100% for fibromuscular dysplasia[72] (Figure 9.3). The outlook after surgery also depends on pathology, with 5-year survival after correction of atheromatous lesions of 79% rising to 95% for fibromuscular dysplasia[71]. No mention has yet been made of nephrectomy; this still has a place if the kidney distal to a functional RAS is significantly damaged and the opposite organ is normal (Figure 9.4).

Two techniques compete with surgery in the treatment of RH: drug therapy and percutaneous transluminal angioplasty (PTA). There is no place in a surgically oriented book for an extended treatise on medical management, but it should be appreciated that new, potent antihypertensive agents now offer strong competition to renovascular operation[8,18]. Today renovascular surgery must be likely to be effective and must carry a very small risk if it is to be an acceptable alternative to drugs for a patient whose problem is solely RH. The problem of the patient with RH *and* incipient or actual renal failure is different and will be dealt with later. RAS affecting a transplanted kidney closely resembles the 'incipient renal failure' situation and this will also be considered later.

Whether PTA is a good option for treating *hypertension alone* depends on a variety

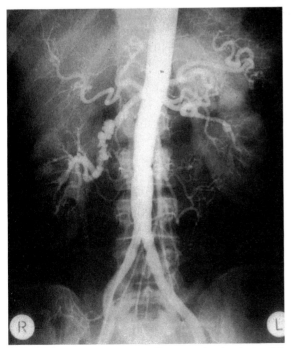

Figure 9.3 Angiogram showing fibromuscular dysplasia of the renal artery. This type of lesion carries a better prognosis after treatment (by PTA or by operation) than the more common atherosclerotic type

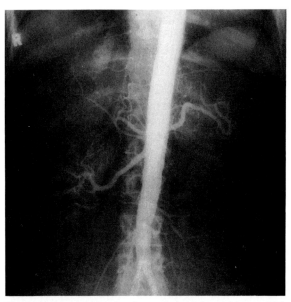

Figure 9.4   Angiogram showing occluded left renal artery. This type of lesion does not respond well to PTA and while in certain circumstances operative revascularization may be appropriate, in this instance hypertension was cured by nephrectomy

of circumstances. It is not risk free; in fact it carries a mortality rate of about 1%, with major complications occurring in 5–10% of patients treated[75–79]. Just as after operation, complications after PTA are more frequent in the elderly with atheroma than in the younger population with fibromuscular dysplasia; if the kidney opposite to that affected by RAS is normal the worry of nephron loss and renal failure due to PTA-induced renal artery thrombosis is reduced. Meta-analysis has suggested that with a 1–5-year follow-up PTA cured or improved 87% of all patients with fibromuscular dysplasia and 92% of those who had a technically successful dilatation – the analagous figures for atherosclerosis were 62% and 75%[80]. Despite previous exhortations by radiologists suggesting that PTA should be recommended for all renal artery lesions with surgery reserved for PTA failure[78], the evidence for such a stance is poor. The most recent and most sophisticated overview of published data describes a total of 670 patients from ten separate publications[81]. PTA was technically successful in 611 (88%). The overall cure rate for hypertension was 24% with a further 43% 'improved'. Those with fibromuscular dysplasia benefited more than those with atherosclerosis and the authors concluded that, while PTA for RH due to fibromuscular dysplasia was worthwhile, the benefit for those with atheroma-tous lesions was 'small'. Fortunately PTA failure does not appear to compromise future surgical correction of the renal artery problem[82].

In summary, for hypertension alone drugs usually offer a safe means of control. Percutaneous transluminal angioplasty and surgery have not yet been adequately compared in clinical trials, but the elderly atheromatous patient is disadvantaged in either case. Certain features make PTA difficult and may tilt the balance in favour of operation if active intervention is deemed necessary. PTA fails most often in patients with ostial stenosis, occlusion, or long atheromatous strictures[80] (Figure 9.5).

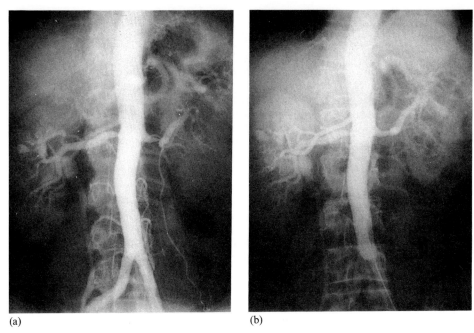

(a)   (b)

Figure 9.5(a)   Angiogram showing ostial stenosis of the right renal artery and non-ostial stenosis of the left renal artery; (b) PTA has been successfully carried out on the left renal lesion. The lesion on the right is much less suitable for PTA; operation is preferred.

Renal failure

Renal failure usually occurs when the second kidney is affected by disease after its partner has been severely compromised or lost, or when a solitary kidney – an allograft is a good example – is affected by disease. When the disease reduces renal blood flow to the extent that exocrine kidney function is affected, medical management is no longer the best option either for hypertension control or for azotaemia, if PTA or operative reconstruction of the arterial supply is feasible. It should not be forgotten that atheroma especially is a progressive disease and that RH regularly precedes renal failure. It is difficult to predict which individuals will be affected but the older the patient, the narrower the stenosis and the more advanced the general atherosclerosis, the more likely that renal failure will supervene during medical management[18]. The angiotensin-converting enzyme inhibitors captopril and enalapril are particularly well known for their propensity to reduce exocrine function in the presence of RAS, but any antihypertensive agent may do this to a degree. Generally, the process is reversible if the drug is *quickly* withdrawn.

The risk of an atheromatous RAS progressing to occlusion is high compared with that for RAS due to fibromuscular dysplasia; this has already been discussed. Frequent serial creatinine estimations are required to detect exocrine failure, and serial ultrasonography is needed to detect loss of renal size in patients who are medically treated for RH. The hypertensive transplant recipient needs particularly careful assessment. In the case of an allograft, gradual stenosis of the renal artery does not result in an increase in capsular and other collateral blood supply. Should the transplant renal artery occlude, a collateral blood flow cannot allow the kidney to survive until elective operation can be performed. It is clear that in certain circumstances great vigilance is essential if the medical treatment of RH is not to lead to irreversible renal failure.

What may we expect of surgery in treating renal failure due to RAS? First, it is technically easier and the results are better when a stenotic but patent, rather than an occluded, renal artery is reconstructed[83], and groups who might be considered for 'prophylactic' surgery have already been mentioned. Secondly, when the aorta is operated on at the same time as the renal artery, the procedure not only carries a combined major morbidity and mortality rare of up to 20%[34], but also only a minority of cases benefit significantly in terms of renal function[73].

Fewer published data exist on the effect of operation on exocrine function than on hypertension. Dean et al.[84] have described a series of 64 patients with a preoperative serum creatinine of over 300 µmol/l who had surgical renal artery reconstruction of whom 58 had atherosclerosis and six had fibromuscular dysplasia. Significant improvement in renal function was noted in only 25 patients, although others were helped to a minor extent. The best predictors of outcome were the state of the vessel beyond the stenosis or occlusion, bilaterality of reconstructable disease, the amount of residual renal mass available for revascularization and the degree of hyperconcentration of non-reabsorbable solutes from the involved kidney. Others have suggested better results from smaller series[13,85], but patients undergoing reconstruction primarily for renal failure often have end-stage atherosclerosis, making long-term benefit unlikely. Even when operation is successful in maintaining long-term blood pressure control, the results in terms of exocrine function are less good[2].

The variation in reported results may well reflect a variation in patient mix as most series are heterogeneous, containing cases of chronic RAS, some of occlusion after RAS and even acute embolic occlusion in an essentially normal renal artery. While the last category is particularly difficult to help, requiring intervention within 24 h at most[59], those with occlusion after chronic stenosis may be helped even after many weeks of occlusion; a long interval between occlusion and revascularization probably decreases the chance of success, but this interval is often unknown. Preoperative renal biopsy does not seem to be worthwhile[18]. It is worth remembering that PTA for RAS causes acute occlusion of the renal artery in about 5% of cases and that urgent surgery in this situation is often successful[86]. Many candidates with occlusion seem unattractive surgical prospects and although success cannot be predicted the results are sometimes remarkable; this is important in a group whose age and disease makes chronic dialysis unattractive and transplantation improbable.

PTA remains a possible method of relieving incipient or actual renovascular renal failure although opinion of its worth in this context is widely divided. Undoubtedly, satisfactory results have been achieved for patients with fibromuscular dysplasia[87], but for those with atherosclerosis the outcome is less good, especially if the renal artery ostium is involved (Figure 9.4)[88]. This last feature not only makes technical success less likely, but even if an apparent satisfactory dilatation is achieved ostial stenosis tends to recur fairly quickly. Even if RH is helped renal failure generally responds poorly to PTA[89]. The problem of renal complications resulting from PTA is greater in patients with pre-existing renal failure than in those with RH alone, because the RAS tends to be more severe and more difficult to instrument in the former group and the injection of potentially nephrotoxic contrast agent is of greater consequence in the kidney whose exocrine function is already compromised.

In summary, for incipient or actual renovascular renal failure the choice of treatment lies between surgery and PTA. No prospective randomized studies comparing these modalities yet exist; indeed it is doubtful if randomization is appropriate. PTA is effective for fibromuscular dysplasia but not so effective for atheroma. Unfortunately, the elderly atheromatous patients are those at greatest risk from aortorenal operation. If the stenosis is non-ostial and short (an example is shown in Figure 9.5) PTA is probably indicated as the initial treatment. If the morphology of the RAS is more complex surgery is preferable; operation is also indicated after PTA failure and for occlusion. It may be that thrombolysis and the newer atherectomy devices will enhance the prospects of percutaneous treatment of such problems in the future.

Renal artery aneurysm (RAA)

The question here is when to operate. The principal technique for managing RAA is conservative watchfulness. Precise, objective indications for elective intervention are lacking but it is generally accepted that symptomatic aneurysms and those associated with apparent RH merit surgical correction with a vascular graft. To these groups must be added pregnant women since they are at special risk of losing not only a kidney but also the fetus and, indeed, their own life. The final group requiring correction are those with aneurysms which appear on serial testing to be enlarging; this is best done by angiography. A diameter of greater than 2.0 cm has been suggested empirically as suitable for operation[90,91]. Anecdotal reports also exist of treatment of RAA by percutaneous transluminal embolization, which may be attractive in the surgically unfit if it can be achieved without excessive loss of nephrons.

Summary

1. The mainstay of treatment for RH is medical therapy.
2. For incipient or actual renal failure PTA is a good choice as first line treatment for fibrodysplastic lesions and for 'suitable' atheromatous lesions.
3. Surgery is indicated to salvage renal function if PTA is unsuitable or if it fails.
4. RAA during pregnancy is a serious threat to the kidney, and to the life of both fetus and mother; in this circumstance especially it merits operative correction.

Concluding remarks

There are many fascinating aspects to the nature, diagnosis and treatment of lesions affecting the renal artery. This chapter has touched, necessarily superficially, on a few of the main points of current interest. While these contemporary issues may be highlighted, definitive answers to many questions are impossible. Although some tentative conclusions have been made it must be said that the quality and quantity of available data in the renovascular field is not as good as in some other areas of vascular surgical endeavour. It is especially to be hoped that the long-term effects of both surgery and – particularly – PTA will be more fully evaluated in the future; it is encouraging that randomized prospective trials are now underway[18].

References

1. Stanley, J. C. and Whitehouse, W. M. (1984) Occlusive and aneurysmal disease of the renal circulation. *Disease-a-Month*, **30**, 1–62
2. Hands, L., Walton, J., Fletcher, E. W., Murie, J. A. and Morris, P. J. (1991) Results of surgical intervention for renal artery disease. *Br. J. Surg.* (in press)
3. Belzer, F. O., Glass, N. and Sollinger, H. (1988) Technical complications after renal transplantation. In *Kidney Transplantation: Principles and Practice* 3rd edition (ed. P. J. Morris) Grune and Stratton, London, pp. 511–532
4. Murie, J. A. and Morris, P. J. (1988) Surgical management of renal hypertension. In *Management of Renal Hypertension* (ed. G. R. D. Catto) MTP Press, Lancaster, pp. 79–111
5. Stanley, J. C., Rhodes, E. L., Gewertz, B. L., Chang, C. Y., Walter, J. F. and Fry, W. J. (1975) Renal artery aneurysms: significance of macroaneurysms exclusive of dissections and fibrodysplastic mural dilatations. *Arch. Surg.*, **110**, 1327–1333
6. Robertson, J. I. S., Morton, J. J., Tillman, D. M. and Lever, A. F. (1986) The pathophysiology of renovascular hypertension. *J. Hypertension*, **4** (suppl. 4), S95–S103
7. Goldblatt, H., Lynch, R. F., Hanzai, R. F. and Summerville, W. (1934) Studies on experimental hypertension, production of persistent elevation of systolic blood pressure by means of renal ischaemia. *J. Exp. Med.*, **59**, 347–379
8. Webster, J. (1988) Modern drug therapy. In *Management of Renal Hypertension* (ed. G. R. D. Catto). MTP Press, Lancaster, pp. 1–39
9. Wilhelmsen, L. and Berglund, G. (1977) Prevalence of primary and secondary hypertension. *Am. Heart J.*, **94**, 543–546
10. Danielson, M. and Dammstrom, B. G. (1981) The prevalence of secondary and curable hypertension. *Acta Med. Scand.*, **209**, 451–455
11. Foster, J. H., Dean, R. H., Pinkerton, J. A. and Rhamy, R. K. (1973) Ten years experience with the surgical management of renovascular hypertension. *Ann. Surg.*, **177**, 755–766
12. Thornbury, J. R., Stanley, J. C. and Fryback, D. G. (1984) Optimising work-up of adult hypertensive patients for renal artery stenosis. *Radiol. Clin. N. Am.*, **22**, 333–339
13. Ying, C. Y., Tifft, C. P., Gavras, H. and Chobanian, A. V. (1984) Renal revascularisation in the azotemic hypertensive patient resistant to therapy. *New Eng. J. Med.*, **311**, 1070–1075
14. Wollenweber, J., Sheps, S. G. and Davis, G. D. (1968) Clinical course of atherosclerotic renovascular disease. *Am. J. Cardiol.*, **21**, 60–71
15. Dean, R. H., Kieffer, R. W., Smith, B. M., Oates, J. A., Nadeau, J. H. *et al.* (1981) Renovascular hypertension. Anatomic and renal function changes during drug therapy. *Arch. Surg.*, **116**, 1408–1415
16. Schreiber, M. J., Pohl, M. A. and Novick, A. C. (1984) The natural history of atherosclerotic and fibrous renal artery disease. *Urol. Clin. N. Am.*, **11**, 383–392
17. Shabanah, F. H., Conolly, J. and Martin, D. C. (1970) Acute renal artery occlusion. *Surg. Gynecol. Obstet.*, **131**, 489–494
18. Bergentz, S. E., Bergqvist, D. and Weibull, H. (1989) Changing concepts in renovascular surgery. *Br. J. Surg.*, **76**, 429–430
19. Weibull, H., Bergqvist, D., Andersson, I., Choi, D. L., Johnsson, K. and Bergentz, S. E. (1990) Symptoms and signs of thrombotic occlusion of atherosclerotic renal artery stenosis. *Eur. J. Vasc. Surg.*, **4**, 159–165
20. Cohen, J. R. and Shamash, F. S. (1987) Ruptured renal artery aneurysms during pregnancy. *J. Vasc. Surg.*, **6**, 51–59
21. Richardson, A. J., Liddington, M., Jaskowski, A., Murie, J. A., Gillmer, M. and Morris, P. J. (1990) Pregnancy in a renal transplant recipient complicated by rupture of a transplant renal artery aneurysm *Br. J. Surg.*, **77**, 228–229
22. Jenkins, A. McL. (1991) Operations for renal ischaemia. In *Surgical Management of Vascular Disease* (eds P. Bell, C. Jamieson and C. V. Ruckley). Baillière Tindall, London, (in press)
23. Stanley, J. C., Whitehouse, W. M., Zelenock, G. B., Graham, L. M., Cronenwett, J. L. and Lindenauer, S. M. (1985) Reoperation for complications of renal artery reconstructive surgery undertaken for treatment of renovascular hypertension. *J. Surg.*, **2**, 133–144
24. Ricotta, J. J. and Williams, G. M. (1980) Endarterectomy of the upper abdominal aorta and visceral arteries through an extraperitoneal approach. *Ann. Surg.*, **192**, 633–638
25. Dubernard, J. M., Martin, X., Gelet, A., Mongin, D., Canton, F. and Tabib, A. (1985) Renal autotransplantation versus bypass techniques for renovascular hypertension. *Surgery*, **97**, 529–534
26. Jordan, M. L., Novick, A. C. and Cunningham, R. L. (1985) The role of renal autotransplantation in paediatric and young adult patients with renal artery disease. *J. Vasc. Surg.*, **2**, 385–392

27. Haddad, M., Barral, X., Boissier, C., Bouilloc, X. and Beraud, A. M. (1989) Extracorporeal repair of renal artery branch lesions. *Eur. J. Vasc. Surg.*, **3**, 435–441
28. Stoney, R. J. and Olofsson, P. A. (1988) Aortorenal arterial autografts: the last two decades. *Ann. Vasc. Surg.*, **2**, 169–173
29. Chilbaro, E. A., Libertino, J. A. and Novick, J. (1984) Use of hepatic circulation for revascularisation. *Ann. Surg.*, **199**, 406–411
30. Brewster, D. C. and Darling, R. C. (1979) Splenorenal arterial anastomosis for renovascular hypertension. *Ann. Surg.*, **189**, 353–358
31. Brendenberg, C. E., Aust, J. C., Reinitz, E. R. and Rosenbloom, M. (1989) Posterolateral exposure for renal artery reconstruction. *J. Vasc. Surg.*, **9**, 416–421
32. Libertino, J. A. and Lagneau, P. (1983) A new method of revascularisation of the right renal artery by the gastroduodenal artery. *Surg. Gynecol. Obstet.*, **156**, 221–223
33. Khauli, R. B., Novick, A. C., Coseriu, G. V., Benen, E. and Hertzer, N. R. (1985) The superior mesenterorenal bypass in patients with infrarenal aortic occlusion. *J. Urol.*, **133**, 188–190
34. van Bockel, J. H., van Schilfgaarde, R., Felthuis, W., Hermans, J. and Terpstra, J. L. (1988) Influence of preoperative risk factors and the surgical procedure on surgical mortality in renovascular hypertension. *Am. J. Surg.*, **155**, 770–775
35. Cooper, G. G., Atkinson, A. B. and Barros D'Sa, A. A. B. (1990) Simultaneous aortic and renal artery reconstruction. *Br. J. Surg.*, **77**, 194–198
36. Havey, R. J., Krumlovsky, F., delGreco, F. and Martin, H. G. (1985) Screening for renovascular hypertension: is renal digital subtraction angiography the preferred noninvasive test? *J. Am. Med. Ass.*, **254**, 388–393
37. Thornbury, J. R., Stanley, J. C. and Fryback, D. G. (1982) Hypertensive urogram: A nondiscriminatory test of renovascular hypertension. *Am. J. Radiol.*, **138**, 43–49
38. Grim, C. E. and Weinberger, M. H. (1983) Renal artery stenosis and hypertension. *Sem. Nephrol.*, **3**, 62–64
39. Evans, G., McClean, A., Young, J., Hilson, A., Sweny, P. and Hamilton, G. (1990) Renal artery stenosis: screening by captopril-enhanced diethylenetriamine penta-acetic acid scan. *Br. J. Surg.*, **77**, A350
40. Meier, G. H., Sumpio, B., Black, H. R. and Gusberg, R. J. (1990) Captopril renal scintigraphy: an advance in the detection and treatment of renovascular hypertension. *J. Vasc. Surg.*, **11**, 770–777
41. Taylor, D. C., Moneta, G. L. and Strandness, D. E. Jr. (1989) Follow-up of renal artery stenosis by duplex ultrasound. *J. Vasc. Surg.*, **9**, 410–415
42. Eidt, J. F., Fry, R. E., Clagett, G. P., Fisher, D. T. Jr., Alway, C. and Fry, W. J. (1988) Postoperative follow-up of renal artery reconstruction with duplex ultrasound. *J. Vasc. Surg.*, **8**, 667–673
43. DeSchepper, A., Parizel, P., Kersschot, E., Degryse, H., Vereycken, H. and van Herreweghe, W. (1983) Digital subtraction angiography in screening for renovascular hypertension: a comparative study of 100 patients. *J. Belg. Radiol.*, **66**, 271–279
44. Gowes, A. S., Pais, S. O. and Barbaric, Z. L. (1983) Digital subtraction angiography in the evaluation of hypertension. *Am. J. Radiol.*, **140**, 179–183
45. Hillman, B. J. (1983) Investigating the presence and significance of renovascular disease. In *Imaging and Hypertension* (ed. B. J. Hillman) W. B. Saunders Co., Philadelphia, pp. 28–48
46. Smith, C. W., Winfield, A. C. and Price, R. R. (1982) Evaluation of digital venous angiography for the diagnosis of renovascular hypertension. *Radiology*, **144**, 51–54
47. Buonocore, E., Meaney, T. F., Borkowsky, G. P., Pavlicek, W. and Gallacher, J. (1981) Digital subtraction angiography in the abdominal aorta and renal arteries. Comparison with conventional angiography. *Radiology*, **139**, 281–286
48. Tifft, C. P. (1983) Renal digit subtraction angiography – a nephrologist's view: A sensitive but imperfect screening procedure for renovascular hypertension. *Cardiovasc. Intervent. Radiol.*, **6**, 231–233
49. Dunnick, N. R., Ford, K. K. and Moore, A. V. (1983) Digital subtraction angiography in the evaluation of renovascular hypertension. *Radiology*, **149**, 51–59
50. Schorner, W., Kempter, H., Bauzer, D., Aviles, C., Weiss, T. and Felix, R. (1984) Venous digital subtraction angiography for diagnosis of renal artery stenosis in arterial hypertrophy: comparison with conventional angiography. *Radiology*, **24**, 171–176
51. Clark, R. A. and Alexander, E. S. (1983) Digital subtraction angiography of the renal arteries: prospective comparison with conventional arteriograms. *Invest. Radiol.*, **18**, 6–10
52. Carmichael, D. J., Mathias, C. J., Snell, M. E. and Peart, S. (1986) Detection and investigation of renal artery stenosis. *Lancet*, **i**, 667–670
53. Nielson, I., Nerstrom, B., Jacobsen, J. G. and Engell, H. C. (1971) The postural plasma renin response in renovascular hypertension. *Acta Med. Sand.*, **189**, 213–220

54. Streeten, D. H. P., Anderson, G. H., Sunderlin, F. S., Mallov, J. S. and Springer, J. (1981) Identifying renin participation in hypersensitive patients. In *Frontiers in Hypertension Research* (eds J. H. Laragh, F. R. Buhler and D. W. Seldin). Springer, New York, pp. 204–207

55. Sellars, L., Shore A., and Wilkinson, R. (1985) Renal vein renin studies in renovascular hypertension: do they really help? *J. Hypertension*, **3**, 177–181

56. Marks, L. S., Maxwell, M. H., Varady, P. D., Lupu, A. N. and Kaufman, J. J. (1976) Renovascular hypertension: does the renal vein renin ratio predict the operative result? *J. Urol.*, **115**, 365–368

57. Pickering, T. G., Sos, T. A., Vaughan, E. D., Case, D. B., Sealley, J. E. *et al.* (1984) Predictive value and changes of renin secretion in patients undergoing successful renal angioplasty. *Am. J. Med.*, **76**, 398–404

58. Marks, L. S. and Maxwell, M. H. (1975) Renal vein renin value and limitations in the prediction of operative results. *Urol. Clin. N. Am.*, **2**, 311–325

59. Ouriel, K., Andrus, C. H., Ricotta, J. J., de Weese, J. and Green, R. M. (1987) Acute renal artery occlusion: when is revascularisation justified? *J. Vasc. Surg.*, **5**, 348–355

60. Mathias, C. J., May, C. N. and Taylor, G. M. (1984) The renin–angiotensin system and hypertension: basic and clinical aspects. In *Molecular Medicine* (ed. A. D. Malcolm). Oxford: IRL Press, Oxford, pp. 178–208

61. Hricik, D. E., Browning, P. J., Kopelman, R., Goorno, W. E., Madias, N. E. and Dzau, V. J. (1983) Captopril-induced functional renal insufficiency in patients with bilateral renal artery stenoses or renal artery stenosis in a solitary kidney. *New Eng. J. Med.*, **308**, 373–376

62. Curtis, J. J., Luke, R. G., Whelchel, J. D., Deithelm, A. G., Jones, P. and Dunstan, H. P. (1983) Inhibition of angiotensin converting enzyme in renal transplant recipients with hypertension. *New Eng. J. Med.*, **308**, 377–381

63. Helmchen, U., Grone, H. J. and Kirchertz, E. J. (1982) Contrasting renal effects of different antihypertensive agents in hypertensive rats with bilaterally constricted arteries. *Kidney Int.*, **12** (suppl.), S198–S205

64. Atkinson, A. B., Brown, J. J., Cumming, A. M., Fraser, R., Lever, A. F. *et al.* (1982) Captopril in renovascular hypertension: long-term use in predicting outcome. *Br. Med. J.*, **284**, 689–693

65. Wenting, G. J., Tan-Tjions, H. L., Derkx, F. H., De Bruyn, J. H., Man in't Weld, A. J. and Schalekamp, M. A. (1983) Split renal function after captopril in unilateral renal artery stenosis. *Br. Med. J.*, **287**, 1413–1417

66. Sfakianakis, G. N., Bourgoignie, J. J., Jaffe, D., Kryiakides, G., Perez-Stable, E. and Duncan, R. C. (1987) Single dose captopril scintigraphy in the diagnosis of renovascular hypertension. *J. Nuc. Med.*, **28**, 1383–1392

67. Chen, C. C., Hoffer, P. B. and Vahjen, G. (1991) A simple method of Tc-99m DTPA captopril renal scintigraphy analysis in patients at risk from renal artery stenosis. *Radiology* (in press)

68. Gruenewald, S. M., Collins, C. T., Antico, V. F., Farlow, D. C. and Fawdry, R. M. (1989) Can quantitative renography predict the outcome of treatment of atherosclerotic renal artery stenosis? *Nucl. Med.*, **30**, 1946–1954

69. Roizen, M. F., Beaupre, P. N., Alpent, R. A., Kremer, P., Cahalan, M. K. *et al.* (1986) Monitoring with two-dimensional transesophageal echocardiography. Comparison of myocardial function in patients undergoing supraceliac, suprarenal-infraceliac, or infrarenal aortic occlusion. *J. Surg.*, **1**, 300–305

70. Mattila, T., Harjola, P. T., Ketonen, P., Vartela, E. and Hekali, P. (1985) Isolated renal artery and combined aortic and renal artery reconstruction for renovascular hypertension. *Ann. Clin. Res.*, **17**, 19–23

71. Morin, J. E., Hutchinson, T. A. and Lisbona, R. (1986) Long-term prognosis of surgical treatment of renovascular hypertension: a fifteen year experience. *J. Vasc. Surg.*, **3**, 545–549

72. van Bockel, J. H., van Schilfgaarde, R., van Brummelen, P. and Terpstra, J. L. (1989) Long-term results of renal artery reconstruction with autologous artery. *J. Vasc. Surg.*, **3**, 515–521

73. Piquet, P., Ocana, J., Verdon, E., Tournigand, P. and Mercier, C. (1988) Atherosclerotic lesions of the aorta and renal arteries: results of simultaneous surgical treatment. *Ann. Vasc. Surg.*, **2**, 319–325

74. Hands, L., Walton, J., Fletcher, E. W., Murie, J. A. and Morris, P. J. (1990) Results of surgical intervention for renal artery disease. *Brit. J. Surg.*, **77**, A351

75. Tegtmeyer, C. J., Kellum, C. D. and Ayers, C. (1984) Percutaneous transluminal angioplasty of the renal artery: results and long-term follow-up. *Radiology*, **153**, 77–84

76. Kuhlmann, U., Greminger, P., Gruntzig, A., Schneider, E., Pouliadis, G. *et al.* (1985) Long-term experience in percutaneous transluminal dilatation of renal artery stenosis. *Am. J. Med.*, **79**, 692–698

77. Millan, V. G., McCauley, J., Kopelman, R. I. and Madias, N. E. (1985) Percutaneous transluminal renal angioplasty in nonatherosclerotic renovascular hypertension: long-term results. *Hypertension*, **7**, 668–674

78. Miller, G. A., Ford, K. K., Braun, S. D., Newman, G. E., Moore, A. V. *et al.* (1985) Percutaneous transluminal angioplasty vs surgery for renovascular hypertension. *Am. J. Roentgenol.*, **144**, 447–450

79. Bell, G. M., Reid, J. and Buist, T. A. S. (1987) Percutaneous transluminal angioplasty improves blood pressure and renal function in renovascular hypertension. *Quart. J. Med.*, **241**, 393–403

80. Tillman, D. M. and Adams, F. G. (1988) Percutaneous transluminal angioplasty in the management of renovascular hypertension. In *Management of Renal Hypertension* (ed. G. R. D. Catto). MTP Press, Lancaster, pp. 113–157

81. Ramsay, L. E. and Waller, P. C. (1990) Blood pressure response to percutaneous transluminal angioplasty for renovascular hypertension: an overview of published series. *Br. Med. J.*, **300**, 569–572

82. McCann, R. L., Bollinger, R. R. and Newman, G. E. (1988) Surgical renal artery reconstruction after percutaneous transluminal angioplasty. *J. Vasc. Surg.*, **8**, 389–394

83. Torsello, G., Szabo, Z., Kutkuhn, B., Kniemeyer, H. and Sandmann, W. (1987) Ten years experience with reconstruction of the chronically totally occluded renal artery. *Eur. J. Vasc. Surg.*, **1**, 327–333

84. Dean, R. H., Englund, R., Dupont, W. D., Meacham, P. W., Plummer, W. D. *et al.* (1985) Retrieval of renal function by revascularisation: a study of preoperative outcome predictors. *Ann. Surg.*, **202**, 367–375

85. Sicard, G. A., Etheredge, E. E., Maeser, M. N. and Anderson, C. B. (1985) Improved renal function after renal artery revascularisation. *J. Cardiovasc. Surg.*, **26**, 157–161

86. Kazmers, A., Moneta, G. L., Harley, J. D., Goldman, M. L. and Clowes, A. W. (1989) Treatment of acute renal artery occlusion after percutaneous transluminal angioplasty. *J. Vasc. Surg.*, **9**, 487–492

87 Tegtmeyer, C. J., Elson, J., Glass, T. A., Ayers, C. R., Chevalier, R. L. *et al.* (1982) Percutaneous transluminal angioplasty: the treatment of choice for renovascular hypertension due to fibromuscular dysplasia. *Radiology*, **143**, 631–637

88. Dean, R. H., Callis, J. T., Smith, B. M. and Meacham, P. W. (1987) Failed percutaneous transluminal angioplasty: experience with lesions requiring operative intervention. *J. Vasc. Surg.*, **6**, 301–307

89. Kim, P. K., Spriggs, D. W., Rutecki, G. W., Reaven, R. E., Blend, D. and Whittier, F. C. (1989) Transluminal angioplasty in patients with bilateral renal artery stenosis or renal artery stenosis in a solitary functioning kidney. *Am. J. Roentgenol.*, **153**, 1305–1308

90. Hageman, J. H., Smith, R. F., Szilagyi, D. E. and Elliott, J. P. (1978) Aneurysm of the renal artery; problems and surgical management. *Surgery*, **84**, 563–572

91. Ernst, C. B. (1989) Renal artery reconstruction. In *Vascular Surgery*, 3rd edition (eds H. Haimovici, A. D. Callow, R. G. DePalma, C. B. Ernst and L. H. Hollier). Appleton and Lange, Norwalk, pp. 763–780

Chapter 10

Iliac artery occlusive disease – what is the role of surgery?

Simon D. Parvin

Introduction

The occluded iliac segment can be treated in a number of different ways but randomized studies to compare them are not yet available. Surgeons have based their practice on a large number of uncontrolled observations in different groups of patients.

Angioplasty is increasingly taking over from surgery in the management of many areas of occlusive vascular disease. This applies particularly to the iliac segment and its optimum role may well be in this area. *Aortoiliac endarterectomy* enjoyed popularity before the routine availability of prosthetic bypass materials and continues to be used by some surgeons. For most, however, it is now largely reserved for the carotid bifurcation and even then its exact role remains uncertain. An *aortic bifurcation graft* provides the most comprehensive surgical approach to the occluded iliac segment, particularly if the disease is bilateral, but may not be suitable for all patients. The very elderly and those with significant cardiac or respiratory disease are usually excluded. This rule does not appear to apply so rigidly to those with aneurysmal disease presumably because of the potentially serious consequences of conservative treatment. With improving intraoperative monitoring and postoperative care it may be that a larger proportion of patients with bilateral iliac occlusion could be managed in this way.

In the patient with unilateral iliac occlusion the surgical options include unilateral iliofemoral, femorofemoral or axillofemoral bypass but there is no consensus about the best approach. There are no studies which directly compare these three methods in a randomized manner.

The questions

A number of questions arise about the management of an iliac occlusion:

1. Should any case of iliac occlusion ever be treated surgically?
2. Does aortoiliac endarterectomy have any role today?
3. Should an aortic bifurcation graft be used in more patients?
4. Which of the surgical options is best in unilateral iliac occlusion?

Should any case of iliac occlusion ever be treated surgically?

Although the first attempts at arterial dilatation were made by Dotter and Judkins in 1964[1], it was not until the introduction of balloon catheters fifteen years ago by Gruntzig and Hopff[2] that the technique became widely available. It is claimed to reduce the need for surgery and to have a lower morbidity, mortality and cost[3].

Angioplasty has been used in almost every vessel. Its use is not confined to arterial disease, being successfully used in venous stenosis, haemodialysis fistula stenosis[4] and in failing vein grafts[5].

In a review article Cole et al.[6] reported the results of iliac angioplasty in 159 cases. Successful angioplasty resulted in a significant rise in the ankle brachial pressure index (ABPI) in both those cases with a patent superficial femoral artery and in those in whom it is occluded. Cumulative patency at three years was 72% (22 cases at risk). Where the indication for surgery was claudication, results were a little better (74%) than for critical ischaemia (66%) but these differences were not significant. All failures occurred early and there were few failures after one month.

Johnston and colleagues[7] reviewed the results of 2257 angioplasty procedures and found a five-year cumulative patency for common iliac lesions of 58%. For external iliac angioplasty the patency rate was 47%. Patients with a stenosis fared significantly better than those with occlusion (65% patency at five years compared with 50% patency at five years for the common iliac group). Where the runoff was poor the results were worse (52% patency in the stenosis group compared with 35% patency for the occlusion group) in the common iliac group.

Beck et al.[8] showed that the late results of angioplasty in the common iliac artery (83% success) were slightly worse than the external iliac group (87.5% success).

Spoelstra et al.[9] showed that iliac angioplasty as an adjunct to femorodistal bypass was successful with a 91.7% three-year patency rate. In these cases angioplasty was performed for stenosis rather than occlusion. In a study of factors affecting outcome, Morin et al.[10] showed by multivariate analysis that in a group of 666 cases, four factors influenced outcome. These were:

- indication for the procedure (claudication/salvage)
- site of dilatation (iliac/femoral)
- runoff
- a history of previous dilatation.

Beck et al. [8] found that stenoses and occlusions over 10 cm in length were associated with comparatively poor long-term results and recommended surgery. Lamerton[11] also suggested that the best results were achieved in occlusions of less than 5 cm in length (Figure 10.1).

These studies suggest that there is considerable variability in the outcome of angioplasty and that surgery may have a role in occlusions rather than stenoses, long stenoses rather than short ones (Figure 10.2), patients with poor runoff in the thigh and in recurrent occlusion of the iliac segment. The complication rate of angioplasty is significantly lower than for surgery. The overall complication rate in 134 iliac and 127 distal angioplasties was 26%[12] but the rate of major complication was 12.6%. Complications included death in three patients, septicaemia in eight and popliteal artery occlusion in two. One patient suffered distal embolization and required toe amputation, and one suffered subintimal dissection in the common iliac artery. Beck et al., however[8], had an overall complication rate of only 2.9% with mortality of 0.007% in 4450 cases. There was arterial dissection in 0.94% requiring surgical

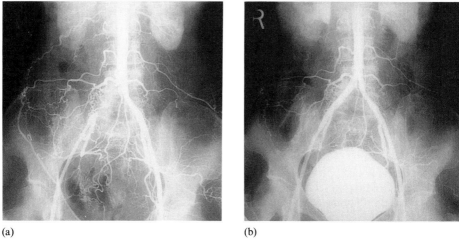

(a)   (b)

Figure 10.1   Short iliac stenosis before (a) and after (b) successful angioplasty

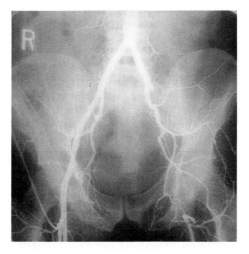

Figure 10.2   Long iliac occlusion unsuitable
for angioplasty

bypass, local arterial thrombosis requiring surgical embolectomy in 0.74% and vessel rupture in 0.31% which required surgical treatment. In 0.16% complications led to amputation and three patients died as a result of pelvic vessel rupture. These rates of complication are again very variable but acceptable when compared with the results of surgery.

Does aortoiliac endarterectomy have any role today?

Before the routine use of prosthetic bypass materials, endarterectomy was one of the mainstays of surgical management in obliterative vascular disease, being first described in 1836 by Astley Cooper. Endarterectomy has now largely disappeared because of the superior results thought to be achievable by bypass surgery. Sonnen-feld[13] reviewed 75 patients with surgery on 85 limbs over a period of eight years from 1973. A retroperitoneal approach was used for the operation and cumulative patency was 94% at three years, with a thirty-day mortality of 3.5%.

Capdevila and co-workers[14] reported excellent results for both the transperitoneal and retroperitoneal approaches: in 47 patients under 50 years of age the four-year patency rate was 78% for the transperitoneal and 79% for the retroperitoneal approaches. In those over 50 years comparable figures were 85% and 82% but the complication rate was higher. In the younger group undergoing transperitoneal surgery there was a 4% mortality with a 28% incidence of postoperative complications. There were no deaths in the retroperitoneal group and the complication rate was 9%. Endarterectomy was said not to be indicated when the lesions were calcific and the arteries kinked, hypoplastic or aneurysmal.

Taylor et al.[15] described the results of endarterectomy in 65 patients. There were three postoperative deaths (4.6%) and five patients had major postoperative complications (7.6%). No occlusions occurred during the follow-up period of up to six years, and late complications were not mentioned.

Willekens and co-workers[16] described their experience with the LeVeen plaque cracker in aortoiliac endarterectomy. In 228 patients the patency rate of 400 limbs was 97% at a mean of 21 months (3–54 months) with a postoperative mortality of 3%. Eight patients required early thrombectomy and there were no late complications related to the technique after a short follow-up period. These results are roughly comparable to those achieved by prosthetic bypass surgery and a small number of surgeons still regularly manage iliac disease in this way. Vascular surgeons in training will only rarely be taught the technique of aortoiliac endarterectomy and it seems likely that it will pass into history unless graft infection becomes a greater problem than it now is.

Should an aortic bifurcation graft be used in a wider group of patients?

Aortic bifurcation grafting is established as the surgical treatment of choice for bilateral aortoiliac occlusion and first reports of the technique go back nearly forty years[17].

Malone et al.[18] reviewed the results of operations upon 277 patients between 1959 and 1974. There was a cumulative patency of 80% at five years; early postoperative mortality was 10% before 1966 but only 1% thereafter. The age range of patients was 34–79 years (mean 52.4). More recently, Harris et al.[19] reported the results of a group of 377 limbs after aortofemoral reconstruction. The mean age of the group was similar, at 56 years, to that in Malone's study and the outcome excellent with a five-year cumulative patency of 91% and a mortality of 3.8%.

Sicard and colleagues[20] compared the outcome of transabdominal and retroperitoneal aortic bifurcation grafts. They found that both groups were of similar age, preoperative cardiac and pulmonary function and had undergone similar procedures. There was a significantly greater blood loss with the transperitoneal approach and both nasogastric intubation and the start of oral feeding were prolonged. Hospitalization in the transperitoneal group was significantly longer than for the retroperitoneal group. Significantly, however, there were no differences in time spent in intensive care, length of endotracheal intubation or mortality. Johnston et al.[21] also compared the trans- and retroperitoneal techniques. The mean age of the whole group studied increased from 48 years in 1961 to 66 years in 1979. Again, there was no difference in mortality or patency between the groups but retroperitoneal surgery led to significantly fewer chest infections, ileus and pulmonary embolism and the operations were quicker. In my own practice no patient has bowel preparation or nasogastric intubation (except after rupture of an aortic aneurysm) and yet there is no significant problem with ileus. All patients are ventilated with air, oxygen and isoflurane which avoids bowel distension at the time of closure and may contribute to a low incidence of ileus. The increasing age of the patients being treated suggests that it may be safe to offer surgical treatment to an older group than has been previously thought possible. Although it may be dangerous to draw parallels, patients with aneurysmal aortic disease are regularly treated surgically into their early eighties with no apparent increase in mortality, and it may be possible to offer aortic bifurcation grafting to the elderly, particularly if it is performed by the retroperitoneal approach.

Which of the surgical options is best in unilateral iliac occlusion?

Most vascular surgeons seem to have a preferred method of achieving revascularization in the patient with a unilateral iliac occlusion but there are no direct randomized trials comparing techniques.

Femorofemoral bypass
In a nine-year follow-up of femorofemoral bypass, Mosley and Marston[22] reported a 90% cumulative patency at five years with a 4.5% operative mortality. The age range of the patients was not stated, but femorofemoral bypass was stated to be the treatment of choice for all patients with unilateral iliac occlusion. Dick et al.[23] reported the results of 133 femorofemoral bypasses with an age range of 47–87 years: cumulative patency was 73% at five years and 64% at ten years with an operative mortality of 6% at thirty days. The higher mortality in this group may be due to the poor condition of some of the patients, many of whom were not fit for transabdominal surgery. Ray et al.[24] reported the results of 67 femorofemoral bypasses with a cumulative patency of 89% at seven years.

There are two potential problems associated with femorofemoral bypass:

1. Graft infection can affect both groins and may lead to bilateral amputations or death, whereas a unilateral iliac bypass only puts the affected leg at risk.
2. Femorofemoral bypass using a stenosed donor iliac segment could lead to a steal syndrome in the donor limb and to a risk of early graft occlusion in the recipient limb. The presence of a steal has been well demonstrated by Nicholson, Beard and Horrocks[25] and should be avoidable if the papaverine test is used to assess the donor limb before bypass[26].

Axillofemoral bypass
Ray et al.[24] reported a four-year patency for unilateral axillofemoral bypass of 74% and for axillobifemoral bypass of 83%. Patients were selected for their lack of fitness and old age (49–84 years). The improved results with the bilateral axillofemoral operation were put down to improved runoff.

The results of 59 axillofemoral bypasses with a mean age of 66 years were reported by Eugene, Goldstone and Moore[27]. The two-year patency rate was only 50% and there were no differences between the unilateral (35) and the bilateral (29) procedures. Moore[28], whose group performed the first reported axillofemoral bypass in 1962, reported the results of 44 cases. Most were elderly and of high risk and only 14% had claudication. The operative mortality was 9% with a poor patency rate and 50% of grafts occluded at 18 months. There was no difference between the unilateral and bilateral groups.

Graham *et al.*[29] suggested a minimum graft flow velocity of 8 cm/sec to maintain patency in axillofemoral grafts. Axillofemoral bypass is not without its risks, with possible steal and donor limb embolism or occlusion[30]. Personal experience suggests that skin erosion and subsequent graft infection are not uncommon complications of axillofemoral bypass, particularly affecting the long descending limb of the graft.

Unilateral iliofemoral bypass

Proponents of unilateral iliofemoral bypass include Kalman *et al.*[31], who has reported the results of 50 cases. The age range was 31–79 years with a patency rate of 92% at two years and no operative mortality. Patients undergoing surgery for claudication had a marginally better outcome than those undergoing surgery for critical ischaemia but the numbers studied were small.

Levinson and co-workers[32] compared the results of 65 unilateral iliac reconstructions with 96 aortobifemoral procedures. Operative mortality in the two groups was similar (3.1% and 2.1% respectively). There were seven early failures in the unilateral group of which three were successfully reopened, and eleven early failures in the aortofemoral group of which three were reopened successfully. The long-term outcome was better in the bilateral group with a 78% patency at five years, compared with a 52% patency in the unilateral group.

Sidawy *et al.*[33] reported the results of retroperitoneal bypass in 57 cases, some of which were bilateral. There was no operative mortality and the two-year patency was 93% irrespective of whether the bypass was unilateral or bilateral. Sidaway emphasized that, unlike axillofemoral bypass where a bilateral procedure was required to achieve a reasonable patency rate, unilateral iliofemoral bypass was as good as the bilateral procedure. It was also emphasized that the procedure was suitable for patients with poor respiratory function whereas aortobifemoral was not[34] and partial aortic or common iliac cross-clamping was unlikely to be associated with the haemodynamic problems of full cross-clamping of the infrarenal aorta[35].

Leicester experience

The results of unilateral iliac bypass in Leicester have been reviewed. During the seven-year period January 1980 to September 1987 69 patients were operated on – ten females and 59 males with a mean age of 61 years (16–84).

Indications for surgery included intermittent claudication in 21 (30%), critical ischaemia in 39 (57%), previously infected graft in seven (10%) and trauma in two (3%). All patients with infected grafts had previously had aortobifemoral or axillobifemoral bypass. One of the patients with trauma was treated acutely and the other presented five years after a bicycle handlebar injury to his left groin. All patients were given a preoperative angiogram to assess the adequacy of inflow, the length of occlusion and the patency of the superficial and profunda femoris arteries. Patients with short occlusions were treated by angioplasty and excluded from the study. Surgery was reserved for patients with long occlusions thought unsuitable for angioplasty and for patients with failed angioplasty.

Associated risk factors included hypertension (20), diabetes mellitus (10), current cigarette smoking (41) and a past history of smoking (20). Associated conditions included myocardial infarction (8), angina (11), and stroke (9). In all cases the aorta or common iliac artery was approached by a muscle-cutting incision in the iliac fossa with retroperitoneal dissection to gain access to the donor vessel. The femoral artery was mobilized through a separate incision in the groin. The graft was routed through the femoral canal to the groin and anastomosed across the junction of the common and profunda femoris arteries where possible. When the graft was performed for a previously infected graft, the new bypass was routed through the obturator foramen to the popliteal artery above the knee. The infected graft was left undisturbed during this part of the procedure. When the new bypass was completed the wounds were closed and covered and the infected prosthesis was removed at groin level. Seven grafts took origin from the aorta, 59 from the common iliac artery and three from a previous aortobifemoral bypass. In 24 cases the graft was inserted across the profunda origin, in 26 into the profunda directly, in four to the common femoral, and in one to the superficial femoral artery. Most distally, nine were inserted into the popliteal artery above the knee. Woven Dacron was used for the bypass in 52 cases and knitted Dacron in one. Most grafts were 10 mm diamater (40), although 8 mm (9) and 12 mm (3) grafts were also used. Polytetrafluoroethylene was used in all cases where the graft was anastomosed to the popliteal artery and in sixteen cases altogether.

Adjunctive femoropopliteal bypass was performed in twelve cases where it was felt that the profunda femoris artery was of poor quality. There were five distal anastomoses to the popliteal artery above the knee, three to the popliteal artery below the knee, one to the tibioperoneal trunk, and two to the posterior tibial artery in the proximal calf. One previously performed femoropopliteal bypass was reanastomosed to the distal end of the iliofemoral bypass. Femorofemoral bypasses were also performed in two other patients.

Results

The thirty-day mortality was 2/69 patients (2.9%). Cumulative patency for the group is shown in Figure 10.3. At one year 94% and at two years 86% of the grafts were patent. Indications for operation did not significantly alter outcome (Figure 10.4). In the infected group, one patient died at 15 months and one graft failed immediately. The remainder were patent at the time of review.

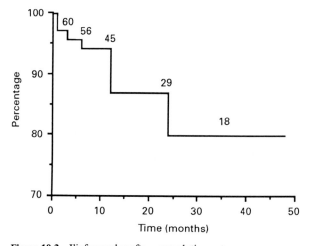

Figure 10.3 Iliofemoral grafts – cumulative patency

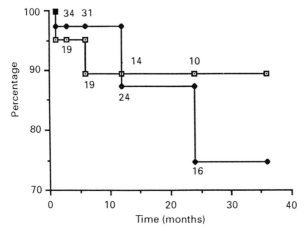

Figure 10.4 Iliofemoral grafts – claudication vs. critical. Indications for operation do not significantly affect outcome. □ claudication; ● critical

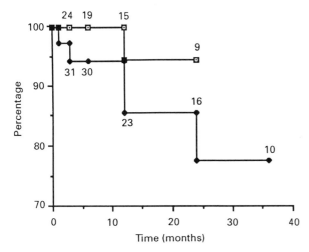

Figure 10.5 Poor runoff in the thigh does not significantly alter outcome. □ superficial femoral artery (SFA) patent; ● SFA occluded

Patency of the superficial femoral artery did not affect the outcome. There were no occlusions in 14 patients with two-vessel runoff. One femoropopliteal graft failure occurred in the twelve additional cases who had an adjunctive femoropopliteal bypass. In contrast there were 9/34 occlusions in the group with a single vessel runoff. These differences do not reach statistical significance (Figure 10.5) (Log rank test).

Twelve grafts failed and four patients died of other causes within two months of graft failure. Two grafts were unblocked, one with the addition of a femoropopliteal bypass. One graft was replaced by a transperitoneal bifurcated graft and three patients with irreversible ischaemia of the foot underwent amputation. The final patient had nothing further done because symptoms were mild.

The best option?

The results of each surgical option including aortic bifurcation grafting are approximately comparable, with the exception of axillofemoral bypass which seems to have a consistently poorer outcome. It must be remembered that none of these studies has randomly allocated patients to the different treatment options. Enthusiasts for axillofemoral bypass who use it in younger, fitter patients with good runoff in the thigh claim it works well.

Each option has its potential disadvantages:

- Axillofemoral bypass seems to have a high failure rate. Infection of the long limb, steal from the arm and occlusion of the axillary artery or embolism into the brachial artery may be a problem.
- Femorofemoral bypass may lead to steal from the donor limb and/or occlusion of the graft. Graft infection is a disaster because both lower limbs are put at risk.
- Aortobifemoral bypass is not regularly performed in the elderly because of worry about mortality rates, but experience with selected cases having aneurysm surgery suggests that this may be unfounded.
- Unilateral iliofemoral bypass requires a patent and reasonable common iliac artery on the right side although on the left aortofemoral bypass is possible. The abdominal incision may be deemed too risky in some high risk cases.

Each option also has its potential advantages:

- Axillofemoral and femorofemoral bypass can both be performed under local anaesthetic. The axillary artery almost always seems to be adequate and inadequacy of other vessels may on occasions rule out all other options.
- Femorofemoral bypass is favoured by many because it is the quickest option and unlike axillofemoral bypass requires only a short tube. Long-term patency is excellent.
- Aortobifemoral bypass has no specific advantages except that it cannot result in steal syndromes and the patency is excellent.
- Unilateral iliofemoral bypass also has this advantage and the graft is physically shorter. Graft infection is a potential problem because, unlike femorofemoral bypass or axillofemoral bypass which can be rescued by iliopopliteal bypass through the obturator foramen, this option is not available except by crossover. The Leicester results suggest that iliofemoral bypass can safely be used for any indication and with any state of runoff.

In conclusion, it is clear that management of unilateral iliac occlusion is riddled with prejudice and that the area is crying out for some randomly controlled trials. It is certainly not possible to draw conclusions from the data we have, even by the sophisticated data manipulation techniques advocated by some authors[36].

References

1. Dotter, C. T. and Judkins, M. P. (1964) Transluminal treatment of arteriosclerotic obstruction. *Circulation*, **30**, 654–670
2. Gruntzig, A. and Hopff, H. (1974) Perkutane rekanalisation chronischer arterieller verschlusse mit einem neuen dilationskatheter. *Dtsch Med. Wochenschr.*, **99**, 2502–2525
3. Doubilet, P. and Abrams, H. L. (1986) The cost of underutilisation. Percutaneous transluminal angioplasty for peripheral vascular disease. *New. Eng. J. Med.*, **310**, 95–102

4. Gordon, D. H., Glanz, S., Butt, K. M., Adamsons, R. J. and Koenig, M. A. (1982) Treatment of stenotic lesions in dialysis access fistulas and shunts by transluminal angioplasty. *Radiology*, **143**, 53–58

5. Parvin, S. D. and Bolia, A. A. (1989) Angioplasty for a failing vein graft. *Eur. J. Vasc. Surg.*, **3**, 283–284

6. Cole, S. E. A., Baird, R. N., Horrocks, M. and Jeans, W. D. (1987) The role of balloon angioplasty in the management of lower limb ischaemia. *Eur. J. Vasc. Surg.*, **1**, 61–65

7. Johnston, K. W., Rae, M., Hogg-Johnston, S. A. *et al.* (1987) 5-year results of a prospective study of percutaneous transluminal angioplasty. *Ann. Surg.*, **206**, 403–413

8. Beck, A. H., Muhe, A., Ostheim, W., Heiss, W. and Hasler, K. (1989) Long-term results of percutaneous angioplasty: A study of 4750 dilatations and local lyses. *Eur. J. Vasc. Surg.*, **3**, 245–252

9. Spoelstra, H., Nevelsteen, A., Wilms, G. and Suy, R. (1989) Balloon angioplasty combined with vascular surgery. *Eur. J. Vasc. Surg.*, **3**, 381–388

10. Morin, J. F., Johnston, W., Wasserman, L. and Andrews, D. (1986) Factors that determine the longterm results of percutaneous transluminal dilatation for peripheral arterial occlusive disease. *J. Vasc. Surg.*, **4**, 68–72

11. Lamerton, A. (1986) Percutaneous transluminal angioplasty. *Br. J. Surg.*, **73**, 91–97

12. Weibull, H., Bergqist, D., Jonsson, K., Karlsson, S. and Takolander, R. (1987) Complications after percutaneous transluminal angioplasty in the iliac femoral and popliteal arteries. *J. Vasc. Surg.*, **5**, 681–686

13. Sonnenfeld, T. (1981) Ileofemoral thromboendarterectomy through retroperitoneal approach. *Surgery*, 390, 868–871

14. Capdevila, J. M., Marco-Luque, M. A., Cairols, M. A. *et al.* (1986) Aortoiliac endarterectomy in young patients. *Ann. Vasc. Surg.*, **1**, 24–29

15. Taylor, L. M., Freimanis, I. E., Edwards, J. M. and Porter, J. M. (1986) Extraperitoneal iliac endarterectomy in the treatment of multilevel lower extremity arterial occlusive disease. *Am. J. Surg.*, **152**, 34–39

16. Willekens, F. G. J., Wever, J., Boeckxstaens, N. C. *et al.* (1987) Extensive disobliteration of the aorta-iliac and common femoral arteries using the LeVeen plaque cracker. *Eur. J. Vasc. Surg.*, **1**, 391–395

17. Voorhees, A. B., Jaretzki, A. and Blakemore, A. H. (1952) The use of tubes constructed from vinyon 'N' cloth in bridging arterial defects. *Ann. Surg.*, **135**, 332–336

18. Malone, J. M., Moore, W. S. and Goldstone, J. (1975) The natural history of bilateral aortofemoral bypass grafts for ischaemia of the lower extremities. *Arch. Surg.*, **110**, 1300–1306

19. Harris, P. L., Cave Bigley, D. J. and McSweeney, L. (1985) Aortofemoral bypass and the role of concomitant femorodistal reconstruction. *Br. J. Surg.*, **72**, 317–320

20. Sicard, G. A., Freeman, M. B., VanderWoude, J. C. and Anderson, C. B. (1987) Comparison between the transabdominal and retroperitoneal approach for reconstruction of the infrarenal abdominal aorta. *J. Vasc. Surg.*, **1**, 19–27

21. Johnston, J. N., McLoughlin, G. A., Wake, P. N. and Helsby, C. R. (1986) Comparison of extraperitoneal and transperitoneal methods of aortoiliac reconstruction. *J. Cardiovasc. Surg.*, **27**, 561–564

22. Mosley, J. G. and Marston, A. (1983) Long term results of 66 femoral-to-femoral by-pass grafts: 19-year follow up. *Br. J. Surg.*, **70**, 631–634

23. Dick, L. S., Brief, D. K., Alpert, J. *et al.* (1980) A twelve year experience with femorofemoral crossover grafts. *Arch. Surg.*, **115**, 1359–1365

24. Ray, L. I., O'Connor, J. B., Davis, C. D. *et al.* (1979) Axillofemoral bypass: A critical reappraisal of its role in the management of aortoiliac occlusive disease. *Am. J. Surg.*, **138**, 117–126

25. Nicholson, M. L., Beard, J. D. and Horrocks, M. (1988) Intra-operative inflow resistance measurement: a predictor of steal syndromes following femorofemoral bypass grafting. *Br. J. Surg.*, **75**, 1064–1066

26. Baker, A. R., Macpherson, D. S., Evans, D. H. and Bell, P. R. F. (1987). Pressure studies in arterial surgery. *Eur. J. Vasc. Surg.*, **1**, 273–283

27. Eugene, J., Goldstone, J. and Moore, W. S. (1976) Fifteen year experience with subcutaneous bypass grafts for lower extremity ischaemia. *Ann. Surg.*, **186**, 177–183

28. Moore, W. S., Hall, A. D. and Blaisdell, F. W. (1971) Late results of axillary-femoral bypass grafting. *Am. J. Surg.*, **122**, 148–154

29. Graham, J. C., Cameron, A. E. P., Ismail, H. I. *et al.* (1983) Axillofemoral and femorofemoral grafts: a 6-year experience with emphasis on the relationship of preoperative flow measurement to graft survival. *Br. J. Surg.*, **70**, 326–331

30. Cushieri, R. J., Vohra, R. and Lieberman, D. P. (1989) Acute ischaemia in the donor limb after occlusion of axillo-femoral grafts. *Eur. J. Vasc. Surg.*, **3**, 267–269

31. Kalman, P. G., Hosang, M., Johnston, K. W. and Walker, P. M. (1987) Unilateral iliac disease: The role of iliofemoral bypass. *J. Vasc. Surg.*, **6**, 139–143
32. Levinson, S. A., Levinson, H. J., Halloran, L. G. *et al.* (1973) Limited indications for unilateral aortofemoral or iliofemoral vascular grafts. *Arch. Surg.*, **107**, 791–796
33. Sidawy, A. N., Menzoian, J. O., Cantelmo, N. L. and Logerfo, F. W. (1985). Retroperitoneal inflow procedures for iliac occlusive vascular disease. *Arch. Surg.*, **120**, 794–796
34. Ali, J., Weisel, R. D., Layug, A. B. *et al.* (1974) Consequences of postoperative alterations in respiratory mechanics. *Am. J. Surg.*, **128**, 376–382
35. Sussman, B. C., Ibrahim, I., Kahn, M. *et al.* (1983) Aortic reconstruction by retroperitoneal approach. *Contemp. Surg.*, **22**, 66–69
36. Niederle, B., Kretschmer, G., Schemper, M. and Polterauer, P. (1990) Extra-anatomic cross over bypass (FF) versus unilateral orthotopic bypass (IF). An attempt to compare results based upon data matching. In *Proceedings of the 4th annual meeting of the European Society for Vascular Surgery*, p. 94
37. Blaisdell, F. W. and Hall, A. D. (1963) Axillary-femoral artery bypass for lower extremity ischaemia. *Surgery*, **54**, 563–568

Chapter 11

Selection of patients for and assessment of femorodistal bypass

Peter R. F. Bell

Bypass grafts to the crural vessels have been performed for some years, but there is disagreement about the success rates which vary between 80% and 25% at three years[1–3]. There is, however, general agreement that artificial grafts are not as good as autologous vein[1]. The wide spectrum of results is perhaps surprising but may be explained by the fact that the margins for success and failure are so small and the number of variables so large (Table 11.1). Unless attention is paid to detail results will be poor and this chapter examines those areas where attention to detail can improve results.

Table 11.1 Factors affecting the success of distal procedures

- The inflow
- The outflow
- Surgical techniques
- The graft used
- Assessment of the procedure at operation
- Postoperative surveillance

Preoperative selection and assessment

Many patients are old and ill but few of them are so unfit that an operation is not possible – a spinal anaesthetic is often all that is required to solve the problem. As these operations are only performed for critical ischaemia, the definition of which has now been agreed[4], the alternative to reconstruction is an amputation which has a high mortality and morbidity[5]. The patient often has ulceration or gangrene of the affected toe (Figure 11.1(a)) or foot (Figure 11.1(b)), and therapy with wide-spectrum antibiotics is essential. Some form of intervention will then be necessary to save the leg as drugs have not been found to be useful with perhaps the exception of iloprost[6] but this remains to be proved. An angiogram will be the next step and will usually adequately outline the crural vessels, allowing the surgeon to choose the best one for possible anastomosis (Figure 11.2). If, however, as does sometimes happen, the arteriogram shows no vessels in the distal part of the leg (Figure 11.3), this does not mean there are none present. It is also important to show the aortoiliac segment in order to exclude an inflow problem. If one is present it should be dealt with first, usually by angioplasty, which may be enough to increase the circulation sufficiently to avoid the need for a bypass graft. If there is no inflow problem and distal vessels

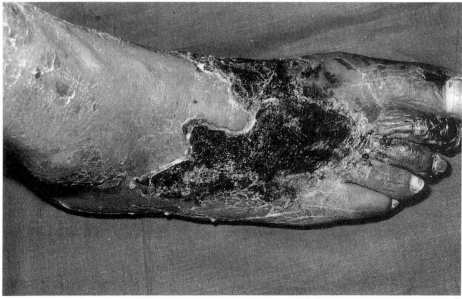

(b)

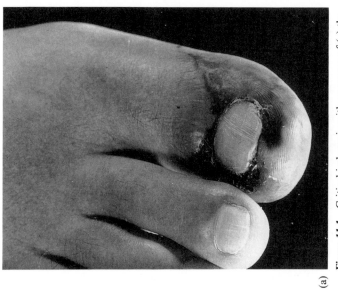

(a)

Figure 11.1   Critical ischaemia with gangrene of (a) the big toe; (b) the foot

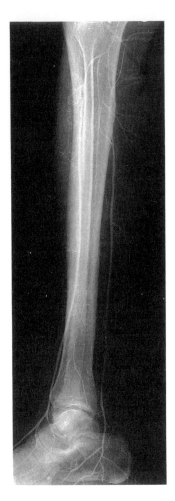

Figure 11.2   Angiogram showing a good anterior and posterior tibial artery suitable for bypass grafting

cannot be seen, alternative methods should be used to find a suitable vessel for exploration. Possible tests to consider are dependent Doppler insonation[7] of the ankle vessels and pedal arch or the use of pressure generated runoff assessment[8].

Inflow assessment

If there is any doubt, either clinical (poor femoral pulse) or radiological (possible plaque or stenosis on a uniplanar angiogram), then a preoperative inflow test should be performed and the lesion dealt with by angioplasty as this will sometimes solve the problem and obviate the need for a distal graft. Unfortunately few non-invasive tests are sufficiently accurate for use in individual cases[9] but the papaverine test[10] has withstood the test of time.

   In order to perform this test, a 21 gauge needle is inserted into the femoral artery on the side to be examined. A second needle to monitor systemic pressure is then inserted into a radial artery at the wrist, local anaesthesia being used for both injections. After baseline readings have been made, 20 mg papaverine is injected into the femoral

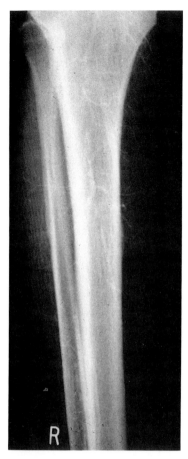

Figure 11.3 Angiogram showing no distal vessels below the knee. This does not mean that none are present

needle and the pressure monitored from both needles for the next 2–3 mins. A significant stenosis of the aortoiliac segment is present if the pressure falls by more than 20% after papaverine has been administered. An at rest pressure difference between the radial and femoral arteries of 10 mmHg or more is equally suggestive.

Dependent Doppler

All three crural vessels at the ankle are examined with a hand-held Doppler for a signal which will usually be faint. This is performed initially with the patient lying flat. If the leg is then lowered over the edge of the bed, a signal will be heard over a patent vessel. All three arteries at the ankle should be examined in this way. If a signal cannot be heard then the leg should be re-examined using the pressure generated runoff test. In this way a patent vessel can nearly always be found in the lower leg or at the ankle.

Pressure generated runoff (PGR)

A cuff is placed above the knee and expanded to between systolic and diastolic pressure to occlude the superficial venous return. A second cuff is placed immediately below the knee around the calf and attached to a compressed air cylinder, via a

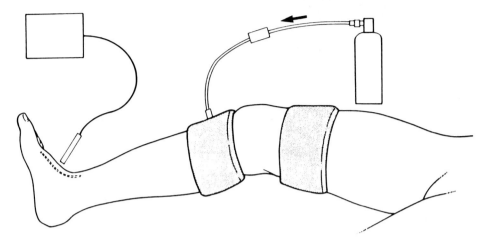

Figure 11.4   Measurement of pressure generated runoff (PGR) using an intermittently inflated cuff

machine which allows intermittent expansion and relaxation of the lower cuff producing intermittent pressure on the calf vessels (Figure 11.4). Each of the calf vessels is then examined with the Doppler, a signal heard at the ankle meaning that the vessel is patent from below the knee to the ankle. In this way the pedal arch can be traced out and the vessel with the best signal explored later. Although this test or the dependent Doppler method can target a patent vessel, neither is able to exclude a stenosis along its course.

Vein mapping

Because autologous vein gives the best results for femorocrural grafting[1] it should always be used if possible. If a Duplex machine is available the long saphenous vein should be mapped to indicate its size, patency and position[11], which takes about 10 min, and the entire course of the vein can be indicated with a suitable marker[12]. Mapping the vein (Figure 11.5) allows the correct incision to be made and thereby avoids wound complications. It always allows the operative procedure to be planned properly in that if the vein is inadequate, alternative sites such as the arm can be examined as a source of suitable vein. Arm veins, although a little thinner, can provide excellent conduits (Figure 11.6) and very good results[13]. The short saphenous vein is usually available and is a good, but short, conduit.

Intraoperative assessment

The artery thought to give the best signal on Doppler insonation or PGR is explored as described in Chapter 12. On exposure, because a picture of the vessel has not been obtained preoperatively and because PGR or dependent Doppler does not necessarily show stenoses in the course of the vessels, a pre-reconstruction angiogram is performed in order to find the best place for the anastomosis. This is done by inserting a butterfly needle into the artery and attaching it to a length of tubing to allow the

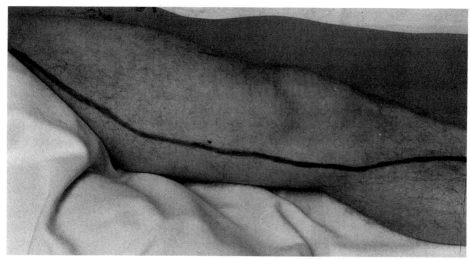

Figure 11.5   Mapping of the long saphenous vein before surgery

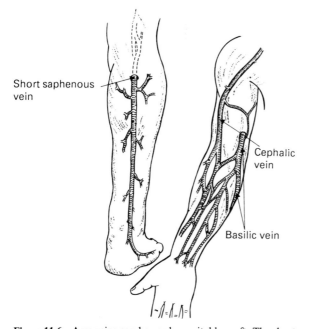

Short saphenous vein

Cephalic vein

Basilic vein

Figure 11.6   Arm veins can be used as suitable graft. The short saphenous vein is also very useful

operator to stand some distance from the table or behind the radiographer in order to avoid irradiation (Figure 11.7). Non-ionized contrast medium is then injected and as the injection continues an X-ray is taken using a film wrapped in a sterile towel and placed under the patient's leg (Figure 11.8). This will give a good picture of the runoff vessel and allow the surgeon to decide exactly where the anastomosis should be, so that the vessel can be exposed at that point. If the resistance is being measured (see below), the angiogram can be taken using the silastic cannulae inserted to measure

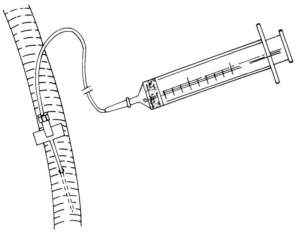

Figure 11.7   Contrast medium is injected into the artery before reconstruction to show the best level for the anastomosis

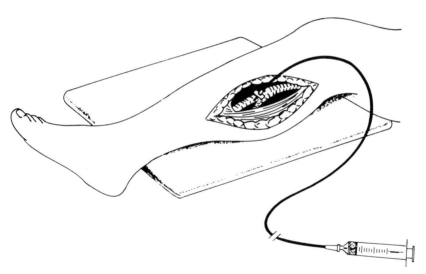

Figure 11.8   A satisfactory angiogram is obtained by placing an X-ray film wrapped in a sterile towel under the area to be examined

resistance. At this point, the surgeon will have most of the information required for a successful procedure (Figure 11.9).

Resistance measurement

The usual way of assessing whether or not the outflow into the foot is adequate is to examine an angiogram taken either before or at the time of surgery. Unfortunately angiography is not adequate to examine all cases, although a good vessel running into a pedal arch is usually a sign that success should be achieved. Measuring the peripheral resistance is another way of objectively assessing outflow and has been shown accurately to predict outcome[15,16]. The resistance is measured by making a

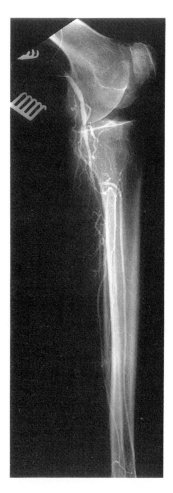

Figure 11.9 Pre-reconstruction on table angiogram showing that the anterior tibial artery would be the best vessel for the distal anastomosis

small arteriotomy in the vessel at a site chosen for the anastomosis and introducing a fine silastic cannula. This is best achieved using magnification with loupes and the surgeon must of course be very careful to avoid damage to the vessel. There is usually no problem if the correct size of cannula is used. Blood is then taken from the patient's femoral artery into a glass syringe and pumped into the cannula at a rate of 100 ml/min using a Harvard Pump or its equivalent. The pressure generated by this flow of blood is measured by a side arm in the system (Figure 11.10). The effect of injected papaverine can also be measured in order to assess the ability of the vascular bed to dilate. The resistance (in arbitrary units) is then calculated by the formula:

$$1\,\text{pru} = \frac{\text{Pressure}}{\text{Flow}}$$

Millipru are found by simply multiplying by 1000

We have found that early (six-month) patency is related to resistance and that

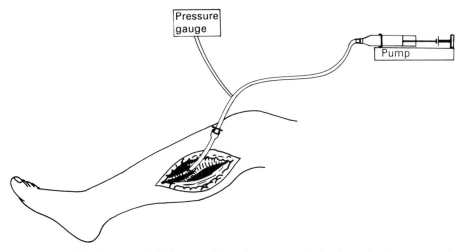

Figure 11.10   Blood at 100 ml/min is pumped into the artery at the site chosen for the anastomosis and the pressure generated measured

patients with a high resistance (greater than 1200 mpru) do significantly worse than those with a low resistance[15,16].

An alternative method of measuring resistance is to use a spring-loaded syringe (Figure 11.11), which is used to inject 20 ml of blood at a constant pressure and the time taken (in seconds) for this volume of blood to enter the artery is noted. The resistance can then be read off the barrel of the syringe. Again using this technique a resistance of higher than 1200 is associated with a poor outcome[17]. The syringe is less accurate than using a pump but possibly simpler.

The cannula can also be used for a pre-reconstruction angiogram, and while the film is being developed, the resistance can be measured. The surgeon will now be in a very good position to decide what to do. If the resistance is low and the vessel reasonable, a reconstruction will almost certainly succeed. If the reverse is the case, then the surgeon must decide to perform either a primary amputation or something else to improve the chances of success. This (something else) can take the form of either an arteriovenous fistula at the distal anastomosis[18] (see Chapter 12) or augmentation of early graft flow using drugs such as Iloprost given directly into the graft at surgery[19]. If the patient has a high resistance and the graft blocks early in

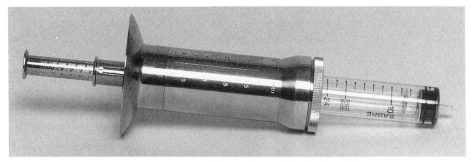

Figure 11.11   Stainless steel syringe used to inject blood into the distal vessel at a constant pressure

the postoperative period (hours) it might be best not to try and re-explore it as a successful outcome is unlikely.

Once all of these tests have been carried out the bypass procedure can be completed. The result will also depend on the graft being used, and the long saphenous vein used *in situ* is probably the best technique, giving superior results in this area[1]. For the distal anastomosis in particular, magnification using loupes will give the best chance of success.

Assessment of the procedure

Once the operation has been completed, a determined effort must be made to ensure that it has been successfully performed and that there are no technical errors. In order to do this, a completion angiogram, with the graft above the lower anastomosis gently clamped (Figure 11.12), will show any technical error at the anastomosis (Figure 11.13) which can be dealt with immediately. If the anastomosis looks all right the surgeon can terminate the operation with confidence (Figure 11.14). If the angiogram is carried out by injecting contrast at the top of the graft it will also be possible to check if any venous branches remain patent (Figure 11.15). Another way of looking for patent branches is to clamp the graft distally and measure flow in the graft moving the clamp progressively upwards. If flow is seen a branch is open above that point. If completion angiography, which is known to improve results[10], is not performed some other method of measuring the adequacy of the operation should be used.

Another assessment technique is to use an electromagnet or Doppler flowmeter to measure volume flow in the graft. If this is 80–100 ml/min it is acceptable, and should increase after the injection of papaverine into the graft. If flow is low or does not increase on papaverine injection then something is wrong[20]. If a needle is placed in the graft below the flowmeter and above the distal anastomosis, flow and pressure can be measured and the peripheral resistance calculated to assess outcome. If the resistance is low the procedure is adequate and the outcome should be good, if not the reverse will be the case[21]. Only when the operators are convinced that the procedure is technically acceptable does nothing further need to be done. It is not good enough to assume that the operation has been performed properly just because it 'looks all right'. Once the vein has blocked it becomes difficult to unblock, particularly if it happens beyond 12 hours postoperatively so everything must be done to ensure that the operation is carried out correctly the first time.

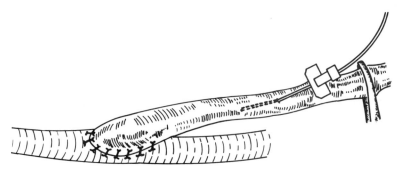

Figure 11.12 A completion angiogram is usually taken by injecting contrast directly into the graft which is first clamped proximally

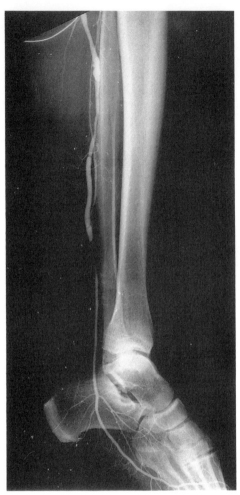

Figure 11.13 Completion angiogram showing a stenosis in the *in situ* vein graft and in the runoff vessel below the anastomosis

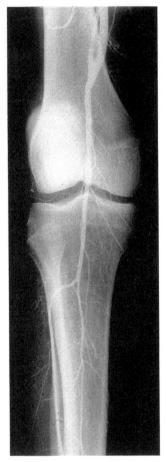

Figure 11.14 Completion angiogram showing above knee PTFE graft with a satisfactory anastomosis

Postoperative period

Early monitoring

It is important to monitor the graft for the first few postoperative hours. This is particularly difficult for the nurses as the patient's pulse may be hard to feel – this can be resolved by covering a portion of the patient's leg wound with a transparent adhesive dressing and placing a specially made Doppler probe (Figure 11.16) over the graft (Figure 11.17). In this way the pulsatility index and velocity can be continuously measured. Any indication of a decreasing mean velocity or increasing pulsatility index suggests that the graft is liable to fail[22] and in this situation if there was a high

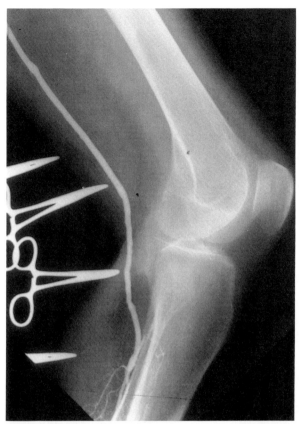

Figure 11.15   Completion angiogram showing no patent branches in an *in situ* vein graft

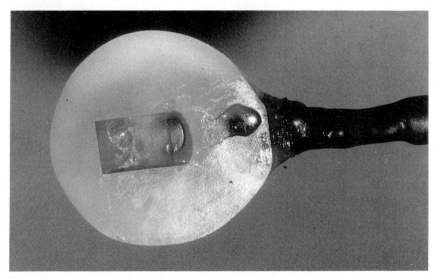

Figure 11.16   Doppler probe which can be placed over the graft for early postoperative monitoring

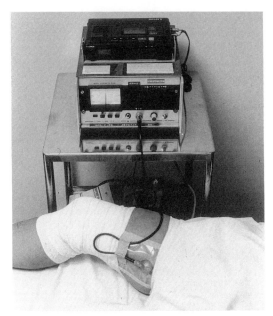

Figure 11.17   The probe shown in Figure 11.16 is placed over an area of the subcutaneous *in situ* vein graft. The wound is covered with a transparent adhesive dressing

resistance at the time of surgery then there is little point in exploring the graft again – an amputation would probably be the best option. If the resistance was low or normal at surgery then early exploration of the graft before it thromboses will be worthwhile: once a vein graft thromboses, it is very difficult to clear completely without intraoperative thrombolysis. In addition, should the pulsatility index be seen to be rising or the frequency doing likewise, then, providing the resistance is low, the patient should be explored. Early monitoring of this kind can predict impending failure and allow early exploration before occlusion of the graft has actually occurred.

Late monitoring

It is now known that up to 30% of vein grafts can develop a fibrous stricture in the first year after surgery, which will lead to thrombosis[2]. Once the graft occludes it may not be possible to unblock it, with unfortunate consequences for the patient. After the first year of surveillance stenoses tend not to occur but grafts can of course occlude with progression of distal disease. For the first year following surgery each graft should therefore be examined at intervals of three months. Examination can be performed by measuring ankle pressure after exercise but a more accurate method is to use duplex scanning, looking for areas of high frequency. If one is found, the patient should have an angiogram or DSA to assess the severity of the stenosis. Although no one is certain, it is likely that the stenosis should be treated first by angioplasty and failing this patched at surgery.

With a surveillance programme it is possible significantly to reduce the incidence of graft occlusion in the first year and to improve patency by 30%.

If all of these precautions are taken before, during or after surgery, the chances of successful femorocrural grafting are good, and patients who are not suitable will be spared an unnecessary operation which has a high chance of failing.

References

1. Rutherford, R. B., Jones, D. N., Bergentz, S. E. *et al.* (1988) Factors affecting the patency of infrainguinal bypass. *J. Vasc. Surg.*, **8**, 236–246
2. Dardik, H., Miller, N., Dardik, I. *et al.* (1988) A decade of experience with the glutaraldehyde tanned human umbilical cord vein graft for revascularisation of the lower limb. *J. Vasc. Surg.*, **7**, 336–347
3. Gardener, G. A., Jr., Harrington, D. P., Koltrun, W. *et al.* (1987) Salvage of occluded arterial bypass grafts by means of thrombolysis. *J. Vasc. Surg.*, **9**, 426–432
4. Norgren, L. (1989) Definition, incidence, epidemiology of critical ischaemia. In *Critical leg ischaemia, its pathology and management* (eds J. Dormandy and G. Stock) Springer-Verlag, pp. 7–13
5. Stoner, H. B., Taylor, L. and Macruson, R. W. (1989) The value of skin temperature measurements in forecasting the healing of a below knee amputation for end stage ischaemia of the leg for peripheral vascular disease. *Eur. J. Vasc. Surg.*, **3**, 355–361
6. Diehm, C., Abri, O., Baitsch, G. *et al.* (1989) Iloprost, ein stabiles prostacycline derivat bei arterieller verschlubkrankheit.im stadium IV. *Dtsch. Med. Wochensch*, **114**, 783–788
7. Shearman, C. P., Gwynn, B. R., Curran, F. *et al.* (1986) Non invasive femoropopliteal assessment: is that angiogram really necessary? *Br. Med. J.*, **293**, 1686–1689
8. Beard, J. D., Scott, D. J. A., Evans, M. *et al.* (1988) Pulse generated run off: a new method of determining calf vessel patency. *Br. J. Surg.*, **75**, 361–363
9. Macpherson, D. S., Evans, D. H. and Bell, P. R. F. (1984) Common femoral artery Doppler waveforms: a comparison of three methods of objective analysis with direct pressure measurements. *Br. J. Surg.*, **71**, 46–49
10. Quin, R. D., Evans, D. H. and Bell, P. R. F. (1975) Haemodynamic assessment of the aortoiliac segment. *J. Cardiovasc. Surg.*, **16**, 586–589
11. Bagi, P., Schroeder, T., Sellesdon, H. *et al.* (1989) Real time B mode mapping of the greater saphenous vein. *Eur. J. Vasc. Surg.*, **3**, 103–107
12. Magee, T. R., Leopold, P. W. and Campbell, W. B. (1990) Vein marking through ultrasound coupling gel. *Eur. J. Vasc. Surg.*, **4**, 491–493
13. Andros, G., Harris, R. W., Dulawi, L. *et al.* (1989) The use of the cephalic vein as a conduit. In *Vascular surgical techniques – an atlas* (ed R. Greenhalgh). W. B. Saunders, London, pp. 235–242
14. Patel, K. C., Semel, L. and Claus, R. H. (1988) Extended reconstruction rate for limb salvage with intraoperative and pre-reconstruction angiography. *J. Vasc. Surg.*, **7**, 531–538
15. Parvin, S. D., Evans, D. H. and Bell, P. R. F. (1985) Peripheral resistance measurement in the assessment of severe peripheral vascular disease. *Br. J. Surg.*, **72**, 751–753
16. Bell, P. R. F. and Parvin, S. D. (1988) Femorodistal bypass or primary amputation – can intraoperative tests help to decide? In *Limb salvage and amputation for vascular disease* (eds R. M. Greenhalgh, C. W. Jamieson and A. W. Nicolaides) W. B. Saunders, London, pp. 153–162
17. Beard, J. D., Scott, D. J. A., Evans, J. M. *et al.* (1988) A simple method of measuring peripheral resistance. In *Conference Proceedings of the Biological Engineering Society* (eds. Price and Evans). **11**, 64–68
18. Harris, P. L. and Campbell, H. (1983) Adjuvant distal arteriovenous shunt with femorotibial bypass for critical ischaemia. *Br. J. Surg.*, **70**, 377–380
19. Shearman, C. P., Hickey, N. C. and Simms, M. H. (1990). Femorodistal flow augmentation with the prostacyclin analogue Iloprost. *Eur. J. Vasc. Surg.*, **4**, 455–459
20. Beard, J. D., Scott, D. J. A., Evans, J. M. *et al.* (1988) Blood flow measurement in clinical diagnosis. In *Conference Proceedings of the Biological Engineering Society* (eds Price and Evans). **11**, 6–12
21. Ascer, E., Veith, F., Martin, L. *et al.* (1984) Quantitative assessment of outflow resistance in lower extremity arterial reconstructions. *J. Surg. Res.*, **37**, 8–15
22. Thrush, A. J. and Evans, D. H. (1990) A simple system for automatic intermittent recording of blood flow in femorodistal bypass grafts using Doppler ultrasound. *Med. Biol. Eng. Comp.*, **28**, 193–195
23. Grigg, M. J., Wolfe, J. H., Tovar, A. *et al.* (1988) The reliability of duplex derived haemodynamic measurements in the assessment of femorodistal grafts. *Eur. J. Vasc. Surg.*, **2**, 177–181

Chapter 12

Operative techniques and adjuvant measures influencing outcome in femorodistal bypass

Peter L. Harris

In a league table comparing the success rate of reconstructive vascular operations femorodistal bypass procedures are to be found at the bottom[1]. Because the results are less than ideal it is universally accepted that these procedures can be justified only for patients with truly critical ischaemia, who are otherwise faced with amputation of their limb. Indeed, very poor patency rates reported with long prosthetic grafts from the groin to the ankle or foot have raised doubts as to whether such procedures have any valid role in clinical practice[2–4]. It is argued that primary amputation might be the better option where the only alternative operation is associated with such a high failure rate. A failed reconstruction will at best yield the same final result, with the added discomfort and distress of multiple operations, a longer hospital stay and probably a significantly increased risk of serious complications including death. However, in the last few years there have been a number of new developments which give cause for rather more optimism regarding distal reconstructive operations.

Some techniques are of proven value while the benefits of others are at present speculative pending the results of properly controlled clinical trials. This chapter includes a description of some of these new techniques, together with a discussion of their potential value based on available clinical evidence.

Choice of graft for femorodistal bypass

An autologous long saphenous vein of good quality is undoubtedly the best conduit for femorodistal bypass. At least one in two vein grafts to the ankle will achieve long-term patency[5]. There are, however, two points regarding the use of vein grafts which warrant further discussion.

First, as a consequence of the excellent results with the *in situ* operation published by Leather and Karmody[6,7], there is a widely held view that this procedure is superior to the reversed operation. That this is not the case for femoropopliteal operations has been demonstrated by a number of authors[8–10], and new clinical trial data suggest that there is no significant advantage for the *in situ* technique at the crural level either (unpublished). Although there are a number of theoretical benefits associated with the *in situ* operation, the only one of practical importance is the alignment of the taper with that of the recipient arteries. Perhaps the best operation may be a non-reversed transposed saphenous vein bypass, which would appear to retain benefits associated with both of the other two methods. However, this operation has not yet been subjected to any comparative trials, and the indications are that provided a meticulous operative technique is employed similar results can be achieved with good saphenous vein grafts by any of the recognized methods.

The second point relates to the quality of the vein. The most objective measure of this is its diameter, and a 4 mm minimum internal diameter seems to be the watershed measurement. Grafts larger than this gives excellent average results, while smaller grafts give very poor results: for example, patency rates of 82.5% and 46.7% respectively at three years were reported in one series of femoropopliteal grafts[8]. Caution is therefore advisable when attempting to construct a bypass from an inadequate vein. It is possible that with the latest techniques the best results with long prosthetic grafts may be superior to those which can be achieved with small or strictured veins.

A number of alternative solutions exist to deal with an absence of adequate ipsilateral saphenous vein, including the use of contralateral saphenous vein, arm veins, superficial femoral veins and composite grafts with various mixtures of autologous and prosthetic materials. All have their advocates and good results can be achieved, but such procedures must be demonstrated to be significantly more effective than a long prosthetic bypass if any are to become widely accepted in preference.

The choice of an artificial substitute continues to be a matter of controversy, which is in itself an indication that none of the prosthetic grafts currently available is ideal. In comparative studies the patency of human umbilical vein grafts (HUV) has proved superior to those constructed from polytetrafluorethylene (PTFE)[11,12]. The problem with HUV grafts is that up to 36% develop aneurysmal dilatation after five or more years[13]. Although there are few data available, there is a general suspicion that all biological substitutes may be prone to the same complication, and until this has been shown not to be the case PTFE grafts will continue to be preferred by most surgeons. There is now clear evidence that externally supported PTFE grafts perform more reliably than non-supported grafts, especially when the knee joint is crossed[14]. The importance of other modifications including thin-walled construction and taper are less clear. It is likely that grafts made from polyurethane may soon become available for clinical use. These grafts differ from all other previous arterial prostheses in that they have compliance which can be matched to that of natural arteries. Assuming that problems associated with the biodegradation of polyurethane and its high level of thrombogenicity have been overcome, such grafts represent an interesting prospect for the future.

Choice and exposure of distal recipient artery

In a critically ischaemic limb the anatomical distribution of the occlusive disease may effectively eliminate any possibility of choice regarding the recipient distal artery, since there may be only one crural vessel patent. That preoperative angiography is an unreliable method for demonstrating the patency of distal arteries under conditions of very low flow is well recognized. It is, therefore, advisable in most cases to employ an additional technique of assessment before any selection of recipient vessels is made (see Chapter 11).

The anterior and posterior tibial arteries enter the dorsal and plantar ends, respectively, of the primary pedal arch. Opinion is divided as to the importance of an intact primary pedal arch, but it is considered advisable wherever possible to graft on to one of the two vessels which supply the arch directly[15]. This may be especially important when there is established necrosis in the foot. Technically the posterior tibial artery is the easiest to expose for an anastomosis, and for this reason it should be the vessel of first choice when patent. The anterior tibial artery requires a lateral approach, but it is not necessary to excise the fibula. It is often accessible at a more proximal level in the calf than the posterior tibial artery. Both of these vessels are readily accessible at the ankle and their primary terminal branches, the lateral plantar and dorsalis pedis arteries, can be exposed in the foot.

The peroneal artery does not run directly into the foot. It terminates just above the ankle by dividing into anterior and posterior communicating branches, which connect with the anterior and posterial tibial arteries respectively. It is also the least accessible of the crural arteries. A lateral approach gives good exposure, but requires fibulectomy, and many therefore prefer to approach it through a medial incision. For reasons unknown, in the presence of severe occlusive disease involving the distal vessels, the peroneal artery is often the one which is least damaged, and it may be the only one of the three to remain patent. Because of its anatomical relationships, the

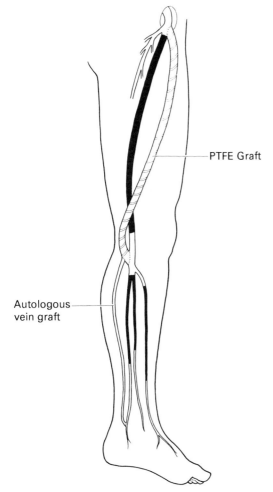

PTFE Graft

Autologous vein graft

12.1 A sequential femoroposterior tibial bypass with a PTFE graft to an isolated popliteal segment and a distal autologous vein graft

difficulty associated with its exposure and the fact that it tends to be selected only in the most severely diseased limbs, the results of peroneal artery reconstruction are generally less favourable than those involving the other two vessels. Nevertheless in expert hands good results can be achieved[16,17].

Occasionally a segment of the popliteal artery is patent in the presence of patent distal vessels, but without any direct continuity between them. A prospective randomized study of such cases has suggested that the chances of success are significantly better with a graft to the isolated popliteal segment than one to the distal vessel[18]. The principle to be followed in such situations, therefore, should be to place a graft to the popliteal artery. A sequential distal graft may then be added if judged appropriate (Figure 12.1).

Choice of proximal recipient artery and length of graft

By tradition the site of origin of distal bypass grafts is the common femoral artery. However, it must now be questioned as to whether this is always the best option. There can be no virtue in bypassing vessels which are healthy or only minimally diseased, and provided that the inflow is adequate almost any vessel may be used for the take-off of a graft. The superficial femoral and popliteal arteries are often suitable alternatives to the common femoral artery, and occasionally the profunda or even a tibial artery may be appropriate.

Longer grafts are associated with a greater risk of occlusion than shorter grafts[19]. This is certainly due in part to the reduced capacity of the runoff from more distal anastomoses, but recent indications that length has an influence on the patency rates of grafts independent of runoff focuses additional attention on the need to consider distal take-off points wherever possible (unpublished data). Where doubt exists about the quality of inflow this should always be tested intraoperatively with pressure measurements under high flow conditions (see Chapter 11).

It is a reasonable assumption that the route taken by the natural arteries in the limb is optimal and under most circumstances it is, therefore, advisable for bypass grafts to take the same route. Only occasionally is an extra-anatomical route likely to be better, for example, in the presence of infection or after multiple previous operations. Prosthetic grafts placed subcutaneously are associated with a risk of erosion of the overlying skin and should therefore be placed in deeper planes wherever possible.

Technique of distal anastomosis – basic principles

Anastomosis of a graft to a tibial artery is a true test of surgical dexterity. The small size of the recipient vessels permits no tolerance of error, and a meticulous technique is therefore essential. A generous length of artery should be exposed so as to ensure that the toe and heel of the anastomosis do not encroach on the limits of the dissection. Care must be taken to avoid damage to concomitant veins with resultant bleeding. Once the dissection has been completed it is advisable to give systemic heparin before manipulation of the artery. Clamps may damage the artery and control should therefore be achieved with soft silastic slings and intraluminal catheters. The size of catheter must be chosen so that it can be accommodated comfortably within the lumen and must not be so large as to impact and cause damage to the flow surface. The artery should be infused proximally and distally with heparinized saline introduced through the catheters, and the site of the anastomosis should also be flushed regularly in order to prevent any deposits of blood clot. Magnification is advisable and excellent illumination essential. For most anastomoses 7.0 sutures are suitable, inserted using a continuous technique. Some surgeons like to place a number of interrupted stitches at the toe and heel of the anastomosis to reduce the risk of stenosis at these critical points. On completion, the anastomosis should be bathed in heparinized saline or the clamps removed immediately to ensure that the suture line and adjacent sites of damaged endothelium are not exposed to static or slowly flowing blood.

Why do distal grafts fail?

In simple terms the unpropitious nature of distal bypass grafts, especially those with prosthetic material, is not difficult to appreciate. A long, relatively large diameter, tube with an artificial and alien flow surface is anastomosed to a very small vessel distally, with an associated high resistance and low runoff capacity. The effects of this arrangement are complex and apparently conflicting so that resolution of all problems is far from simple. Consider first the question of blood flow velocity: the volume of blood carried by the conduit and therefore its velocity, tend to be low. In experimental studies with a canine model Sauvage et al. demonstrated that all prosthetic conduits had a characteristic thrombotic threshold of velocity of blood flow below which thrombotic occlusion was likely to occur[20]. This study accords with clinical data showing that grafts with a high runoff resistance and low rates of flow are associated with the highest risk of occlusion[21–23]. Natural conduits including autologous vein grafts have a very low thrombotic threshold velocity, and therefore tolerate much lower rates of flow than prosthetic grafts[20]. These observations have led to attempts being made using various adjuvant measures to accelerate blood flow in prosthetic grafts in excess of their thrombotic threshold levels (see below).

A second factor to be considered is the exposure of the blood to the artificial flow surface. The greater the contact of the blood elements with this surface the greater the risk of thrombosis, both within the graft itself and at the anastomosis through changes initiated by platelets. The amount of contact is increased by a high circumference:cross-sectional area ratio within the conduit, and is therefore greater in tubes of small diameter. In normal laminar flow the blood elements are protected from contact with the flow surface by an acellular marginal zone. This breaks down under conditions of high velocity. The point at which blood flow within any conduit is likely to become turbulent with increasing velocity is determined by Reynold's number ($Re = \rho U d / v$ where ρ = density of blood, U = blood velocity, d = the diameter of the lumen and v = viscosity of the blood), and the mean Reynolds number above which turbulent transition is likely to occur can be described as the critical Reynolds number. Under normal conditions the critical Reynold's number may be exceeded at peak systolic velocity but not at other stages of the cardiac cycle, and any flow disturbance which occurs tends to be very transient. In order to avoid persistent turbulence it is necessary to ensure that the average blood velocity is well below that of the critical Reynold's number. Consider, for example, a long straight PTFE graft of 5 mm internal diameter (Figure 12.2). In the central portion of the graft laminar flow tends to become unstable when the Reynold's number exceeds 2000, which equates to an average blood velocity of approximately 160 cm/s or a volume flow of

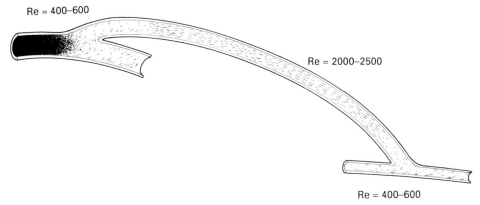

Re = 400–600

Re = 2000–2500

Re = 400–600

Figure 12.2   Sites of turbulence in a bypass graft with end-to-side anastomoses. Reynolds number $Re = \rho U d / v$ where $U =$ blood viscosity, $d =$ diameter of graft, $\rho =$ density of blood and $v =$ viscosity of blood

1880 ml/min. Such flow rates are never likely to be attained in practice in distal bypass grafts; however, at each end of the graft, owing to the complex geometry of the anastomoses flow disturbance is generated at much lower Reynold's numbers (in the order of 400–600). A Reynold's number of 400 equates to an average blood velocity of approximately 32 cm/s or a volume flow rate in the order of 370 ml/min. If flow rates occur in excess of this flow disturbance generated at the proximal anastomosis will persist for a variable distance into the graft, resulting in inexpedient contact between platelets and the artificial flow surface. Experimental studies of thrombotic threshold velocity (TTV) in dogs[20] and sheep[24] suggest that the TTV for such a graft is approximately 7 cm/s, which equates to a flow of 82 ml/min. From these data it would appear that for optimum conditions blood velocity should be maintained at a level well in excess of 7 cm/s and considerably less than 32 cm/s, that is to say within a fairly narrow and specific range.

Undoubtedly the most critical point of a distal bypass graft is the distal anastomosis itself. The small size of the recipient artery is the principal source of failure, but there are additional aggravating factors. End-to-side junctions do not occur naturally in the circulation. The geometry of an anastomosis of this type leads to gross flow disturbance with areas of both high and low wall shear. The result is likely to be adhesion of platelets, which have already been activated by contact with the artificial flow surface of the graft. The final outcome may be immediate thrombosis within the anastomosis or the later development of subintimal hyperplasia mediated by platelet-derived factors acting on arterial smooth muscle cells. In either circumstance failure of the bypass is very likely because the small cross-sectional area of the recipient artery is intolerant of any encroachment upon its lumen. Unfortunately, the obvious solution to this problem, the construction of an end-to-end anastomosis, is not normally practical, especially where prosthetic grafts are concerned, because of the considerable disparity in the size between the graft and the recipient artery and the need to preserve some flow in the proximal direction.

It is thought that an added factor with regards to the development of subintimal hyperplasia may be a mismatch in compliance between the prosthetic graft and the recipient artery[25]. Although the size and nature of the recipient artery cannot be changed, it is possible to modify the junctional zone between the graft and the artery, that is the distal anastomosis, in order to ameliorate the consequences associated with its less than ideal geometrical form.

Whether a graft occludes soon after operation due to thrombosis or later due to the effects of subintimal hyperplasia it seems to be the case that interaction between blood constituents and the artificial flow surface is an important step in the process. By careful design of the bypass it may be possible to minimize contact between the two reactants with beneficial effects on patency rates. At the same time measures may be applied to modify more directly this potentially damaging interaction and its immediate effects. This might be achieved by altering the physical and chemical properties of the flow surface to make it more acceptable or by changing the behaviour of the blood elements themselves in order to modify their response to contact with any abnormal surface.

Collectively technical procedures or other treatments which are undertaken in addition to the basic bypass operation with the intention of improving patency rates are described as adjuvant measures. Because of poor patency rates achieved with unmodified femorotibial prosthetic grafts, much interest has been focused recently on the role of adjuvant measures in association with these operations.

Adjuvant measures to influence the patency rates of femorodistal grafts

The theories described above regarding the reasons for the high failure rate of femorodistal bypass grafts form the basis of a number of adjuvant measures which have been applied in an attempt to improve results. None are yet of proven value and all continue to be under the process of evaluation. This is a difficult task since, because of the multifactorial nature of graft failure, it is unlikely that any single measure alone could have a dramatic effect. For the best results it will be necessary to optimize blood flow velocity, mitigate the effects of the unfavourable geometry at the distal anastomosis, overcome the enhanced thrombogenicity of the artificial flow surface and suppress the thrombogenic activity of platelets exposed to such a flow surface.

Adjuvant arteriovenous shunt

This is a technique designed to increase the blood flow velocity within a graft above the thrombotic level. An arteriovenous shunt is constructed at or close to the distal anastomosis in order to create an additional runoff channel and thereby to reduce runoff resistance[26–28]. Two techniques of construction have been used most frequently.

In the first, known as a common ostium shunt, the recipient artery and one of its concomitant veins are opened longitudinally, and the adjacent walls are sutured together to create a common ostium. The graft is then anastomosed to this common ostium (Figure 12.3). This technique produces a shunt of large capacity, the actual volume of flow being limited only by the size of the vein.

An alternative method, the preanastomotic shunt, involves a smaller side-to-side anastomosis between the artery and its concomitant vein approximately 0.5 cm proximal to the graft-to-artery anastomosis (Figure 12.4). The short section of host artery between the graft and the shunt serves to limit the volume of flow through it, with the intention of maintaining velocities within an optimal range.

In practice no significant difference in performance has been demonstrated between those two methods. Adjuvant arteriovenous shunts have been shown to be free from side effects, and fears that 'steal' from the distal part of the limb may occur have

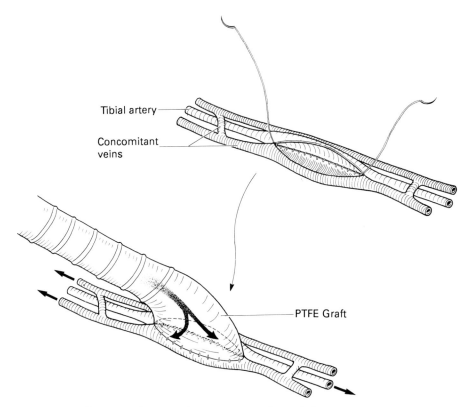

Figure 12.3 Adjuvant arteriovenous shunt; common ostium technique

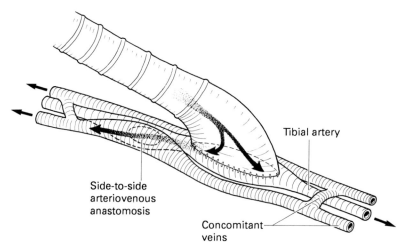

Figure 12.4 Preanastomotic adjuvant arteriovenous shunt

proved unfounded. However, there is to date little convincing evidence of real benefit from their use. In a series of HUV grafts with arteriovenous shunt reported by Dardik *et al.* a 42% patency rate was obtained at one year[28], while in a similar series of 80 grafts from Liverpool the patency rate was 39% at one year (unpublished data). Both series included only operations which would normally be considered to carry a very poor chance of success. Without a properly controlled prospective trial it is difficult to be certain whether or not an adjuvant arteriovenous shunt confers any benefit, but on current evidence it does not so far seem to have been a very effective antidote to the high early occlusion rate of distal grafts. There is a possibility in some cases that excessive augmentation of flow with too high velocities in the graft, together with the added complexity of the distal anastomosis may paradoxically have increased the risk of thrombosis. Benefits may be outweighed by disadvantages, and without further refinement of technique the overall effect could be detrimental. The fact remains, however, that grafts fail if the velocity of blood flow through them is inadequate, and the objective of ensuring that thrombotic threshold levels are exceeded seems to be rational. The essential trick would seem to be containment of blood velocity within the optimum range.

Venous interposition grafts, patches and cuffs

Technically the construction of an anastomosis between a non-compliant prosthetic conduit and a fragile tibial vessel can be exceedingly difficult. This is in contrast to an anastomosis of an autologous vein graft to a tibial artery, which is relatively less demanding. In order to overcome this difficulty with prosthetic grafts autologous vein inserts have been employed in different ways including interposition or sequential grafts[29], patches[14] and cuffs[30]. Some excellent results have been reported for femorotibial grafts with these techniques.

Britton and Leveson[29] reported 65% cumulative patency at a mean follow-up period of 19 months with a bicomposite graft of PTFE and a distal segment of autologous vein. Taylor, McFarland and Cox[14] reported 78% cumulative patency of PTFE grafts at three years with a diamond-shaped autologous vein patch at the distal anastomosis (Figure 12.5). Miller *et al.*[30] constructed a complete cuff of autologous vein at the distal anastomosis (Figure 12.6) and achieved a 72.4% cumulative patency rate of PTFE grafts at eight months using this technique. A modification of the Miller Cuff technique to incorporate some benefits of the Taylor patch (Figure 12.7) has been proposed by Wolfe (unpublished data).

Evidence is accumulating that there may be benefits associated with these techniques other than that of simply facilitating the operation. Most importantly there is a possibility that the incidence of occlusion associated with subintimal hyperplasia may be reduced. The reasons why this might be the case must be speculative at this stage, but it has been suggested that a segment of vein interposed between the graft and the artery may buffer the effects of compliance mismatch. Undoubtedly a vein patch as applied by Taylor and a Miller Cuff (especially with a Wolfe modification) produces a tapering or funnel-shaped anastomosis, which is likely to be conducive to better flow characteristics and may therefore mitigate some of the damaging effects of an end-to-side anastomosis. Furthermore, if platelet deposition and subintimal hyperplasia should occur the more spacious anastomosis is better able to accommodate it without disastrous consequences.

Prospectively randomized clinical trials are required to establish with certainty the effect of these new techniques, but the evidence to date of benefit from uncontrolled

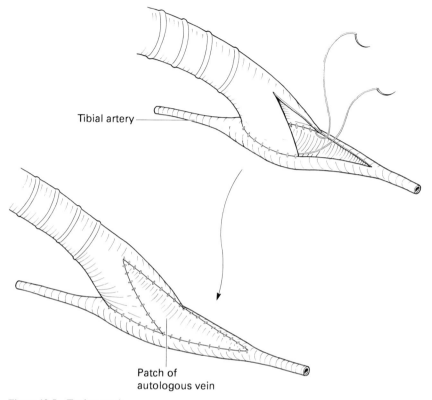

Tibial artery

Patch of
autologous vein

Figure 12.5   Taylor patch

data is becoming increasingly persuasive, and as understanding of the mechanism involved increases so further refinements may be developed. An interesting possibility is that a vein cuff or patch at the distal anastomosis may offset some of the detrimental effects of an adjuvant arteriovenous shunt.

Endothelial seeding of prosthetic grafts

Natural blood vessels are lined by a monolayer of endothelial cells which is non-thrombogenic by virtue of the fact that it does not cause activation of platelets, largely owing to its ability to produce prostacyclin. Prosthetic grafts in humans become endothelialized only for short distances at each anastomosis, and most of the luminal surface remains relatively thrombogenic[31]. Such observations have given rise to the concept of endothelial seeding by which autologous endothelial cells are harvested and 'seeded out' onto the entire flow surface of the graft, with the aim of producing a complete and confluent monolayer. In canine studies autologous endothelial cell seeding of prosthetic grafts leads to a confluent monolayer within 4–6 weeks, with a concomitant improvement in graft patency rates even in situations of relatively low blood flow[32,33]. In humans, however, two main obstacles to practical cell seeding have been encountered: first the relatively small number of autologous endothelial

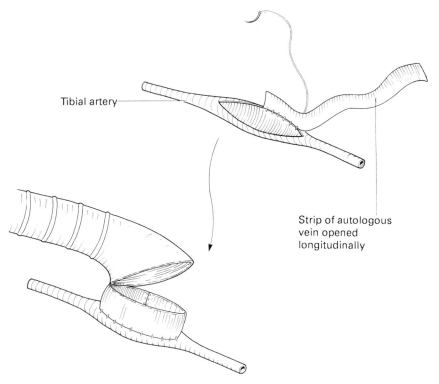

Tibial artery

Strip of autologous
vein opened
longitudinally

Figure 12.6   Miller Cuff. A short length of autologous vein is opened longitudinally to form a strip
which is then sutured to the margins of the arteriotomy. A vertical row of sutures completes the
formation of the cuff to which the prosthetic graft is anastomosed as illustrated

cells available, and secondly a low rate of retention of seeded cells due to poor
attachment to the surface of the graft[34]. Cells are normally harvested from segments
of autologous vein. It has been shown that omentum can be used to increase the yield
of cells but this has practical limitations[35]. Mesothelial cells have also been tried and
found to be less effective than endothelial cells[36]: fortunately, endothelial cells can
be grown in tissue culture and the most effective seeding is achieved by incubating
grafts in a suspension of previously harvested cells[37].

Attachment of the endothelial cells is enhanced considerably by pretreatment of the
graft to prepare the luminal surface. Coatings of fibrin preclot, fibronectin, gelatin,
poly-l-lysin and various types of collagen have all been tried and of these fibrin
preclot[36] and fibronectin[37] appear to be the most effective.

To date no advantage has been demonstrated from the application of endothelial
cell seeding in clinical practice, and it is apparent that a number of technical problems
remain to be resolved. However, there are indications from published experimental
data that with persistence the potential benefits for patients may eventually be
realized.

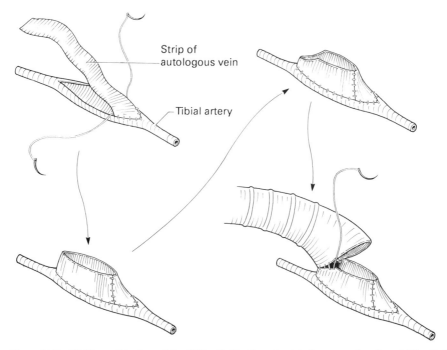

Figure 12.7   Wolfe modification of the Miller Cuff – the vein strip is prepared as for a Miller Cuff. Suturing commences at the point of the arteriotomy to which a corner of the vein strip is joined. The short margin of vein is then sutured to one side of the arteriotomy following which the longer margin is sutured to the remaining circumference of the arteriotomy. The cuff is completed as shown and the posterior end of the cuff is trimmed before anastomosis with the PTFE graft

Adjuvant pharmacotherapy

Platelets play a major role in graft occlusion at whatever stage after operation it occurs and the terminal process is always thrombosis. There are therefore strong theoretical grounds for employing pharmacological agents which modify platelet activity and thrombogenesis.

Evidence of benefit from clinical trials is scarce, but Clyne et al.[38] demonstrated improved patency of prosthetic distal grafts when the patients were given a combination of aspirin and Persantin for three months postoperatively. Antiplatelet therapy of this type, either low-dose aspirin alone or in combination with Persantin should ideally be commenced at least 48 hours preoperatively. There is no clear guidance on the optimum duration of therapy and opinions vary between giving short courses only and maintaining treatment for life. New, more powerful agents, such as the stable prostacyclin analogue Iloprost which is now undergoing clinical trials, may have a role in the future[1].

Most surgeons use heparin anticoagulation perioperatively, but there is less agreement about the use of long-term oral anticoagulants. In one study the effect on graft patency was minimal, but there were other benefits in that the incidence of associated vascular complications, including fatal myocardial infarction, was reduced[39]. In selective cases the use of long-term oral anticoagulation may be justified despite the not inconsiderable inconvenience for the patient. For the highest risk grafts a combination of oral antiplatelet and anticoagulant drugs is possibly the most effective adjuvent therapy despite the risk of haemorrhagic complications.

Conclusions

Despite the difficulties associated with femorodistal bypass grafting such procedures remain probably the best option for most patients with truly critical ischaemia of the limb. Saphenous vein grafts give the best results provided that the quality of the vein is adequate, and the method chosen (reversed, *in situ* or non-reversed transposed) is probably less important than the application of a meticulous surgical technique. The use of prosthetic grafts remains problematical, but there are grounds for optimism in that the application of adjuvant procedures may improve the prospects for future patients.

Since the failure of femorodistal grafts is multifactorial a single adjuvant measure in isolation cannot be expected to have a dramatic effect on patency rates. In order to achieve the best possible results all of the known elements which combine to culminate in graft failure may need to be addressed by application of appropriate adjuvant measures.

References

1. European Consensus Document on Critical Limb Ischaemia (1990) In *Critical Leg Ischaemia: Its pathophysiology and management* (Eds J. Dormany and G. Stock). Springer-Verlag, Berlin
2. Charlesworth, D., Brewster, D. C., Darling, R. C., Robinson, J. G. *et al.* (1985) The fate of polytetrafluorethylene grafts in lower limb surgery: a six-year follow up. *Br. J. Surg.*, **72**, 896–899
3. Bell, P. R. F. (1985) Are distal vascular procedures worthwhile? *Br. J. Surg.*, **72**, 335–339
4. Harris, P. L. and Campbell, H. (1986) Femoro-distal bypass for critical ischaemia: is the use of prosthetic grafts justified? *Ann. Vasc. Surg.*, **1**, 67–72
5. Harris, P. L. and Moody, P. (1989) The natural history of arterial bypass grafts with special reference to distal reconstructions. In *Pharmacological intervention to increase patency after arterial reconstructions* (eds D. Bergqvist and B. Lindblad). ICM AB, Malmo, Sweden
6. Leather, R. P., Shah, D. M. and Karmody, A. M. (1979) A reappraisal of the 'in-situ' saphenous vein arterial bypass. Its use in limb salvage. *Surgery*, **86**, 453–461
7. Leather, R. P., Shah, D. M. and Karmody, A. M. (1981) Infrapopliteal arterial bypass for limb salvage: Increased patency and the utilisation of the saphenous vein used 'in-situ'. *Surgery*, **90**, 1000–1008
8. Harris, P. L., How, T. V. and Jones, D. R. (1987) Prospectively randomised clinical trial to compare in-situ and reversed saphenous vein grafts for femoropopliteal bypass. *Br. J. Surg.*, **74**, 252–255
9. Watalet, J., Chacysson, E., Poels, D., Menhard, J. F., Papion, H. and Testart, J. N. (1986). In situ versus reversed saphenous vein for femoropopliteal bypass: a prospective randomised study of 100 cases. *Ann. Vasc. Surg.*, **1**, 441–452
10. Porter, J. M. (1988) In-situ versus reversed vein graft: Is one superior? *J. Vasc. Surg.*, **7**, 79–80
11. Eickhoff, J. H., Buchardt-Hansen, H. J., Bromme, A., Kordt, K. F., Mouritzen, C. *et al.* (1983) A randomised clinical trial of PTFE versus human umbilical vein for femoropopliteal bypass surgery. Preliminary results. *Br. J. Surg.*, **70**, 85–88
12. Eickhoff, J. H., Bromme, A., Ericsson, B. F., Buchardt-Hanson, H. J. *et al.* (1987) Four years results of a prospectively randomised clinical trial comparing polytetrafluoroethylene and modified human umbilical vein grafts for femoropopliteal bypass. *J. Vasc. Surg.*, **6**, 506–511
13. Dardik, H., Ibrahim, I. M., Sussman, B., Kahn, M., Sanchez, M. *et al.* (1984) Biodegradation and aneurysm formation in umbilical vein grafts: observations and a realistic strategy. *Ann. Surg.*, **199**, 61–68
14. Taylor, R. S., McFarland, R. J. and Cox, M. I. (1987) An investigation into the causes of failure of PTFE grafts. *Eur. J. Vasc. Surg.*, **1**, 335–345
15. Simms, M. H. (1988) Is pedal arch patency a pre-requisite for successful reconstruction? In *Limb*

Salvage and Amputation for Vascular Disease (Eds R. M. Greenhalgh, C. W. Jamieson and A. N. Nicolaides). W. B. Saunders Co., London

16. Dardik, H., Ibrahim, I. M. and Dardik, I. (1979) The role of peroneal artery for limb salvage. *Ann. Surg.*, **189**, 189–198
17. Karmody, A. M., Leather, R. P., Shah, D. M., Corson, J. D. and Naraynsingh, V. (1984) Peroneal artery bypass: A reappraisal of its value in limb salvage. *J. Vasc. Surg.*, **1**, 809
18. Darke, S. G., Lamont, P., Chant, A., Barros D'Sa A. A. B., Clyne, C. *et al.* (1989) Femoro-popliteal versus femoro-distal bypass grafting for limb salvage in patients with an 'isolated' popliteal segment. *Eur. J. Vasc. Surg.*, **3**, 203–207
19. Harris, P. L. and Campbell, H. (1986) Femoro-distal bypass for critical ischaemia: Is the use of prosthetic grafts justified? *Ann. Vasc. Surg.*, **1** (1), 66–72
20. Sauvage, L. R., Walker, M. W., Berger, K. E., Robel, S. B., Lischko, M. M. *et al.* (1979) Current arterial prostheses: Experimental evaluation by implantation in the carotid and circumflex coronary arteries of the dog. *Arch. Surg.*, **114**, 687–691
21. Ascer, E., Veith, F. J., Morris, L., Lesser, M. L., Gupta, S. K. *et al.* (1984) Components of outflow resistance and their correlation with graft patency of lower extremity arterial reconstructions. *J. Vasc. Surg.*, **1**, 817–828
22. Vos, G. A., Rauwerds, J. A., Van den Broek, Th. A. A. and Bakker, F. C. (1989) The correlation of per-operative outflow resistance measurements with patency in 109 infra-inguinal arterial reconstructions. *Eur. J. Vasc. Surg.*, **3**, 539–542
23. Cooper, C. G., Austin, C., Fitzsimmons, E., Brannigan, P. D., Hood, J. M. and Barros D'Sa, A. A. B. (1990) Outflow resistance and early occlusion of infra-inguinal bypass grafts. *Eur. J. Vasc. Surg.*, 279–283
24. Carson, S. N., Demling, R., Esquivel, C., Talken, L., Tillman, P. *et al.* (1981) Testing and treatment of arterial graft thrombosis. *Am. J. Surg.*, **142**, 137–143
25. Kidson, I. G. (1983) The effect of wall mechanical properties on patency of arterial grafts. *Ann. R. Coll. Surg. Eng.*, **65**, 24
26. Dardik, H., Sussman, B., Ibrahim, I. M., Kahn, M., Svoboda, J., Mendes, D. and Dardik, I. (1983) Distal arteriovenous fistula as an adjunct to maintaining arterial and graft patency for limb salvage. *Surgery*, **94**, 478–486
27. Harris, P. L. and Campbell, H. (1983) Adjuvant distal arteriovenous shunt with femorotibial bypass for critical ischaemia. *Br. J. Surg.*, **70**, 377–380
28. Dardik, H., Miller, N., Dardik, A., Ibrahim, I. M., Sussman, B. *et al.* (1988) A decade of experience with the glutaraldehyde-tanned human umbilical cord vein graft for revascularisation of the lower limb. *J. Vasc. Surg.*, **7**, 336–346
29. Britton, J. P. and Leveson, S. H. (1987) Distal arterial bypass – bicomposite graft. *Br. J. Surg.*, **74**, 249–251
30. Miller, J. H., Foreman, R. K., Ferguson, L. and Faris, I. (1984) Interposition vein cuff for anastomosis of prosthesis to small artery. *Aust. NZ J. Surg.*, **54**, 283–285
31. Berger, K., Sauvage, L. R., Rao, A. M. and Wood, S. J. (1972) Healing of arterial prostheses in man: its incompleteness. *Ann. Surg.*, **175**, 118–127
32. Kempczinski, R. F., Rosenman, J. E., Pearce, W. H., Roedersheimer, L. R., Berlatzky, U. and Ramalangjaona, G. (1985) Endothelial cell seeding of a new PTFE vascular prosthesis. *J. Vasc. Surg.*, **2**, 424–429
33. Schmidt, S. P., Hunter, T. J. and Hirko, M. (1985) Small diameter vascular prosthesis: two designs of PTFE and endothelial cell seeded and non-seeded Dacron. *J. Vasc. Surg.*, **2**, 292–297
34. Foxall, T. L., Auger, K. R., Callow, A. D. and Libby, P. (1986) Adult human endothelial cell coverage of small diameter Dacron and polytetrafluoroethylene in vitro. *J. Surg. Res.*, **41**, 158–172
35. Jarrell, B. E., Williams, S. K. and Stokes, G. (1986) Use of freshly isolated capillary endothelial cells for the immediate establishment of a monolayer on a vascular graft at surgery. *Surgery*, **100**, 392–399
36. Thomson, G. J. L., Vohra, R. and Walker, M. G. (1989) Cell seeding for small diameter PTFE vascular grafts: comparison between adult human endothelial and mesothelial cells. *Ann. Vasc. Surg.*, **3**, 140–145
37. Budd, J. S., Bell, P. R. F. and James, R. F. L. (1989) Attachment of indium-111 labelled endothelial cells to pretreated polytetrafluoroethylene vascular grafts. *Br. J. Surg.*, **76**, 1259–1261
38. Clyne, C. A. C., Archer, T. J., Atuhaine, L. K. *et al.* (1987) Random controlled trial of a short course of aspirin and dipyridamole (Persantin) for femoro-distal grafts. *Br. J. Surg.*, **74**, 246–248
39. Kretschmer, G., Wenzl, E., Schimper, M. *et al.* (1988) Influence of post-operative anticoagulant treatment on patient survival after femoropopliteal vein bypass surgery. *Lancet*, **i**, 797–799

Chapter 13

Vascular surgical sepsis – challenges in prevention

Jonathan D. Beard and Colin C. Wilmshurst

Vascular reconstructive surgery is classified as a clean procedure, yet wound infection is surprisingly common. This may cause considerable prolongation of hospital stay[1]. Infection of the prosthetic graft itself is much more serious. Although graft infection is rare it is associated with a high morbidity and mortality. Amputation rates of 17–79% and mortality rates of 17–26% after prosthetic graft infection have been reported[2–4].

Incidence of infection

There is a wide variation in the reported wound infection rates after vascular surgery, ranging from less than 1% to 22%. Much of this variation can be explained by differences in the case mix and risk factors. For instance, many studies of infection after vascular surgery exclude patients with distal skin necrosis which is known to be a significant risk factor[5–7]. The reported incidence of graft infection is lower, at 1–6%. Differences in the definition of wound and graft infection have also contributed to the difficulty in assessing true incidence. Szilagyi et al.[8] introduced a grading system for infections which has been used to standardize other series. Grades I and II were confined to the dermis and subcutaneous tissues and Grade III involved the prosthesis itself. For Grade III infections, incidence of less than 1% for aortoiliac grafts, 1.5% for aortofemoral grafts and 3% for prosthetic femoropopliteal grafts have been reported.

The variation in the time of onset of a clinical graft infection also makes assessment of the true incidence more difficult. For femoropopliteal grafts, the time lapse before infection becomes clinically obvious is usually short, often within one month, whereas aortic graft infections may manifest themselves many months or even years after the initial surgery[9].

Microbiology

Many bacteria have been implicated in prosthetic graft infections[3,8,10–16]. These series have been combined to produce the 'league table of bacteria' in Table 13.1. Staphylococci accounted for almost half of all graft infections. Coagulase-positive staphylococcal infections tend to present fairly soon after the initial operation

Table 13.1   Bacteria implicated in prosthetic graft infection

Organism	Incidence in graft infections (%)
Staphylococci (coagulase + ve and − ve)	44
Proteus	11
Escherichia coli	10
Streptococcus faecalis	8
Pseudomonas	7
Serratia marcescens	5
Klebsiella and Corynebacterium	4
Bacteroides	3
Streptococcus viridans	1
Diphtheroides	1
Salmonella	1

whereas the coagulase-negative species tend to present later. This may reflect their lower virulence.

It is dangerous to assume that because a culture has been reported as negative for bacterial growth, pathogenic organisms are not present. Positive culture in suspected graft infection depends on how hard it is sought: most vascular surgeons have encountered the persistent 'sterile' graft seroma which eventually reveals itself as an infection. The difficulty in obtaining a positive culture may be due to the protective effect of the bacterial glycocalyx[17] which consists of a mass of polysaccharides projecting from the surface of the bacteria and binds the bacteria to the graft so that there may be few free bacteria in the perigraft fluid (Figure 13.1). Several reported

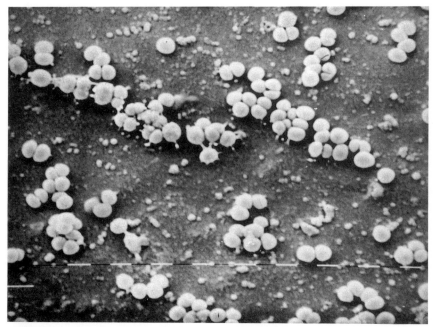

Figure 13.1   Scanning electron photomicrograph showing staphylococci adhering to a smooth surface. The bacteria initially adhere by means of visible pseudopodia and subsequently by production of mucus

series of infected grafts record an incidence of up to 20% 'no bacterial growth' from swabs. Aspiration of fluid or tissue from around the graft rather than simple culture swabs improves the detection rate. Ultrasonic disruption of the glycocalyx with subsequent release of organisms can also aid identification.

Origin of infection

The possible sources of graft infection are listed in Table 13.2. Although there are many possible sources of infection the most common mechanism appears to be implantation at the time of surgery of organisms from the patient's skin. The groin is particularly prone to infection because it is commonly contaminated with bowel organisms related to the anogenital region. An alternative theory is that groin infections are due to bacteria arising from divided lymphatics in patients with distal skin sepsis[18]. However, clinical studies do not support this theory[19,20].

Non-sterility of prosthetic grafts must be exceedingly rare. Two studies of intraoperative bacterial contamination of grafts have not shown a single contaminated dry graft ([21]; Barrie, 1990, personal communication) which is not surprising, as most prosthetic graft materials, being non-biological, are easily sterilized. Once the graft is wetted and handled it is a different story, as 55–80% of grafts become contaminated ([21]; Barrie 1990, personal communication). Coagulase-negative staphylococci consistent with the patient's skin flora are the most frequent contaminants. Wooster et al.[21] were able to reduce the contamination rate to 35% by changing gloves before handling the graft. Barrie (1990, personal communication) was unable to correlate glove punctures with graft contamination, again implicating the patient's own skin flora as the source of the contamination.

The other less common, but well-recognized, source of infection is the artery to which the graft is sutured. Although the mycotic aneurysms that occur in Salmonellosis and intravenous drug abusers are well recognized, there is increasing evidence that the walls of atherosclerotic arteries can also harbour bacteria[22]. The organism most prevalent in the aortic wall is again the coagulase-negative staphylococcus. This is an aerobic bacterium, but can also be a facultative anaerobe and lie deep in the atherosclerotic arterial wall for many years. Figures for positive arterial wall cultures vary from 20–80%. The higher figure reflects the sophisticated techniques employed by some surgeons and microbiologists to detect bacteria that may be scanty and difficult to culture.

The postoperative outcome for a patient with a positive arterial wall culture may be compromised. Malone et al.[23] found that five out of seven patients with positive aortic wall cultures who received short-term broad-spectrum antibiotics for less than

Table 13.2   Possible sources of prosthetic graft infection

Unsterile graft
Infected artery
Patient's skin
Surgeon's hands
Perforated viscera
Severed lymphatics
Recent arteriography
Blood-borne

ten days died of aortic disruption and haemorrhage. None of the six patients with positive cultures treated with high dose culture-specific intravenous antibiotics for six weeks, followed by oral antibiotics for six months died. There were no cases of infected grafts in patients with negative aortic wall cultures. It is interesting to note that organisms in the aortic wall and subsequent graft infections only matched in 48% of cases.

A more recent study again isolated bacterial pathogens from the aortic wall during aneurysm repair in 28 of 90 patients, but this was not a significant risk factor for subsequent graft infection[24]. All patients received routine broad-spectrum antibiotic prophylaxis and prolongation beyond 24 hours did not appear necessary.

Most aortic graft infections by bowel organisms are probably caused by contamination at the time of surgery. A likely source of this contamination is an inadvertent needlestick injury to the bowel, especially the duodenum. Although this is unlikely to cause leakage of bowel contents, the needle might well be a source of infection if used to suture the graft. The greatest risk appears to arise when the retroperitoneum is repaired after insertion of the graft. The duodenum is also at particular risk of damage during repair of an inflammatory aneurysm as there is often no easy plane of dissection between the two. The use of plastic bags to contain the small bowel during aortic surgery is common but the transudate can harbour bacteria[25].

Most patients undergoing vascular surgery will have received an arteriogram, usually via the femoral artery, sometimes beforehand. Landrenau and Raju[26] found an increased rate of wound infection after bypass surgery following femoral arteriography. They recommended that if the same femoral vessel used for arteriography is to be the site of anastomosis using prosthetic material, then the operation should be carried out within 24 hours or delayed until the puncture wound is healed. However, Bunt[27] could find no correlation between groin infection following peripheral revascularization and ipsilateral transfemoral arteriography.

Early graft infection often follows local wound sepsis[28], and even late graft infection may be due to prolonged infection by an organism of low virulence implanted at the time of surgery. Blood-borne graft infections are not often documented but may be another cause of late graft sepsis.

Canine experiments[29] have shown that prosthetic grafts challenged at progressive time intervals with a single intravenous infusion of *Staphylococcus aureus* were nearly all infected up to one month postoperatively. The incidence then fell but was still 30% at one year. The grafts were examined three weeks after the infusion, and every graft with complete pseudoendothelial coverage was free from infection.

Risk factors

Many of the risk factors for the development of wound or graft infection after vascular surgery have already been mentioned. In general terms, the risk factors can be related to:

- The patient
- The operation
- The graft

Elderly, malnourished and diabetic patients have been shown to have an increased susceptibility to infection[3]. Earnshaw *et al.*[30] studied the risk factors for sepsis after vascular surgery in 100 patients with lower limb ischaemia. Wound infections occurred in 19% overall and was significantly higher in patients with rest pain or necrosis than those with claudication or aneurysms. Pathogenic organisms on the skin were also found more commonly in patients with rest pain and necrosis. In a review of 163 femoropopliteal vein grafts, Wengrovitz[31] found that positive patient-related risk factors for wound infection included women, diabetes, steroid therapy and an ipsilateral leg ulcer.

Deficient surgical technique is probably the most important operative factor, although the incidence of prosthetic graft infection does appear to be higher for aortofemoral and femoropopliteal grafts than for aortic or aortoiliac grafts[8]. This difference is probably explained by the groin dissection but in the femoropopliteal group there are other factors such as the larger proportion of patients with diabetes, rest pain and necrosis. Hazards of surgery associated with increased wound infection rates are listed in Table 13.3[2,3,31–34].

Views differ on the risk of abdominal aortic aneurysm repair combined with biliary or gastrointestinal surgery. Bickerstaff et al.[35] reviewed 563 aortic aneurysm repairs at the Mayo clinic and found only one graft infection out of 113 patients who had undergone an additional non-vascular procedure including cholecystectomy, appendicectomy and small bowel resection. However, there was a trend in the group towards a higher rate of complications related to the additional procedure. In a recent review, Tennant and Baird[36] reported no graft infections in a series of 247 aortic aneurysm repairs which included 13 combined cholecystectomies and one gastronomy. However, the incidence of other complications, especially haemorrhage related to heparinization, was high.

Most series of graft infections report a far higher risk for prosthetic than for vein grafts. Not only are the hazards of infection greater in patients with prosthetic grafts, but the artificial material itself may enhance bacterial infectivity[1]. Autologous vein grafts are remarkably resistant to infection even in the presence of a major wound infection. Although the vein itself is resistant, the same may not be true of the material used to ligate the tributaries. It is important to use non-absorbable ligatures or clips as absorbable materials degrade more quickly in the presence of infection and may result in secondary haemorrhage.

Adherence of bacteria to prosthetic materials has been studied recently[37,38]. Woven and knitted Dacron prostheses have rough surfaces which enable bacteria to adhere to them more easily than to the relatively smooth surface of polytetrafluoroethylene (PTFE) grafts. PTFE is more hydrophobic than Dacron which tends to reduce bacterial adherence. When PTFE, woven and knitted velour Dacron grafts were inoculated with *Staphylococcus aureus*, *Staphylococcus epidermidis*, mucin-secreting

Table 13.3 Operative risk factors associated with an increased infection rate after vascular surgery

Groin incision
Simultaneous gastrointestinal or biliary surgery
Skin flap necrosis
Haematoma/heparin
Seroma/lymph leak
Inaccurate skin apposition
Long leg incision
In situ/distal grafts
Reoperative surgery
Early graft thrombosis

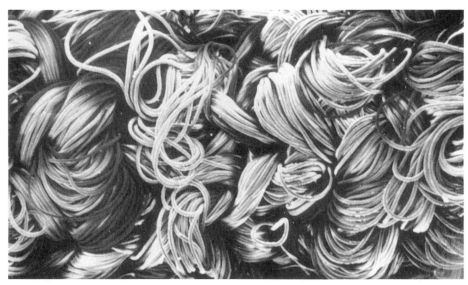

Figure 13.2   Scanning electron photomicrograph of a velour Dacron graft. The large surface area aids tissue incorporation but may also permit easier colonization by bacteria. (Reproduced by permission of Vascutek Ltd)

Staphylococcus epidermidis and *Escherichia coli*, all four species adhered more readily to Dacron than to PTFE[37]. *E. coli* and *Staph. aureus* adhered in greater numbers to knitted velour than to woven Dacron (Figure 13.2). The secretion of mucus enables *Staph. epidermidis* to adhere much more easily to both PTFE and Dacron grafts. Bacterial adherence to untreated knitted velour Dacron is greater than to clotted or albumin-coated Dacron[38].

Once bacteria, protected by their glycocalyx are established in the interstices of a graft, it seems unlikely that they could be eradicated by antibiotics alone.

Prevention of infection

Just as the aetiology of infection is multifactoral, there is no single solution to the prevention of vascular surgical sepsis. If the major cause is endogenous infection then reducing the number of skin pathogens should be beneficial. Several studies have demonstrated a reduction in bacterial skin colonization and wound infection rates after preoperative chlorhexidine baths or showers[39–41]. However, Earnshaw *et al.* did not confirm this benefit in a small UK trial of patients undergoing vascular surgery[20].

The best method of skin preparation immediately before surgery is also unclear, although there is some evidence that povidone–iodine is more effective than chlorhexidine and ethanol preparations[5,42]. The use of iodine-impregnated incise drapes and impervious disposable drapes may also reduce the risk of prosthetic contamination by endogenous skin pathogens. Biogel gloves (LRC Products Ltd) as well as being powder-free, also contain an antiseptic, cetylpyridinium chloride. This has been shown to reduce significantly the postoperative bacterial counts from the hands and gloves compared with plain gloves[43].

The use of prophylactic antibiotics during vascular surgery seems entirely justified because of the documented risk of preoperative bacterial contamination of a prosthesis ([21]; Barrie, 1990, personal communication), and the dire consequences of any subsequent infection. Many randomized trials of various parenteral prophylactic antibiotics have shown a reduction in wound, but not graft infections. Agents shown to be effective include cephazolin[5], cefotaxime[43a], cefuroxime[33], netilimicin plus methicillin[44] and amoxycillin/clavulanate[45].

No trial has shown any one agent to be superior, but a broad-spectrum agent with activity against coagulase-negative staphylococci seems appropriate[46]. It is unlikely that the effect of prophylactic antibiotics on graft sepsis will ever be known as studies would require thousands of patients followed over many years. However, as antibiotic prophylaxis has been shown to reduce wound infection, a major risk factor for graft infection it is logical to expect it to be beneficial.

Many vascular surgeons in the UK employ a regime of cefuroxime or amoxycillin/ clavulanate at induction of anaesthesia followed by two postoperative doses. However, the use of more than one dose of antibiotic for prophylaxis has recently been criticized[47]. There is little evidence that multiple doses have any benefit and in fact they may result in the proliferation of resistant organisms[33]. Continuation of therapy with culture-specific antibiotics does seem indicated if the patient has severe sepsis and if an aortic wall culture is positive[23]. Antibiotic prophylaxis may be less vital where autogenous vein is used[7]. Direct perioperative instillation of antibiotic solutions seems to be of no additional benefit[6] but antibiotic-bonded prosthetic grafts appear an attractive proposition for the future[48].

Patients with prosthetic grafts should be considered 'at risk' from bacteraemia for life and should receive prompt treatment of any pyogenic infections and antibiotic prophylaxis for invasive procedures in a similar manner to those with heart valve replacements[49]. A single oral dose of a cephalosporin or amoxycillin/clavulanate before the procedure seems appropriate.

Careful surgical technique is probably an important factor in avoiding sepsis after vascular surgery but this is extremely difficult to prove. It seems sensible to use a no-touch technique when handling prosthetic grafts and to avoid allowing them to touch the skin. Bowel should be handled gently and if a bowel bag is used the transudate should not be returned to the peritoneal cavity as it can contain bacteria[25]. Haemostasis is also important, as a haematoma around the graft, like a seroma, predisposes to infection and prolongs the time to tissue incorporation of the graft.

It is worth remembering that oxidized cellulose haemostatic sponge has an antibacterial action whereas gelatin sponge does not[50]. Vacuum drains are often employed in the groin wound after vascular surgery to reduce the risk of haematoma and seroma; however, a recent randomized trial of drainage versus no drainage showed no difference in lymph leakage, haematoma or wound infection[51]. It is also common practice to wrap the graft in the aneurysm sac after aortic aneurysm repair, the aim being to reduce the incidence of secondary aortoduodenal fistula. The wisdom of wrapping a potentially infected aortic wall around the graft ought to be questioned: covering the graft with omentum could be a better alternative.

Autogenous vein must be regarded as the graft of choice for infrainguinal reconstruction if graft infection is a major consideration. However, this must be balanced against a higher rate of wound infections which accompany the necessarily larger incision and longer operation. When only small patches of graft are required, as for a profundoplasty, it also seems sensible to use vein if possible. If a prosthetic graft is required then PTFE appears to be more resistant to infection than Dacron[37] but it is less suitable for suprainguinal reconstruction. Coated Dacron may also be more resistant to infection

The risk of concomitant biliary or upper gastrointestinal surgery appears small, but is probably best avoided unless it is absolutely necessary, and Thomas[52] gives excellent guidelines on this subject. There is also some evidence that aneurysm rupture can be precipitated postoperatively if the other coexisting pathological problem is dealt with first[53].

In summary, the causes and prevention of infection after vascular surgery are multifactorial. Because of this, and the low incidence of graft infection, it is difficult to come to any definite conclusions. However, prophylactic antibiotics and careful surgical techniques are probably the keys to a successful outcome.

References

1. Johnson, J. A., Cogbill, J. J., Strutt, P. J. and Grundersen, A. L. (1988) Wound complications after infrainguinal bypass: Classification, predisposing factors and management. *Arch. Surg.*, **123**, 859–862
2. Lorentzen, J. E., Nielsen, O. M., Arendrup, H., Kimose, H. H., Bille, S. (1985) Vascular graft infection: An analysis of sixty two graft infections in 2411 consecutive implanted synthetic vascular grafts. *Surgery*, **98**, 81–86
3. Edwards, W. H., Martin, R. S., Jenkins, J. M., Edwards, W. H. and Mulherin, J. L. (1987) Primary graft infections. *J. Vasc. Surg.*, **6**, 235–239
4. Kitka, M. J., Goodson, S. F., Bishara, R. A., Meyer, J. P., Schuler, J. J. and Flanigan, D. P. (1987) Mortality and limb loss with infected infrainguinal bypass grafts. *J. Vasc. Surg.*, **5**, 566–571
5. Kaiser, A. S., Clayson, K. R., Mulherin, J. L., Roach, A. C., Allen, T. R. *et al.* (1978) Antibiotic prophylaxis in vascular surgery. *Ann. Surg.*, **188** (3), 283–287
6. Pitt, H. A., Postier, R. G., MacGowan, A. W., Frank, L. W., Surmak, A. J. *et al.* (1980) Prophylactic antibiotics in vascular surgery. Topical, systemic or both? *Ann. Surg.*, **192**, 356–364
7. Walker, M., Litherland, H. K., Murphy, J. and Smith, J. A. (1984) Comparison of prophylactic antibiotic regimes in patients undergoing vascular surgery. *J. Hosp. Infect.*, **5**, (suppl. A), 101–106
8. Szilagyi, D. E., Smith, R. F., Elliot, J. P. and Vrandecic, M. P. (1972) Infection in arterial reconstruction with synthetic grafts. *Ann. Surg.*, **176**(3), 321–333
9. Lieweg, W. G. and Greenfield, L. J. (1977) Vascular prosthetic infections: collected experience and results of treatment. *Surgery*, **81**, 335–342
10. Reinaerts, H. (1985) Infection in vascular grafting In *Proceedings of the 3rd Vascutek International Symposium*, pp. 168–175
11. Conn, J. H., Hardy, J. D., Chavez, C. M. and Fain, W. R. (1970) Infected arterial grafts. *Ann. Surg.*, **171** (5), 705–714
12. Jamieson, G. G., DeWeese, J. A. and Robb, C. G. (1975) Infected arterial grafts. *Ann. Surg.*, **6**, 850–852
13. Bandyk, D. F., Berni, G. A., Thiele, B. L. and Towne, J. B. (1984) Aortofemoral graft infection due to Staphylococcus epidermidis. *Arch. Surg.*, **119** (1), 102–108
14. Doscher, W., Kristinasastry, K. V. and Deckoff, St. L. (1987) Fungal graft infections: Case report and review of the literature. *J. Vasc. Surg.*, **6**, 398–402
15. Mannion, P. T., Thom, B. T., Reynolds, C. S. and Strachan, C. J. L. (1989) The Acquisition of antibiotic resistant coagulase-negative staphylococci by aortic graft recipients. *J. Hosp. Infect.*, **14**, 313–323
16. Wakefield, T. W., Pierson, C. L., Schaberg, D. R., Messina, L. M., Lindenauer, S. M. *et al.* (1990) Artery, periarterial adipose tissue and blood microbiology during vascular reconstructive surgery: perioperative and early post operative observations. *J. Vasc. Surg.*, **11** (5), 624–629
17. Costerton, J. W., Geesey, G. G. and Cheng, K. J. (1978) How bacteria stick. *Scientific American*, **238**, 86–95
18. Bunt, T. J. and Mohr, J. D. (1984) Incidence of positive inguinal lymph node culture during peripheral re-vascularisation. *Am. Surg.*, **50** (10), 522–523
19. Weaver, P. C., Chattopadhyay, B. and Angel, J. (1973) An investigation into the spread of bacterial infection in lower-limb amputations. *Br. J. Surg.*, **60**, 723–729
20. Earnshaw, J. J., Berridge, D. C., Slack, R. C. B., Makin, G. S. and Hopkinson, B. R. (1989) Do pre-operative chlorhexidine baths reduce the risk of infection after vascular reconstruction? *Eur. J. Vasc. Surg.*, **3**, 323–326

21. Wooster, D. L., Louch, R. E. and Krajden, S. (1985) Intraoperative bacterial contamination of vascular grafts: a prospective study. *Can. J. Surg.*, **28**, 407–409

22. Lalka, S. G., Malone, J. M., Fisher, D. F., Bernhard, V. M., Sullivan, D. *et al.* (1989) Efficiency of prophylactic antibiotics in vascular surgery: An arterial wall microbiologic and pharmacokinetic perspective. *J. Vasc. Surg.*, **10**, 501–509

23. Malone, J. M., Lalka, S. G., McIntyre, K. E., Bernhard, V. M. and Pabst, T. S. (1988) The necessity for long-term antibiotic therapy with positive arterial wall cultures. *J. Vasc. Surg.*, **8**, 262–267

24. Brandimarte, C., Santini, C., Venditti, M., Baiocchi, P., Serra, P. *et al.* (1989) Clinical significance of intra-operative cultures of aneurysm walls and contents in elective abdominal aortic aneurysmectomy. *Eur. J. Epidemiol.*, **5**, 521–525

25. Russell, H. E., Barnes, R. W. and Baker, W. H. (1975) Sterility of intestinal transudate during aortic reconstructive procedures. *Arch. Surg.*, **110**, 402

26. Landreneau, M. D. and Raju, S. (1981) Infections after elective bypass surgery for lower limb ischaemia: the influence of preoperative transcutaneous arteriography. *Surgery*, **90**, 956–961

27. Bunt, T. J. (1986) Sources of Staphylococcus epidermidis at the inguinal incision during peripheral revascularisation. *Am. Surg.*, **52**, 472–473

28. Moore, W. S. (1982) Pathogenosis of vascular graft sepsis. In *Extra-anatomic and secondary arterial reconstruction* (ed. R. M. Greenhalgh). Pitman, London, pp. 1–9

29. Malone, J. M., Moore, W. S., Campagna, G. and Bean, B. (1975) Bacteremic infectability of vascular grafts: the influence of pseudointimal integrity and duration of graft function. *Surgery*, **78**, 211–216

30. Earnshaw, J. J., Slack, R. C. B., Hopkinson, B. R. and Makin, G. S. (1988) Risk factors in vascular surgical sepsis. *Ann. R. Coll. Surg. Eng.*, **70**, 139–143

31. Wengrovitz, M., Atnip, R. G., Gifford, R. R., Neumyer, M. M., Heitjan, D. F. and Thiele, B. L. (1980) Wound complications of autogenous subcutaneous infrainguinal arterial bypass surgery; predisposing factors and management. *J. Vasc. Surg.*, **11**, 156–161

32. Goldstone, J. and Moore, W. S. (1974) Infection in vascular prostheses. Clinical manifestations and surgical management. *Am. J. Surg.*, **128**, 225–233

33. Hesselgren, P. O., Invarsson, L., Risberg, B. and Seeman, T. (1984) Effects of prophylactic antibodies in vascular surgery. A prospective, randomised, double-blind study. *Ann. Surg.*, **200**, 86–92

34. Durham, J. R., Malone, J. M. and Bernhard, V. M. (1987) The impact of multiple operations on the importance of arterial wall cultures. *J. Vasc. Surg.*, **5**, 106–169

35. Bickerstaff, L. K., Hollier, L. H., Van Peenen, H. J., Melton, L. J., Pairolero, P. C. and Cherry, K. J. (1984) Abdominal aortic aneurysm repair combined with a second surgical procedure – Morbidity and Mortality. *Surgery*, **95**, 487–491

36. Tennant, W. G. and Baird, R. N. (1990) Second intra-abdominal pathology: Concomitant or sequential surgery? In *Care and Management of Aneurysms* (eds R. M. Greenhalgh and J. A. Mannick). Saunders, London, pp 321–326

37. Schmitt, D. D., Bandyk, D. F., Pequet, A. J. and Towne, J. B. (1986) Bacterial adherence to vascular prosthesis. *J. Vasc. Surg.*, **3**, 732–740

38. Siverhus, D. J., Schmitt, D. D., Edmiston, C. E., Bandyk, D. F., Seabrook, G. R. *et al.* (1990) Adherence of mucin and non mucin producing staphylococci to preclotted and albumin-coated velour knitted vascular grafts. *Surgery*, **107**, 613–619

39. Hayek, L. J., Emerson, J. M. and Gardner, A. M. N. (1987) A placebo controlled trial of the effect of two preoperative baths or showers with chlorhexide detergent on postoperative wound infection rates. *J. Hosp. Infect.*, **10**, 165–172

40. Newson, S. W. B. and Rowland, C. (1988) Studies of perioperative skin flora. *J. Hosp. Infect.*, **11** (suppl. B), 21–26

41. Holm, J. (1985) Wound and graft infection. Clinical aspects and prophylaxis. *Acta Chir. Scand.*, **529** (suppl.), 37–39

42. Rotter, M., Koller, W. and Wewalka, G. (1980) Providone–iodine and chlorhexidine gluconate-containing detergents for disinfection of hands. *J. Hosp. Infect.*, **1**, 149–158

43. Newsom, S. W. B. (1987) Microbiological aspects of surgical practice. In *Risks and complications. The patient and Surgeon in theatre*, The Medicine Group, Oxford, pp. 14–15

43a. Salzmann, G. (1983) Perioperative infection prophylaxis in vascular surgery – a randomised prospective study. *Thorac. Cardiovasc. Surg.*, **31**, 239–242

44. Worning, A. M., Frimodt-Møller, N., Ostri, P., Nilsson, T., Højholdt, K. and Frimodt-Møller, C. (1986) Antibiotic prophylaxis in vascular reconstructive surgery: a double-blind placebo-controlled study. *J. Antimicrob. Chemother.*, **17**, 105–113

45. Dieterich, H. J., Groh, J., Behringer, K., Lauterjung, L. and Martin, E. (1989) The prophylactic activity of amoxycillin/clavulanate and cefoxitin in vascular surgery – a randomized clinical study. *J. Antimicrob. Chemother.*, **24** (supp. B), 209–211

46. Pollock, A. V. (1988) Surgical prophylaxis – the emerging picture. *Lancet*, 225–229
47. Daschner, F. D. (1986) Single or multiple dose antibiotic prophylaxis? *J. Hosp. Infect.*, **7**, 307–308
48. Webb, L. X., Myers, R. T., Cordell, A. R., Hobgood, C. D., Costerton, J. W. and Gristina, A. G. (1986) Inhibition of bacteria adhesion by antibacterial surface pre-treatment of vascular prostheses. *J. Vasc. Surg.*, **4**, 16–21
49. Working Party of the British Society for Antimicrobial Chemotherapy (1982) The antibiotic prophylaxis of infective endocarditis. *Lancet*, **ii**, 1323–1326
50. Dineen, P. (1976) Antibacterial activity of oxidised regenerated cellulose. *Surg. Gynecol. Obstet.*, **142**, 481
51. Dunlop, M. G., Fox, J. N., Stonebridge, P. A., Clason, A. E. and Rockley, C. V. (1990) Vacuum drainage of groin wounds after vascular surgery: a controlled trial. *Br. J. Surg.*, **77**, 562–563.
52. Thomas, J. H. (1989) Abdominal aortic aneurysmorrhaphy combined with biliary or gastrointestinal surgery, (1989) *Surg. Clin. N. Am.*, **69** (4) 807–815
53. Swanson, R. J., Littooy, F. N. and Hunt, T. K. (1980) Laparotomy as a precipitating factor in the rupture of intra abdominal aneurysms. *Arch. Surg.*, **115**, 299

Chapter 14

The popliteal artery – sinister harbinger of pathology

P. Michael Perry

The popliteal artery measures 15–20 cm and is the continuation of the femoral artery. It traverses the popliteal fossa, commencing at the adductor magnus opening and dividing into the anterior tibial and posterior tibial arteries at the lower border of the popliteus. The peroneal artery arises 2.5 cm below the lower border of the popliteus as a branch of the posterior tibial artery. The popliteal artery is relatively fixed at its origin and at its termination as the anterior tibial artery penetrates the interosseous membrane. Further restriction in mobility occurs because of geniculate and muscular branches. With the knee joint in extension the popliteal artery runs parallel to the long axis of the femur and tibia, but with flexion the artery becomes lengthened relative to the posterior surface of the bones, and, allowing for its position in the popliteal fossa, the redundant artery will become tortuous. During the process of ageing, atheromatous arteries lose their elasticity and do not bend so easily, thus being more liable to kinking and luminal obstruction. It is this constant knee flexion–extension which encourages turbulent blood flow in a diseased vessel, facilitating the presence of thrombus. Atheromatous stenoses of the femoral artery are common at the site of the adductor hiatus and may be followed by a post-stenotic dilatation, which can conceivably lead to aneurysmal formation. The popliteal artery is also vulnerable to trauma, entrapment due to a congenital anatomical variation, cystic disease of the adventitia or subject to rare tumours.

Popliteal aneurysm

Introduction

Popliteal aneurysm surgery has a long history[1]. As long ago as the 3rd century AD Antyllus, of ancient Greece, ligated the artery above and below the lesion and then evacuated its contents. A century later Philagrius of Macedonia excised the sac after tying both ends of the artery. As the years went by the technique was gradually improved and in 1875 Desault left the sac untouched, having tied the upper pole of the aneurysm. Six months later John Hunter, in his famous operation, ligated the superficial femoral artery in the subsartorial canal and left the aneurysm alone. It is true to reflect that Hunter did not appreciate the importance of the development of a collateral circulation, particularly to the extent of preserving an adequate blood supply to preserve a limb.

Hunter, curiously, remained reticent concerning his famous case. Only just before his death were the details of the patient published by his brother-in-law assistant, Everard Home. A 45-year-old coachman had noticed an enlarging swelling for three years, and under tourniquet application (not tightened so as to leave the parts in their natural position) a double ligature was passed and tied just enough to compress the sides together. A similar application was made lower down. The patient died of unrelated causes 15 months later.

In the next century Matas[2] drew attention to a 10% incidence of distal gangrene after Hunterian ligation; his own contribution being that of endoaneurysmorrhaphy. In this operation the aneurysm is incised and all the vessel apertures opening into it are obliterated without actually damaging the vessels themselves.

Dissatisfaction with all these procedures prompted Pringle to try vein grafting, and in 1913 he described two cases of vein bypass below the aneurysm with good results[3]. The present results of vein grafting have been successful due to aseptic technique, antibiotic cover, use of heparin and improved anaesthesia.

General aspects

Aneurysms of the popliteal arteries are predominantly diseases of men[4]. They have an atherosclerotic aetiology but may be caused by bacterial infections, syphilis or associated with Marfan's syndrome[5]. Most patients present between 50–80 years of age and may have associated extrapopliteal aneurysms[6]. Aneurysms vary in size between 1 and 15 cm[6,7] and most patients are heavy cigarette smokers[6]. Between 1964 and 1979 in Detroit[8] 62 patients with 87 popliteal aneurysms were admitted: this represents one admission for popliteal artery aneurysm for 5000 general patient admissions per year and one popliteal for every 15 aortic aneurysms. During 1989 (Table 14.1) only four patients with popliteal aneurysms were admitted to a district general hospital in Portsmouth, with a district population of 550 000. Fifty-one patients with abdominal aortic aneurysms were admitted during this time.

The clinical diagnosis is based on a high index of suspicion. The physical findings of an aneurysm are often missed. Unless the popliteal arteries are carefully palpated and the widening of the pulse noted, the diagnosis will not be considered on routine physical examination. Even when the patient presents with an ischaemic leg, diagnosis may not be apparent in men with small thrombosed aneurysms[7]. Patients with bilateral popliteal aneurysms are more likely to have an associated abdominal aortic aneurysm than those with a solitary popliteal lesion (69% compared with 32%)[9]. The presence of extrapopliteal aneurysmal disease may be a good prognostic factor, as patients with generalized arteriomegaly carry a lower risk of thrombosis[9].

The diagnosis of a popliteal aneurysm usually arises as a result of increased clinical suspicion, particularly when the patient has generalized arteriomegaly or has presented with symptoms or signs referrable to a thrombosed limb artery. B-Mode ultrasound scanning is an accurate method of determining the size of the aneurysm in addition to confirming the diagnosis[8]; Duplex scanning will give more information

Table 14.1   Patients admitted with arterial disease to surgical wards, Portsmouth 1989

Disease type	No. admitted
All arterial disease	429
Aortic aneurysm (hot and cold)	51
Popliteal aneurysm	4

about the nature of clot in the aneurysm (Figure 14.1). The delineation of the anatomical relations of the artery may be better served by MRI or CT, especially in complicated large aneurysms. Arteriography[10] and digital subtraction angiography may be misleading as in demonstrating the diameter of the lumen of the aneurysm, reduced to near normality by intra-aneurysmal thrombus, the very presence of the aneurysm will remain unrecognized.

Symptomatic popliteal aneurysms

Popliteal aneurysms have a reputation for causing limb-threatening complications. They have been aptly described as 'sinister harbingers of sudden catastrophe'[11], and 60% present symptomatically as a result of acute thrombosis with resultant distal ischaemia or chronic ischaemia with intermittent claudication[7]. Less frequently the patient complains of the effects of pressure from an enlarging aneurysm or even rupture[7]. Distal embolization gives rise to progressive occlusion of the tibial vessels or may be asymptomatic until critical ischaemia occurs (Figure 14.2). Symptomatic patients may be conveniently divided into six clinical groups:

1. acute thrombosis
2. chronic thrombosis
3. acute embolism
4. chronic embolism
5. local pressure symptoms
6. rupture

These patient groups are diagnosed clinically, by ultrasound, by arteriography or latterly by CT or MRI. All major studies[1,6–8,11–16] have indicated an amputation rate of at least 20% but the advent of treatment by thrombolysis has been encouraging[17–21].

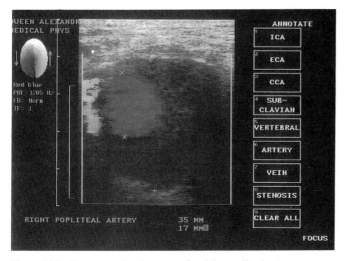

Figure 14.1 Transverse Duplex scan of a right popliteal artery aneurysm measuring 35 mm diameter, with an eccentric lumen of 17 mm diameter

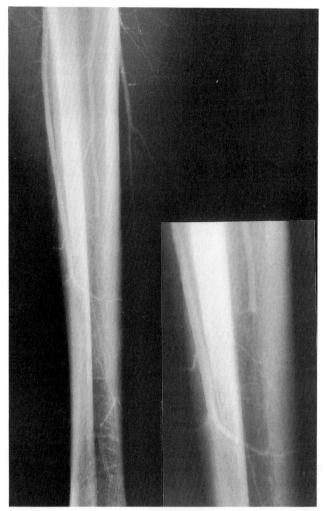

Figure 14.2   Angiogram demonstrating embolization of distal vessels

Group 1: acute thrombosis

The aneurysm presents as a complete occlusion of the popliteal artery with little or no distal runoff. Operative mortality in this group may be 5%[16] but the best results are obtained by using autologous long saphenous vein grafts giving a patency rate of at least 70%. This is best achieved by an end-to-end anastomosis after ligation of the aneurysm[16]. Dacron grafting does not give as good a five-year patency and the amputation rate in this group is high, 20–50%[16,21]. The size of the aneurysm may preclude an end-to-end anastomosis and distal segment *in situ* vein grafting may be indicated. Division of the medial head of gastrocnemius and an inlay type of anastomosis may be helpful in a tight popliteal fossa.

The successful management of thrombosed popliteal aneurysms by arteriography and low dose intra-arterial streptokinase was first described in 1984[17]. A 61-year-old man was admitted with a four-day history of sudden onset of coldness in his left foot. Ultrasound confirmed a 4 cm swelling and a femoral ateriogram showed total occlusion of the popliteal artery just above the knee joint. An infusion of 5000 units/h streptokinase was started and within 14 hours the runoff vessels were open and the popliteal aneurysm was seen to contain residual clot. A further four-hour infusion of streptokinase resulted in all the clot being lysed. Six hours after stopping the streptokinase, heparin was given intravenously at 600 units/h. The following day the patient underwent successful reversed small saphenous vein bypass after surgical repair of the aneurysm. The patient was discharged with a warm leg and a good dorsalis pedis pulse. Since then other groups have had similar good results[18–22].

Group 2: chronic thrombosis
In these patients who are claudicating the aneurysms are usually thrombosed, but arteriography will demonstrate a distal circulation which may be amenable to bypass grafting although the results are disappointing. These patients fare better with autologous vein grafting, although the success of surgery depends greatly on the quality of the distal arteries. In a study in Boston of 23 patients[16], 15 were reconstituted employing 12 vein grafts and three Dacron grafts. There was also one elective resection without reconstruction, which failed and led to amputation. Among those with vein grafts, two had unrelieved claudication and one of these had an amputation. The late treatment failures were five vein grafts and one Dacron graft.

Group 3: acute embolism
Unusually the patient presents with an acute distal embolism: in a series of 244 aneurysms[16] only 13 presented in this way. These patients may have generalized arteriomegaly and it may be impossible to know whence the embolism originated[9]. An embolectomy should be performed immediately, and reconstruction with ligation of the aneurysm and vein bypass with an end-to-end anastomosis is the preferred option. Eight vein grafts were used in 13 patients but two early and one late treatment failure resulted in amputations[16].

Group 4: chronic embolism
The patient has claudication, the aneurysm is patent and there is clinical and radiological evidence of previous embolization. Among 19 patients who presented in this way, 12 had reconstruction with vein grafts, five Dacron grafts and two extirpations with primary end-to-end anastomoses[16]. Early treatment failures occurred from two vein grafts, one ending in amputation. One Dacron graft failed but resulted only in unrelieved claudication. There was one late treatment failure following the use of a Dacron graft.

Group 5: local symptoms
Less than 10% of patients will present as a result of pressure symptoms due to the size of the aneurysm[7,16]. Hunterian ligation without bypass will result in a 10% amputation rate[2]. In 11 patients treated by ligation and bypass, three vein grafts were successful but three of the six Dacron grafts failed.

Group 6: rupture
Aneurysm rupture is rare[6,7], although in one study four out of 147 popliteal aneurysms presented with rupture during a 20-year period[14]. Three of the four patients required amputation; the single reconstituted patient maintained a patent graft.
    The medial incision is preferred for most patients. In order to avoid embolization,

it is important to ligate the aneurysm distally, as closely to the dilated segment as possible to allow access to the lower part of the popliteal fossa for bypass. When thrombus is present below the aneurysm, this is removed by an embolectomy catheter[12]. If the aneurysm is large, it should be incised, evacuated and obliterated by suture[12]. Excision of the aneurysm may be dangerous, destroying collateral vessels and damaging the popliteal vein and nerves. One-half of patients on presentation may have complications of the aneurysm itself[6]. Of 233 aneurysms diagnosed between 1961 and 1968, 111 had complications – 65 patients had thromboses, 30 venous occlusion, 28 ulceration or gangrene, 23 peripheral embolism, 15 compression of the popliteal nerves, 11 thrombophlebitis, six had ruptured and two had severe infection. Many had more than one complication.

With the advent of reconstructive arterial surgery, treatment consists ideally of ligation of the aneurysm followed by end-to-end bypass grafting. Patency of at least one tibioperoneal segment has a profound influence on the outcome of surgery and the late patency rate. Postoperative pulse recovery reflects the quality of outflow that can be re-established at the time of popliteal reconstruction and this parameter influences the long-term result of graft replacement more than any other[14]. In this study the 10-year patency was 64% when one or both pedal pulses were restored and the limb salvage rate was 85% when one was restored and 96% when both were restored. In comparison, the late patency rate was 32% for all grafts then available for consideration in extremities that received only an isolated popliteal pulse. Fourteen of 123 limbs managed by graft replacement required amputation during the early postoperative period or within 10 years, and nine of these occurred in the patients who had only received an isolated popliteal pulse. Cumulative patency was significantly superior in extremities with pedal pulses but the value of a good outflow was also reflected in few limbs being lost even after graft occlusion. The collateral circulation is better able to cope after occlusion when there was a good initial outflow.

Good results have been reported using Dacron graft[23], but most studies have shown better 10-year patency rates and limb salvage using autologous vein grafts[4,9,14,16,24]. Of 95 aneurysms, 90% were successfully treated with an amputation rate of 5%[9]. Thirty-two patients had autologous vein grafts with five graft occlusions compared with 60% occlusion of 14 Dacron and nine PTFE grafts. There was one failure of aneurysms treated by excision and end-to-end anastomosis. In a Boston series[16] the cumulative patency of saphenous vein bypass grafting was 77% over a five-year period compared with 29% for Dacron, whereas a 40% total amputation rate was reported, associated with 17 failures of 52 vein grafts and 12 failures of 39 Dacron grafts. In another series[14] there were eight occlusions in 13 PTFE grafts.

Symptomatic aneurysms which are complicated by acute thrombosis with little or no runoff should be investigated by arteriography and treated by intra-arterial infusion of streptokinase, especially if managed within 72 hours of occlusion[22]. Elective reconstruction will give good results in these patients. The aneurysm uncomplicated by acute thrombosis will be appropriately managed by ligation and autologous vein bypass grafting. In the absence of a suitable vein, the use of a venous cuff may well make the use of a prosthetic material justifiable, although in a limb-threatening situation prosthetic grafts *must* be tried as the patency rates are moderately good, depending to a large extent on the patency of the tibial and peroneal vessels.

The operative mortality following bypass surgery after ligation of the aneurysm is low, varying from 1 to 7%[4,15]. However, the late mortality, usually with associated arterial disease, is disappointing: of 87 patients in one series 33 had died within a 14 year period[14]. Lymphoedema was the major complication but was alleviated by leg elevation and prophylactic compression stockings[7]. Graft infection rate is less than 1%[9,15]. False aneurysms have been reported following the use of silk sutures, but recurrence of the disease was not unknown[15].

Asymptomatic popliteal aneurysms

There is considerable conflict in the debate on the need for treatment in the asymptomatic patient. Most authors stress the need for surgery to prevent the onset of limb-threatening complications, but surgery itself may be seen to be harmful and unnecessary[25]. As a policy, why not wait for symptoms to occur and then treat them by thrombolysis[22]? The success of prophylactic surgery in this group must be measured by the operative morbidity on the one hand and the likelihood of symptoms developing if the aneurysm is left untreated on the other. The overall death rate for patients with popliteal aneurysm is greater than for the general population[14], although the myocardial and cerebral morbidity must be considered low for peripheral surgical procedures. Of 147 popliteal aneurysms presenting over a 20-year period, 49 were asymptomatic and 26 were untreated[14]. Eighteen remained asymptomatic but eight (31%) developed limb-threatening complications, four had successful bypasses, two required amputations and two were symptomatic with rest pain but refused surgery[14]. Anton et al.[4] described 77 asymptomatic patients but only 15 were placed under observation and 13 remained asymptomatic, two patients having mild claudication. In another study[9], 46 asymptomatic aneurysms were divided into 20 surgically treated and 26 observed. In this latter group, only two developed thromboses but were successfully treated.

Wychulis et al.[6] studied 94 asymptomatic patients, 27 of whom became symptomatic within seven years with a 3% limb loss. They noted that smaller aneurysms were less likely to cause symptoms. Within seven years, 31 patients had died, four harbouring complicated aneurysms. The remaining 23 of the original 94 became complicated; four were successfully treated by grafting, three remained asymptomatic and the rest had symptoms but were not treated surgically. Szilagyi et al. have recommended that aneurysms of 2 cm or less may be observed, but that aneurysm size may not be a good prognostic indicator, many arteries being smaller than this when complicated by thrombus[7,8]. Reilly et al.[16] described 112 asymptomatic aneurysms of 244 patients during 24 years; 72 were reconstituted with a 97.2% patency. Three patients required amputation following treatment failures. Seventeen patients out of a total of 79 with palpable aneurysms in Dallas, Texas, were asymptomatic[15]. The patients who underwent bypass surgery had a 1.3% mortality and the patency rate was 75%. Between 1975 and 1987, 35 popliteal aneurysms were noted in Oxford[25], 12 of which were symptomless. Equal numbers of symptomless and symptomatic aneurysms were treated surgically. Five symptomless aneurysms were treated conservatively: all remained asymptomatic whereas only four of the asymptomatic group treated surgically remained symptomless within a 2-year period. It was suggested that surgery was harmful in this group. Intra-arterial streptokinase has been used successfully in the treatment of thrombosed popliteal aneurysm[17–21].

Since 1981 a prospective study in Guildford has been carried out in the management of asymptomatic popliteal aneurysm[22]. Since the outset of this study nine patients have presented with acute thrombosis of their aneurysms, all have been evaluated by arteriography and treatment commenced with low dose intra-arterial streptokinase. Early treatment is preferable and if thrombolysis is employed within 72 hours of onset of the arterial occlusions 70–100% lysis may be observed – however, in this study streptokinase was ineffective if attempted 10 or more days after the thrombosis. Three of the six patients treated by thrombolysis had successful elective reconstruction. Significant lysis occurred in one patient, resulting in spontaneous intrapelvic haemorrhage and shock which caused aspiration of vomit. The ensuing Mendelson's syndrome proved fatal. This was the only death in 100 patients treated in that unit[20]. Two other patients were later anticoagulated and patency was maintained. Four of the lysed patients developed complications: two had minor haematomas, one a major haematoma which required evacuation and the fourth patient died. Two of the patients in this study who did not respond to thrombolysis due to their late presentation died at five years without leg ischaemia and the foot ulcer of a ninth patient healed after PFTE grafting and forefoot amputation. Since Schwarz et al. published their first successful case[17], good results have been reported from Australia[18]. In this latter series of 102 patients treated with intra-arterial streptokinase, 37 had occluded vascular grafts and 65 had no previous vascular surgery. Ten patients had thrombosed popliteal aneurysms, only three of whom had been diagnosed previously. The other seven became evident after streptokinase had cleared thrombus from their aneurysms. Three patients lost their legs and seven limbs were saved: five had subsequent elective bypass surgery with aneurysm exclusion and the other two had viable legs without surgery.

The controversy surrounding the management of popliteal aneurysms has been maintained on review of the literature! While it is true that meddlesome surgery can be dangerous the best series suggest that surgery is very successful, with a cumulative patency rate of 96% and no mortality, provided that the aneurysm is ligated and reconstitution is feasible with an autologous vein graft and a patent tibioperoneal trunk[4,25]. The protagonists of a 'watch' policy have to show that their management is utterly feasible. Immediate access to expert personnel for thrombolysis and subsequent surgical management is clearly not the forte of every district general hospital. Conservative management of the patient with an asymptomatic popliteal aneurysm must include regular surveillance, particularly by ultrasound, with expert attention available at short notice for arteriographic and surgical attention. Conservative management must demonstrate a 90% or more patency rate to be a viable alternative to elective surgery. The other question, of course, is what is the place of informed consent if the patient is placed in a study of this sort? However, the natural history of the disease is largely unknown and various risk factors such as aneurysm size have not been studied accurately. A study is being undertaken by the Joint Vascular Research Group UK to evaluate the different sizes of popliteal aneurysm, with particular attention to the likelihood of thrombosis in the larger lesions and to the rate of growth of the smaller ones. It is hoped that this study will help to determine those patients particularly at risk although it is highly likely that the combination of thrombolysis and surgery will be required treatment in most symptomatic patients.

Trauma to the popliteal artery

The popliteal artery is vulnerable to trauma particularly associated with femoral fracture or civil strife[26,27]. Delay in diagnosis of a vascular injury because of the more obvious long bone fracture results in a decreased limb salvage rate. Almost one-third of major military arterial injuries complicate fractures[28].

Because of the need to restore the circulation, arterial repair appears most logical but early fixation of the bone ensures stability of the limb and allows the accurate measurement of the appropriate length of vein graft required for vascular repair. Furthermore, if the bone fragments are not stable, excessive vascular damage will occur even after repair of the artery. The conflict, therefore, is to balance early successful bone stabilization against the need for vascular repair to avoid muscle ischaemia in the limb. Intra-arterial shunting has been shown to allow an adequate circulation during transfer of patients and also during stabilization of the fracture[29]. Indeed, a routine policy of arterial and venous shunting has been adopted in Northern Ireland, with encouraging results[30]. Arterial shunting revitalizes the limb after the artery has been severed and lessens the urgent need to undertake vascular repair. Venous shunting is encouraged when there is combined arterial and venous damage. With massive destruction, reperfusion accomplished by shunting allows demarcation to occur, enabling accurate assessment of the need for debridement; also, if perfusion is adequate, bleeding points will become apparent and better haemostasis will be achieved. The presence of a shunt will allow more time for the use of a suitable vein graft. This may be achieved through a composite vein graft as time may well permit this technique.

If the risk of muscle ischaemia is recognized it is safer to undertake fasciotomy. With major trauma to the leg, it may be sensible to excise the middle third of the fibula to allow decompression of all the muscular compartments of the lower leg. Fasciotomy itself may be complicated by infection and poor healing and there is some evidence that shunting of the artery and vein may decrease the necessity for fasciotomy in some cases[30].

Popliteal artery entrapment

An anomalous course of the popliteal artery may be associated with intermittent claudication, especially in young people, and was first recognized in 1979[31]. In this anomaly whole or part of the medial head of the gastrocnemius compresses the popliteal vessels, bilaterally in 25% of cases[32]. Usually the popliteal artery is the only vessel affected but occasionally both artery and vein are involved. The popliteal artery may be similarly compressed by trauma[33] or previous bypass surgery[34]. As a result of entrapment of the popliteal artery thrombosis, aneurysm formation or vessel sclerosis may occur.

The presentation of intermittent claudication in a young male under 40 years of age should alert the clinician. Rest pain and gangrene are the result of arterial thrombosis. Arteriography will show a medial deviation of the artery, though this may not be conclusive[35]. Computed tomography defines the vascular and muscular anatomy and will demonstrate thrombosed vessels. Investigations of both popliteal fossae in young adults is mandatory[36].

Surgical treatment is concerned with division of the medial head of gastrocnemius with resultant freeing of the popliteal artery and attention to the artery if there are vessel changes. Excision of the thrombosed or aneurysmal vessel and replacement with a vein graft is adequate. The popliteal fossa is best approached posteriorly although a suitable vein is not always in this position.

Early detection of this abnormality is essential. Symptoms may be present for months and the complications of thrombosis and aneurysm formation will result in limb loss[37]. Division of the medial head of gastrocnemius in the asymptomatic limb is recommended to prevent potentially serious complications, but no long-term prospective study has been carried out in asymptomatic patients.

Cystic adventitial disease of the popliteal artery

This unusual disease was first described in 1946 by Atkins and Key[38], although they reported a 'growth' on the external iliac artery. The popliteal artery was first implicated in 1953[39] and up to 1979, 115 cases had been identified throughout the world[40]. This group was followed up by correspondence and 105 patients were studied in detail. The age range was 11–70 years, with a mean of 42 years, there were 83 men and 18 women, the sex not being stated in the remaining four.

The aetiology of this disease remains obscure but repeated trauma to the adventitia by stretching, leading to release of enzymes and the production of acid mucopolysaccharides, may result in the formation of a cystic lesion. Other theories include an embryological origin, of mucin-secreting cells which over the years secrete mucus to eventually cause an arterial stenosis. Shute and Rothnie[41] demonstrated a connection between the cyst and the neighbouring knee joint. They suggested that the pathogenesis is similar to that of a simple ganglion.

The presentation is unilateral claudication which runs a progressive course. As the lesion is represented by stenosis rather than occlusion distal pulses will disappear when the affected patient's knee is sharply flexed. Diagnosis may be difficult but a loss of ankle pressure unilaterally on exercise will indicate a stenosis. Duplex scanning is superior to arteriography in the identification of a cystic mass in the wall of the artery[42] and the choice of treatment is dependent on the operative findings.

Evacuation of the cyst alone may be effective when the artery has not occluded and when the arterial wall has not degenerated. Intraoperative aspiration, evacuation or excision of the cyst can be performed as necessary to restore normal arterial flow through the untouched lumen of the vessel – intraoperative documentation of perfect arterial flow is a requirement of this procedure[40]. Angioplasty, vein patch or direct suture alone do not cure this condition. Total occlusion should be treated by resection of the affected artery and autologous vein bypass grafting which carries a 94% success rate[40].

Tumours of the popliteal artery

Tumours of the popliteal artery are rare and only two recorded cases are present in the world literature[43]. Leiomyosarcomata do occur in the inferior vena cava where 60 cases have been reported[44], but other venous sites of origin of this tumour are less common.

Both reported cases of popliteal artery leiomyosarcoma presented with a tender swelling in the popliteal fossa. The arteries had thrombosed and were totally occluded with tumour but neither patient had ischaemic symptoms. One patient was treated with a mid-thigh amputation and the other by wide excision and radiotherapy. Both patients had evidence of distant metastases within a short time of presentation.

In most cases of leiomyosarcoma of large vessels, little correlation has been made between their microscopic features and surgical outcome, although the higher the mitotic count, the greater the possibilities of the patient developing metastatic disease[44].

The favoured management of a vascular tumour is wide, local excision to include the structures in the immediate region of the tumour. In the case of popliteal vessel involvement, the correct option would therefore be that of above-knee amputation in the absence of metastatic disease.

References

1. Schecter, D. C. and Bergan, J. J. (1986) Popliteal aneurysm: A celebration of the bicentenial of John Hunter's operation. *Ann. Vasc. Surg.*, **1**, 118–126
2. Matas, R. (1920) Endoneurysmorrhaphy. *Surg. Gynecol. Obstet.*, **30**, 456–458
3. Pringle, J. H. (1913) Two cases of vein grafting for the mainenance of a direct arterial circulation. *Lancet*, **ii**, 1795–1796
4. Anton, G. E., Hertzer, N. R., Beven, E. C., O'Hara, P. J. and Krajewski, L. P. (1986) Surgical management of popliteal aneurysms. *J. Vasc. Surg.*, **3**, 125–134
5. Bonds, J. W. and Fabian, T. C. (1985) Surgical treatment of mycotic popliteal artery aneurysm: A case report and review of the literature. *Surgery*, **98**, 979–982
6. Wychulis, A. R., Spittell, J. A. and Wallace, R. B. (1970) Popliteal aneurysms. *Surgery*, **68**, 942–952
7. Inahara, T. and Toledo, A. C. (1978) Complications and treatment of popliteal aneurysms. *Surgery*, **84**, 775–783
8. Szilagyi, D. E., Schwartz, R. C. and Reddy, D. J. (1981) Popliteal arterial aneurysms. *Arch. Surg.*, **116**, 724–728
9. Schellack, J., Smith, R. B. and Perdue, G. D. (1987) Non operative management of selective popliteal aneurysms. *Arch. Surg.*, **122**, 372–375
10. Downing, R., Ashton, F., Grimley, R. P. and Slaney, G. (1985) Problems in diagnosis of popliteal aneurysms. *J. R. Soc. Med.*, **78**, 440–444
11. Gifford, R. W., Hines, E. A. and Janes, J. M. (1953) An analysis and follow up of one hundred popliteal aneurysms. *Surgery*, **33**, 284–293
12. Bouhoutoutsos, J. and Martin, P. (1974) Popliteal aneurysm: a review of 116 cases. *Br. J. Surg.*, **61**, 469–475
13. Gaylis, H. (1974) Popliteal arterial aneurysms. A review and analysis of 55 cases. *S. A. Med. J.*, **48**, 75–81
14. Vermilion, B. D., Kimmins, S. A., Pace, W. G. and Evans, W. E. (1981) A review of one hundred and forty-seven popliteal aneurysms with long-term follow up. *Surgery*, **90**, 1009–1014
15. Towne, J. B., Thompson, M. D., Patman, D. D. and Persson, A. V. (1976) Progression of popliteal aneurysmal disease following popliteal aneurysm resection with graft. A twenty year experience. *Surgery*, **80**, 426–432
16. Reilly, M. K., Abbott, W. M. and Darling, R. C. (1983) Aggressive surgical management of popliteal artery aneurysms. *Am. J. Surg.*, **145**, 499–502
17. Schwarz, W., Berkowitz, H., Taormina, V. and Gatti, J. (1984) The pre-operative use of intra-arterial thrombolysis for a thrombosed popliteal artery aneurysm. *J. Cardiovasc. Surg.*, **25**, 465–468
18. Ferguson, L. J., Faris, I., Robertson, A., Lloyd, J. V. and Miller, J. H. (1986) Intra-arterial streptokinase therapy to relieve acute limb ischaemia. *J. Vasc. Surg.*, **4**, 205–210
19. Earnshaw, J. J., Gregson, R. H. S., Makin, G. S. and Hopkinson, B. R. (1987) Early results of low-dose intra-arterial streptokinase therapy in acute and subacute lower limb arterial ischaemia. *Br. J. Surg.*, **74**, 504–507
20. Walker, W. J. and Giddings, A. E. B. (1988) A protocol for the safe treatment of acute lower limb ischaemia with intra-arterial streptokinase and surgery. *Br. J. Surg.*, **75**, 1189–1192
21. Kissin, M. W., Pullan, R., Scott, D. J. A., Horrocks, M. and Baird, R. N. (1989) Popliteal aneurysms presenting as acute limb ischaemia. *Br. J. Surg.*, **76**, 416
22. Bowyer, R. C., Cawthorn, S. J., Walker, W. J. and Giddings, A. E. B. (1990) Conservative management of asymptomatic popliteal aneurysm. *Br. J. Surg.*, **77**, 1132–1135
23. McCollum, C. H., DeBakey, M. E. and Myhre, H. O. (1983) Popliteal aneurysms: Results of 87 operations performed between 1957 and 1977. *Cardiovasc. Res. Cent. Bull.*, **21**, 93–100
24. Guvendik, L., Bloor, K. and Charlesworth, D. (1980) Popliteal aneurysm: sinister harbinger of sudden catastrophe. *Br. J. Surg.*, **67**, 294–296
25. Hands, L., Collin, J. and Morris, P. J. (1989) A warning from 12 years of popliteal aneurysm treatment. *Br. J. Surg.*, **76**, 416
26. Smith, R. F., Szilagi, D. E. and Elliot, J. P. (1969) Fracture of the long bones with arterial injury due to blunt trauma. *Arch. Surg.*, **99**, 315–324

27. Barros D'Sa, A. A. B., Hassard, T. H., Livingston, R. H. and Sinclair Irwin, J. W. (1980) Missile induced vascular trauma. *Injury*, **12**, 13–30
28. Rich, N. M., Baugh, J. H. and Hughes, C. W. (1970) Acute arterial injuries in Vietnam: 1,000 cases. *J. Trauma*, **10**, 359–369
29. Eger, M., Golcman, L., Goldstien, A. and Hirsch, M. (1971) The use of a temporary shunt in the management of arterial vascular injuries. *Surg. Gynecol. Obstet.*, **132**, 67–70
30. Barros D.Sa, A. A. B. (1981) A decade of missile induced vascular trauma. *Ann. R. Coll. Eng.*, **64**, 37–44
31. Stuart, T. P. A. (1979) Note on a variation in the course of the popliteal artery. *J. Anat. Physiol.*, **13**, 162–165
32. Rich, N. M. (1982) Popliteal entrapment and adventitial cystic disease. *Surg. Clin. N. Am.*, **62**, 449–465
33. Evans, E. W. and Bernhard, V. (1971) Acute popliteal artery entrapment. *Am. J. Surg.*, **121**, 739–740
34. Baker, W. H. and Stoney, R. J. (1972) Acquired popliteal entrapment syndrome. *Arch. Surg.*, **105**, 780–782
35. Rich, N. M., Collins, G. J., McDonald, P. T., Kozloff, L., Clagett, G. P. and Collins, J. T. (1979) Popliteal vascular entrapment. *Arch. Surg.*, **114**, 1377–1384
36. Ferrero, R., Barile, C. and Bretto, P. (1980) Popliteal artery entrapment syndrome: Reports on seven cases. *J. Cardiovasc. Surg.*, **21**, 45–52
37. Sieunarine, K., Prendergast, F. J., Paton, R., Goodman, M. A. and Ibach, E. G. (1990) Entrapment of popliteal artery and vein. *Aust. NZ. J. Surg.*, **60**, 533–537
38. Atkins, H. J. B. and Key, J. A. (1946) A case of myxomatous tumour arising in the adventitia of the left external artery. *Br. J. Surg.*, **34**, 426–427
39. Hierton, T., Lindberg, K. and Rob, C. (1957) Cystic degeneration of the popliteal artery. *Br. J. Surg.*, **44**, 348–351
40. Flanigan, D. P., Burnham, S. J., Goodreau, J. J. and Bergan, J. J. (1979) Summary of cases of adventitial cystic disease of the popliteal artery. *Ann. Surg.*, **189**, 165–175
41. Shute, K. and Rothnie, N. R. (1973) The aetiology of cystic arterial disease. *Br. J. Surg.*, **69**, 397–400
42. Schöllorn, J., Arnolds, B., von Reutern, G. M. and Schlosser, V. (1985) Cystic adventitial degeneration as a cause of dynamic stenosis of the popliteal artery: A case report. *Angiology*, **36** (11), 809–814
43. Basu, S. K., Scott, T. D., Wilkhurst, C. C., MacEachern, A. C and Clyne, C. A. C. (1988) Leiomyosarcomata of the popliteal vessels: Rare primary tumours. *Eur. J. Vasc. Surg.*, **2**, 423–425
44. Varela-Duran, J., Oliva, H. and Rosai, J. (1979) Vascular leiomyosarcoma. The malignant counterpart of vascular leiomyoma. *Cancer*, **44**, 1684–1691

Chapter 15

The diabetic foot – how can it be saved?

John Chamberlain

Patients with diabetes are particularly prone to vascular complications, and of these vascular insufficiency and neuropathy involving the foot may cause severe disability and may lead ultimately to major amputation.

In England and Wales inpatients who are referred for the fitting of artificial limbs, 20% of all amputations, and just under one-third of all 'vascular amputations', are undertaken in diabetics[1]. The true figure for amputation in diabetics is likely to be somewhat higher as not all patients are referred for limb fitting. The outlook for the diabetic amputee is poor with a higher mortality than for the non-diabetic patient, and over half of diabetic amputees come to amputation of the opposite leg within five years. The high mortality is related particularly to cardiac and renal disease and many patients do not live long enough to undergo this second amputation. The incidence of diabetes in the elderly population continues to rise, together with an increasing liability to circulatory problems in these patients. The situation is further compounded because many of these patients have multiple medical conditions.

The diabetic patient is at great risk, from an increased incidence of occlusive disease of the large arteries of the cerebral, coronary and peripheral circulation; also altered tissue metabolism and abnormal microvascular pathology exacerbate the effect of large vessel disease. In the younger patient, microvascular disease itself may lead to local lesions which, together with altered blood flow and superimposed infection, result in extensive ulceration and necrosis.

This chapter will review current thoughts on the pathophysiology of the 'diabetic foot', its evaluation and management. However, it cannot be over-emphasized that these patients require support, advice and treatment from a multi-specialist team including physicians, surgeons, nurses, chiropodists and appliance fitters. This multi-specialty approach is needed if the problems related to the diabetic foot are to be prevented and correctly managed when they do occur.

Pathophysiology

Peripheral neuropathy

Peripheral neuropathy in diabetes involves both the anatomical and peripheral nerves, with microvascular changes and the development of arteriovenous shunts[2]. It is suggested that there is reduced capillary flow with oedema and subsequent impaired tissue nutrition. These metabolic effects are also associated with an absence of sympathetic vasoconstrictor tone so that many patients do not respond further to sympathectomy. A dry skin may result from this and lead to superficial fissuring which allows infection.

The pathogenesis of neuropathy has not been conclusively established but there appears to be a strong correlation between the clinical diabetic state, the level of blood glucose and the degree of neuropathy. There is considerable evidence that hyperglycaemia is important in this pathogenesis[3]. The neuropathy is associated with demyelination of nerves due to the metabolic alterations associated with hyperglycaemia, and also with axonal degeneration which complicates microangiopathy resulting in ischaemia of the nerve. There is also decreased sweating, loss of sensation and subsequent weakening of the intrinsic muscles, especially the interossei, lumbricals and extensor digitorum brevis of the foot, resulting in a cavus deformity of the foot with claw toes and atrophy of the skin. Subsequently, submetatarsal callosities develop over pressure points and these areas are likely to ulcerate. The diabetic foot also appears to undergo autosympathectomy with vasomotor denervation, resulting in arteriolar dilatation with increased local blood flow and arteriovenous shunting.

Blood flow in the foot in diabetes

The main arteries supplying the foot are the posterior tibial and dorsalis pedis arteries leading to the pedal arches which in turn, give rise to the digital vessels supplying the arterioles and the capillary circulation. There are also numerous arteriovenous anastomoses, particularly towards the plantar surface of the foot. Blood flow to the skin is controlled by the sympathetic nerves which control the arteriolar tone and arteriovenous anastomotic shunts.

In addition there is a local axon reflex whereby local injury results in the release of a vasodilatory peptide and a so-called veni vasomotor reflex, probably mediated through a local axon reflex, which controls capillary pressure and prevents the development of dependent oedema.

It is commonly believed that arteriolar occlusion is the main factor in the development of diabetic ischaemia. However, a number of studies[4,5] show that the extent of small vessel occlusion in diabetic patients is the same as in non-diabetics. In these studies, the severity of ischaemia compares best with the degree of large vessel disease. The larger vessels most often involved are those below the inguinal ligament that is the femoral, popliteal and tibial arteries. The effects of this large vessel disease in diabetics are compounded by three other factors:

Local tissue factors
   Impaired collagen synthesis
   Hyperglycaemia
   White cell dysfunction
Abnormalities of the microcirculation
   Capillary wall thickening
   Increased permeability of the capillaries
Local sepsis
   Decreased capillary perfusion, local tissue destruction, digital artery thrombosis, tissue necrosis

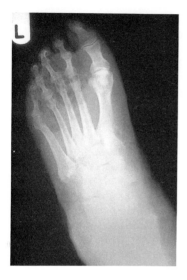

Figure 15.1   Diabetic gas gangrene

Infection

Most infections in the diabetic foot involve a mixture of both aerobic and anaerobic bacteria. The most common anaerobic organisms are *Bacteroides fragilis,* anaerobic streptococci and clostridia. *Staphylococcus aureus* and the coliforms are the most common aerobes, especially *Escherichia coli* and proteus.

Microbial cultures should be obtained from all lesions and the specimens should be taken from the deepest area possible in ulcers or from areas of necrosis. Not infrequently there may be underlying bone infection with osteomyelitis of the phalanges or metacarpals. This may be revealed on a plain X-ray of the foot. Gas may be produced in the soft tissues by anaerobic organisms (Figure 15.1), often associated with severe systemic upset and infection ketoacidosis.

Clinical presentation

Complications of the diabetic foot can occur at any age. Patients may present with predominantly neuropathic signs and these are usually younger patients who are insulin dependent or with ischaemic lesions and evidence of peripheral vascular disease (older patients). There may be a mixture of these signs.

Diabetics suffer a high incidence of atherosclerosis with a worse prognosis both for the limb and for life. Up to 50% of diabetics have evidence of peripheral arterial disease 10–15 years after the onset of the disease. The arterial lesion tends to be at multiple levels, particularly in the femoral and popliteal segments and in two or three of the tibial vessels. Lesions are also commonly seen in the main arteries in the foot. Disease in the arteries below the knee is commonly associated with calcification making arterial reconstruction difficult, if not impossible[6].

Diabetic patients may present with the ischaemic symptoms of intermittent claudication or rest pain, as in non-diabetic atherosclerosis, and are more likely to have ulceration or gangrene[7]. Ischaemic ulcers are usually painful and associated with a previous history of claudication and rest pain. However, if there is some degree of neuropathy, the ulcers may be painless and occur over bony prominences such as the heel, metatarsal heads or the plantar aspect of the big toe (Figure 15.2).

Foot lesions occur in both insulin dependent and non-insulin dependent diabetic patients. Boulton[8] has classified such lesions (Table 15.1, adapted from Wagner[9]).

Grade 1 lesions mainly consist of a superficial ulcer due mostly to pressure. These ulcers may respond to conservative management such as footwear inserts to remove pressure, or walking plaster casts.

Grade 2 lesions are deeper, penetrating through the subcutaneous fat down to deeper structures, with associated local infection and cellulitis. These patients require control of their diabetes, local antiseptic dressings and appropriate antibiotic therapy. If the ulcers become clean, they can be treated as a Grade 1 ulcer. If there is any evidence of proximal arterial disease, the patient should be considered for surgical revascularization.

Grade 3 lesions are characterized by deep infection with abscess formation, and are often associated with osteomyelitis (Figure 15.3). These lesions require local treatment with bed rest, antibiotic therapy, possibly local surgical debridement if appropriate, and full investigation for proximal arterial disease. Local amputations may be required.

Grade 4 lesions present as gangrene of the heel, toes or a larger part of the forefoot. These patients require urgent vascular investigation, vascular reconstruction if possible, local amputation and debridement. If a single gangrenous toe is dry and not

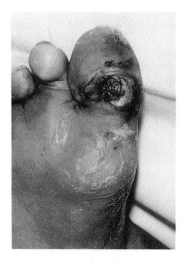

Figure 15.2   Neuropathic ulcer of plantar aspect of the big toe

Table 15.1   Classification of ischaemic foot lesions

Grade 0	At risk foot. No obvious ulcer, but thick callus, prominent metatarsal heads, claw toes, or any bony abnormality
Grade 1	Superficial ulcer, not clinically infected
Grade 2	Deeper ulcer, often infected, but no bone involvement
Grade 3	Deep ulcer, abscess formation, bony involvement
Grade 4	Localized gangrene (for example, toe or forefoot)
Grade 5	Gangrene of whole foot

Adapted from [9]

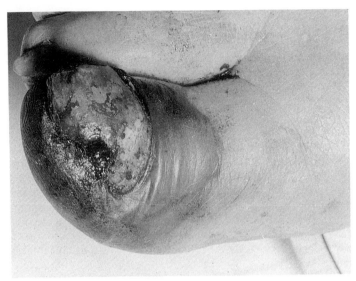

Figure 15.3   Local gangrene with osteomyelitis

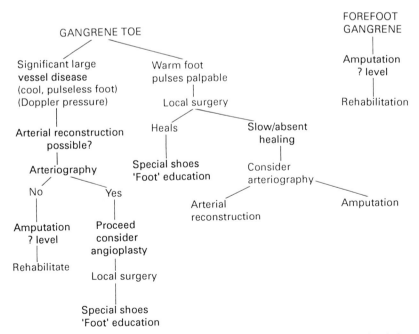

Figure 15.4   Algorithm for the management of a patient presenting with a grade 4 lesion of the foot (From reference 8)

infected, then it may be left to separate spontaneously. In all of these patients, good control of the diabetes is essential. An algorithm for the management of a patient presenting with a Grade 4 lesion is described by Boulton[8] (Figure 15.4).

Grade 5 lesions include patients presenting with major gangrene of the foot and who therefore require a major amputation.

Investigation

In addition to general assessment, all diabetic patients should have a careful examination of the peripheral vascular system, particularly in the lower limbs. Any patient newly presenting with symptoms of peripheral vascular disease should be tested for diabetes. On clinical examination there may be signs of vascular impairment, including brittle and deformed toenails, and skin atrophy with loss of hair from the foot or lower leg. There may be frank evidence of severe ischaemia with skin breaks, ulceration or even gangrene. The gangrene may be dry or infected. Buerger's test may show evidence of ischaemia with pallor of the foot on elevation and typical rubor with delayed filling on dependency.

All pulses should be palpated, especially the popliteal, posterior tibial, dorsalis pedis and peroneal: the peroneal artery is the only patent vessel in the lower limb in many diabetics. Auscultation may reveal a bruit over a larger vessel, suggesting proximal stenosis.

The use of Doppler ultrasound has revolutionized bedside assessment: it can be used to detect blood flow in the pedal vessels and allows the systolic pressure to be measured in these individually. Diabetic arteries may be rigid and incompressible with considerable mural calcification and a misleadingly high systolic pressure may be measured, however the pressures may still give a guide to the degree of disease in the peripheral arteries.

Exercise testing and transcutaneous oxygen measurements in claudicants may be carried out for further assessment of the degree of ischaemia.

In any patient with critical ischaemia (i.e. rest pain, ulceration or gangrene) angiography is mandatory for assessment of the peripheral circulation in order to determine whether reconstruction can be used to improve the blood supply to the limb. It is, however, likely that some form of amputation will still be required. In diabetics with claudication, the indications for angiography are the same as those in a non-diabetic and are dependent on the severity of the patient's symptoms. If the patient has a compelling disability, perhaps a younger patient unable to work or an older patient whose lifestyle is severaly inhibited, angiography is indicated.

Appropriate microbial swabs should be taken from any infected lesions. Plain X-rays of the abdomen, pelvis and limbs are very helpful as they may show up extensive calcification, which may indicate whether or not a reconstructive procedure is possible (Figure 15.5).

Transcutaneous oxygen measurements ($Tcpo_2$)

Hauser and colleagues[10] compared the measurement of $Tcpo_2$ with other non-invasive diagnostic tests in diabetic and non-diabetic patients. A significantly higher diagnostic accuracy was found with $Tcpo_2$ than with other commonly used measurements including Doppler ankle pressures, pressure index, pulse volume recording and

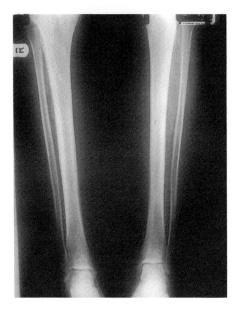

Figure 15.5   Tibial artery calcification

toepulse reappearance times. The authors suggested that this should be the initial non-invasive test for diabetic peripheral vascular disease.

Angiography

It is extremely important, particularly in diabetics, that full imaging of the peripheral arterial tree is obtained from the level of the renal arteries down to the ankle and foot vessels. This has become easier in recent years with the development of computerized digital vascular imaging equipment and subtraction angiography which enable all vessels to be visualized. There may be arterial disease at multiple sites although diabetics are particularly prone to disease below the inguinal ligament. Significant proximal lesions may be present requiring treatment by surgery or by balloon dilatation in order to improve the inflow so that a more distal procedure, if needed, may succeed. If there is any doubt about the haemodynamic significance of a lesion above the inguinal ligament, papaverine testing[11] will often determine if this requires intervention.

Transluminal angioplasty in the diabetic patient

Localized stenoses may be suitable for treatment by balloon angioplasty, which may be carried out at the same time as angiography. Percutaneous transluminal angioplasty was first carried out in 1964 by Dotter and Judkins[12], who showed that an arterial stenosis could be dilated by passing a series of Teflon catheters of increasingly larger diameter through a narrowed vessel. Although the technique succeeded, there were many technical problems and the long-term success was poor resulting in discontinuation of the procedure. In 1974 Gruntzig[13] introduced a dilating balloon catheter for the procedure, and radiologists now have available balloon catheters which can be inflated to predetermined diameters and pressures, reducing the risks of complications. Percutaneous transluminal angioplasty is most appropriate for short lesions in non-calcified large or medium-sized arteries, a pattern of disease frequently occurring in diabetics. The multiple arterial lesions occurring in the femoral, popliteal, and particularly in the tibial arteries are not so readily treated by transluminal angioplasty; just as this distribution of disease is not easy to treat by surgery.

The indications for transluminal angioplasty are little different from those for a non-diabetic patient with atherosclerotic disease. Patients considered unsuitable for surgical intervention because of poor general medical condition or because of the nature and distribution of their disease may be treated by this method. It is important that these procedures are undertaken only after discussion between radiologist and surgeon, who should work very closely together. Transluminal angioplasty should not normally be undertaken in the asymptomatic patient. A worthwhile advantage of transluminal angioplasty is that if it fails surgery is still an option in many patients.

For patients with short stenoses or occlusions in the iliac arteries, angioplasty is as successful as in non-diabetics: for iliac angioplasty the primary success rate may be as high as 95% with a two-year patency rate of up to 90%. This compares well with a primary sucess rate of 95% for bypass surgery with a normal runoff.

In the femoropopliteal segment initial patency after angioplasty is 80%–90%, falling to 70%–80% after two years. It is in the femoral, popliteal and more distal segments that angioplasty may give considerable benefits in diabetic patients. Transluminal angioplasty is an acceptable alternative to surgery in short stenotic lesions or occlusions up to 10 cm in length (Figures 15.6 and 15.7) although multiple short stenoses do not seem to do as well. Spence and colleagues[14] compare the results of transluminal dilatation of the iliac and femoral vessels in diabetics and non-diabetics. The two-year patency rates in the iliac arteries was 92% in diabetics and

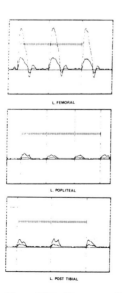 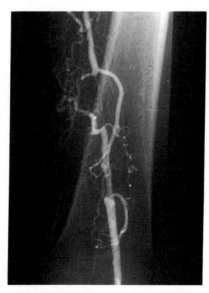

Figure 15.6   Femoropopliteal occlusion before balloon dilatation. Note the damping of distal pulse waves (left)

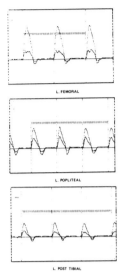

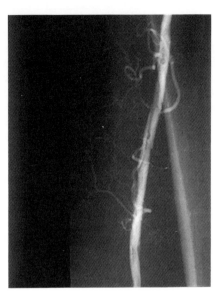

Figure 15.7 Femoropopliteal occlusion after balloon dilatation. Note that the distal pulse wave (shown on the left) has now returned to normal

78% in non-diabetics. In the femoral vessels the two-year patency was much better in the non-diabetics at 85.4% with only 54% of vessels patent in the diabetic group. Long-term studies of the results of angioplasty are awaited. Initial results would suggest that angioplasty in the diabetic patient, who often has more widespread disease with calcified arteries, may not be so effective in the smaller arteries. It is also recognized that if the patient continues to smoke, the results are worse. It would still seem reasonable to carry out transluminal angioplasty of discrete lesions in the distal arteries, but widespread disease and multiple stenoses might be better treated by surgical bypass if the patient is otherwise fit enough. Evidence suggests that bypass surgery gives equally good results in diabetics as non-diabetics for a similar distribution of disease.

The smaller the vessel opened up by balloon angioplasty the less likely it is to stay patent. There have unfortunately been no adequate controlled trials comparing angioplasty with bypass surgery.

If occlusive disease is so extensive that no available surgical technique would be possible and amputation seems inevitable, recannulization with a balloon catheter combined with thrombolytic therapy may be attempted. Infusion of streptokinase or the more recently introduced Thromboplastin Activator can be directed into the thrombus via an arterial catheter, and may be effective even after a number of weeks. This therapy may also lyse thrombus in small vessels in the foot which are not amenable to surgery. However, if it is possible, bypass surgery in a critically ischaemic leg may be preferred as thrombolytic therapy may take too long to save the limb.

Lumbar sympathectomy

Many diabetics, particularly insulin-dependent diabetics, already have maximum sympathetic vasodilatation. Lumbar sympathectomy therefore has little to offer, and there is no evidence that sympathectomy has ever saved a limb with critical ischaemia.

Reconstructive arterial surgery in diabetics

Aortoiliac stenotic disease is rarely an isolated lesion in diabetics and is treated in the same way as in non-diabetics. Long-term patency rates for such reconstructions depend on the runoff: if runoff in the superficial femoral and profunda arteries is good, 100% patency over five years can be expected, provided that arterial disease does not progress further distally.

If the patient is considered unfit for major abdominal surgery, then an extra-anatomic bypass, either axillobifemoral (for bilateral lesions) or a crossover femoral graft (if one iliac artery is free from disease) is applicable.

Femoropopliteal occlusion, if unsuitable for angioplasty, should be treated by bypass. Little difference has been reported between the patency rates for above-the-knee bypass in diabetics and non-diabetics, although the five-year patency rate for infrapopliteal grafts tends to be a little lower in diabetics. Rosenblatt[15] studied 150 patients, 75 diabetic and 75 non-diabetic, with 171 vein grafts. No established difference was found in the primary patency for patients with or without diabetes. Diabetic patients operated on for limb salvage because of critical ischaemia, ulceration or gangrene, showed an increased patency of the vein graft over the non-diabetic. There was a higher incidence of minor amputations in these patients and a greater requirement for reconstruction to distal tibial or pedal arteries. Rosenblatt's paper shows that an aggressive approach to reconstruction can preserve the foot even in patients with severe ischaemia.

Pomposelli and colleagues[16] recently reported on the efficacy of the dorsal pedal bypass for limb salvage in diabetic patients, reviewing their experience in 96 patients, 94% of whom had diabetes, who had 97 bypasses placed to the dorsal pedal artery for limb salvage. Superimposed infected lesions were present in 42.3% of these patients. Digital subtraction angiography was used to visualize the artery for bypass in 92 patients. In 12 cases, the artery was found by Doppler examination. The procedures utilized vein for the bypass graft, inflow being taken from the femoral artery in 48, the popliteal artery in 45, the tibial artery in two, and from a femorotibial graft in two. There was a low perioperative mortality of 1.92% and the graft patency, limb salvage, and patient survival were 82%, 87% and 80% respectively at 18 months. Consequently, these authors also recommend an aggressive approach to reconstruction to preserve the diabetic foot. A third of their patients required additional procedures, such as digital ray amputation (17), transmetatarsal amputation (1), and debridement and split thickness skin grafts (15). The procedure carried out depends largely on good angiography to visualize the vessels. The authors emphasize the importance of the use of magnification during surgery, the use of 7/0 or 8/0 Prolene sutures, and of taking the inflow from the most distal vessel possible.

These more aggressive approaches suggest that a great deal can be done to preserve the ischaemic foot in the diabetic, avoiding the need for amputation.

Local treatment and amputation without revascularization

Some patients will require either local surgery or amputation. Those patients who have widespread disease, particularly with ulcers overlying the heel and widespread gangrene in the forefoot, will require major amputation and usually do well with a below-knee procedure. Every effort should be made in these patients to retain the knee joint to improve rehabilitation, which is usually more often possible in diabetics than in non-diabetics. In a series of 117 below-knee amputations (personal data), the conversion rate to above-knee for diabetics was one-half of that for non-diabetics (Table 15.2). In those patients with fewer gross lesions it is important to control any local infection with appropriate use of systemic antibiotics, with provision of free local drainage and excision of all necrotic tissue. If bone is involved this also should be removed because healing will not usually occur with continuing underlying osteomyelitis. In such instances, local amputations leaving the wound open may succeed, repeated if necessary and excising digital bone or the distal part of a metatarsal. If infection is present, no attempt should be made to suture these wounds which may heal by secondary intention or may require subsequent skin grafting. Debridement should be carried out for local lesions, especially if there is any necrotic tissue. Cellulitis requires aggressive antibiotic therapy, rest and elevation. Plantar spaces are inspected for infection and necrotic plantar fascia removed. Tendons should be examined where indicated during amputation of any necrotic toes and ray amputations of metatarsals.

A paper by Francis and colleagues[17] reintroduced the Syme's amputation for diabetics with palpable ankle pulses. The average age of their patients was 60 years, of whom 26 underwent either a one-stage (23 patients) or a two-stage (3 patients) Syme's amputation which was successful in twenty patients (77%). The authors suggest that the single most important feature for success is to limit this operation to those patients with a palpable posterior tibial pulse. Local amputation may succeed when the pedal pulses are present or after revascularization by a previous reconstruction, and particularly in the neuropathic foot with good inflow. Gasivoda and colleagues[18] advocate investigation, including standard X-rays, 99Tc^m diphosphate bone scans, and ^{67}Ga citrate scans to determine the extent of soft tissue and bony involvement, in order to determine the degree of local tissue involvement.

Unfortunately the outlook in these patients is poor. Bose[18] reviewed 300 consecutive patients with diabetic foot complications, of whom 80% had an abscess in the foot, 8% had cellulitis of the dorsum and 12% had perforated ulcers. Also, 40% of these patients had a high amputation, above or below the knee. Only 16.7% of patients with a malperforens ulcer required a high amputation and local drainage and excision of necrotic fissure or distal amputation salvaged the foot, or portions of it, in 180 cases. In another study in Oxford[20], 15% of patients died during their stay in hospital, 8% required reamputation and only 25% were alive four years later. In this series the contralateral limb amputation rate was over 50% in diabetic patients.

It is evident that in order to retain and heal the diabetic foot careful management is required. Foot conservation may be achieved avoiding local pressure and treating infections aggressively, with the prompt removal of dead tissue and avoidance of pressure on other exposed parts of the foot. Unfortunately, there is a high rate of reamputation after local procedures but there is, at present, no method of adequately evaluating the circulation to provide a good guide to amputation level.

Table 15.2 Outcome of below-the-knee amputation in 117 operations

Outcome	No. patients
Operative mortality	13 (11.1%)
Conversion to above-knee amputations	21 (17.9%)
Non-diabetic	14 (11.9%)
Diabetic	7(6.0%)

Conclusion

Peripheral ischaemic problems in the diabetic remain difficult to manage. Patients now tend to be older, have multiple medical conditions, and remain a high risk for surgery. It is vital that every effort is made to prevent complications by the use of appropriate footwear and careful chiropody. Accurate control of the diabetic state is essential.

In the neuropathic patient, foot lesions often respond to conservative treatment with aggressive management of infection and local surgery. In the patient with coexistent vascular disease local treatment of ischaemic lesions together with revascularization either by interventional radiology or bypass surgery, can often preserve a foot and avoid more major amputation. It is to be stressed that a team approach is essential in the management of these patients, involving physician, surgeon, chiropodist and appliance fitters.

References

1. *On the State of the Public Health 1986.* Department of Health and Social Security, London
2. Edmonds, M. E., Roberts, V. C. and Watkins, P. J. (1982) Blood flow in the diabetic neuropathic foot. *Diabetologia,* **22,** 9–15
3. Pirart, J. (1977) Diabetes mellitus and its degenerative complications: A prospective study of 4,400 patients observed between 1947 and 1973. *Diabetes Metab.,* **3,** 245–256
4. Nielsen, P. R. (1973) Does diabetic microangiography cause the development of gangrene? *Scand. J. Clin. Invest.,* **31** (suppl. 128), 229–234
5. Strandness, D. E. Jr., Priest, R. E. and Gibbon, G. E. (1964) Combined clinical and pathological study of diabetics and non-diabetics peripheral arterial disease. *Diabetes,* **13,** 366–372
6. Ferrier, T. M. (1967) Comparative study of arterial disease in amputated lower limbs from diabetics and non-diabetics. *Med. J. Aust.,* **1,** 5–11
7. Steer, H. W., Cuckle, H. S., Franklin, P. M., Morris, P. J. *et al.* (1983) The influence of diabetes mellitus upon peripheral vascular disease. *Surg. Gynecol. Obstet.,* **157,** 64–72
8. Boulton, A. J. M. (1988) The diabetic foot. *Med. Clin. N. Am.,* **72,** 6
9. Wagner, F. W. (1983) Algorithms of diabetic foot care. In *The Diabetic Foot* (eds M. E. Levin and F. W. O'Neal). C. V. Mosby, St. Louis
10. Hauser, C. J., Appel, P. and Shoemaker, W. C. (1984) Atherophysiologic classification of peripheral vascular disease by positional changes in regional transcutaneous oxygenation. *Surgery,* **95,** 689–693
11. Quin, R. O., Evans, D. H. and Bell, P. R. F. (1975) Haemodynamic assessment of the aorto-iliac segment. *J. Cardiovasc. Surg.,* **16,** 586–589
12. Dotter, C. T. and Judkins, M. P. (1964) Transluminal treatment of arteriosclerotic obstruction. *Circulation,* **30,** 654–670
13. Gruntzig, A. and Hopff, H. (1974) Percutane rekanalisation chronescher arterielter vesschuese mit einem neuen dilatations. *Kathetes. Deutsch. Med. Wochenschr.,* **99,** 2502–2505
14. Spence, R. K., Freiman, D. B., Bagatnby, R., Hobbs, C. and Markus, E. F. (1981) Long term results of transluminal angioplasty of the iliac and femoral arteries. *Arch. Surg.,* **116,** 1377–1386
15. Rosenblatt, M. S., Quist, W. C., Sidaway, A. N., Paniszyn, C. C., LoGerfo, F. W. *et al.* (1990) Result of vein graft reconstruction of the lower extremity in diabetes and non-diabetic patient. *Surg. Gynecol. Obstet.,* **171,** 331–335
16. Pomposelli, F. B. Jr., Jepson, S. J., Gibbons, G. W., Gottschalk, F., Fisher, D. F. *et al.* (1990) Efficacy of the dorsal pedal bypass for limb salvage in diabetic patients: short term observations. *J. Vasc. Surg.,* **11,** 745–752
17. Francis, H., Robert, R., Clagett, J. P. *et al.* (1990) The Syme amputation: success in elderly diabetic patients with palpable ankle pulses. *J. Vasc. Surg.,* **12,** 237–240
18. Gasivoda, P. L., Sollitto, R. J., and Slamowitz, H. (1990) Diabetic foot amputations: Part I Digital. *J. Foot Surg.* **29** (1), 72–78
19. Bose, K. A. (1979) A surgical approach for the infected diabetic foot. *Int. Orth.,* **3,** 177–181
20. Finch, D. R. A., MacDougal, M., Tibbs, D. J. and Morris, P. J. (1980) Amputation for vascular disease: the experience of a peripheral vascular unit. *Br. J. Surg.,* **67,** 233–237

Recommended further reading

Greenhalgh, R. M., Jamieson, C. W. and Nicholaides, A. N. (eds) (1988) *Limb Salvage and Amputation for Vascular Disease*. W. B. Saunders,

Levin, M. E. and O'Neal, L. W. (eds) (1988) *The Diabetic Foot*, 4th edition. C. V. Mosby, St Louis

Conner, H., Boulton, A. J. M. and Ward, J. D. (eds) (1987) *The Foot in Diabetes*. John Wiley and Sons

Chapter 16

Lower limb amputation – time for critical appraisal

C. Vaughan Ruckley

The objective evaluation of surgical procedures by clinical trial is in its infancy. In particular, critical analysis has rarely been applied to amputation operations or the care of the amputee, so the topic abounds with unanswered questions.

Some of the most interesting and difficult aspects of care of the amputee relate not so much to surgical technique but to less tangible issues such as decision making, rehabilitation, psychological factors and quality of life. These issues are seldom discussed.

What are the current trends in amputation surgery? The great majority of amputations are performed for arterial disease and were formerly very much a part of the routine experience of any general surgical unit. This is no longer the case for two reasons. First, although not officially separate from general surgery (in the UK at least) vascular surgery is increasingly becoming a separate specialty. Secondly it is now recognized as inappropriate for any limb with arterial insufficiency to be amputated without specialist referral and usually angiography. When it transpires that active intervention such as thrombolysis, angioplasty or reconstruction is of no avail, the task of amputation generally falls to the vascular surgeon.

Are more limbs being saved? Undoubtedly they are, although this assertion is difficult to prove except by indirect evidence. The overwhelming majority of reconstructions are performed for limb salvage, and even the most problematic reconstructions such as synthetic below-knee femoropopliteal grafts or vein femorodistal bypasses carry a three-year patency of 20% or better[1]. We know that in follow-up there is a high mortality from cardiac or cerebral vascular disease before graft occlusion can occur[2]. National data are available on the number of procedures performed but not on their outcomes. The number of arterial reconstructions per annum in Scotland, as shown by Scottish Hospital In-patient Statistics (SHIPS) data, has doubled over the past eight years (Figure 16.1). Reliable figures for angioplasty do not appear to be available, but there is no doubt that the increase here is even more spectacular.

Are fewer amputations being performed as a result of this massive increase in arterial reconstruction and angioplasty? Figure 16.1 shows that there has been a more than 30% increase in annual amputations in the last eight years. It appears therefore that although improvements in radiological intervention and arterial reconstruction protect individuals from amputation, the increasing elderly population and the prevalence of obliterative arterial disease ensure that overall more limbs are being lost. The deferment of amputation by angioplasty and reconstructive surgery and the progressive rise in the average age at which amputation is being performed must have

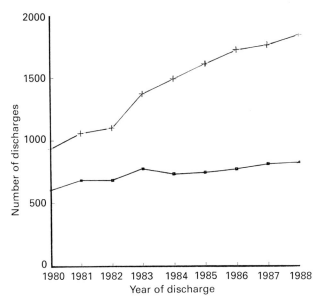

Figure 16.1 Trends in major amputations and total arterial reconstructions, Scotland, 1980–1988. ■, Amputations; +, bypass grafts

inevitable consequences for its outcome. These factors must lead to a reduction in the proportion of amputees who can be successfully rehabilitated, at least to independence. We can also forecast that in the older population, including those with failed bypass grafts, the proportion of amputees in whom it is either possible or worthwhile to preserve the knee joint is also likely to decrease.

The techniques of commonly performed amputations are well described in the literature and will not be rehearsed in detail here. However, it is often the small aspects of technique which make large differences in the success or failure of an operation so, in the second part of this chapter, attention will be drawn to a number of technical points which might help the surgical trainee to achieve better results.

Whether to amputate?

In pathological terms it is not difficult to decide when to consider amputation, but there may be a difficult humane or ethical decision. This is one of the most common questions in vascular surgery. There are two principal areas of doubt.

The first is the choice between amputation or reconstruction. The latter involves double discomfort and hazard since the decision hinges on angiography. Furthermore, the more borderline the patient in terms of age and fitness the lower the probability that the angiogram will demonstrate vessels suitable for reconstruction. Some purists would argue that no critically ischaemic leg should be amputated without the patient being offered angiography and the chance of reconstruction. This is not a policy to be dogmatically applied in every case. It is tempting to justify aggressive policies of arterial reconstruction by comparing their outcomes with those of amputation, but no such comparison can be valid and it would be impossible to mount a randomized trial. Happily the trend over the last decade has been for more reconstruction, grafts being carried down to the ankle or even to the foot. The ability to perform such procedures is now expected of all vascular trainees.

Having performed an angiogram and demonstrated an arterial tree of borderline operability in an elderly and unfit patient, the dilemma now arises: amputation, or attempted reconstruction with a probability of later amputation?

Do we know what the success rates are in very elderly and debilitated patients? This is where surgical audit has a role to play. It matters not what triumphs of limb salvage have been reported from other centres where, in all probability, different demographic factors, referral practices and selection criteria apply. Overall patency or complication rates may be entirely misleading when considering what to do for a patient who is at the extreme end of a population spectrum. What counts is the surgeon's own experience and record of success in a time-consuming and technically demanding area: it is an individual decision for the patient and for the surgeon.

The second category of difficult choices is one that in the author's experience, is becoming more common, and arises in respect of the critically ischaemic leg in the very elderly and debilitated patient, in whom arterial reconstruction is either inappropriate or impossible. Do we amputate or do we simply provide care, comfort and analgesia and let nature take its course? Critical ischaemia is often a terminal, albeit gradual, event. Amputation, at this stage of life, may be an unwarranted assault. Major amputation carries an operative mortality of 10–25% and a subsequent mortality of 10–20% per year. In the category of patient we are considering, mortality is much higher and life expectancy much worse. And what will be the quality of life? Severe pain should not be regarded as an indication for amputation in this circumstance, since effective analgesia can be achieved by modern methods such as continuous intravenous infusion of opiate.

Who decides?

Of course the patient normally decides, after receiving medical advice. Some elderly patients with vascular disease, however, are too ill, incapable or uncertain as to whether they wish to undergo amputation. In these circumstances it is not unusual for medical staff to ask relatives whether they think an amputation should be performed. This wish to involve relatives in decision making is often kindly and humanely meant, but it may amount to an inappropriate and unfair transfer of responsibility. It is medical responsibility to obtain information from relatives as to the patient's previous medical and psychiatric state (where this cannot be fully ascertained from the patient) and to garner all the details concerning social circumstances, level of support and quality of life which must colour the decision. If relatives offer opinions they must be carefully heeded. But it must be clear to all, particularly to the relatives, if later feelings of guilt are to be avoided, that the decision whether or not to recommend amputation is finally taken by the surgeon – otherwise what is medical training for?

We can be very sure that different surgeons apply different ethical arguments and different policies of selection for arterial reconstruction, amputation or the withholding of amputation. The implications of these differences for the evaluation of results are important and will be discussed later.

When to amputate?

It is customary to allow necrotic tissue to demarcate before amputating, a sound principle in most instances. Certainly premature operation, before it is clear that an ischaemic or septic process has stabilized, may result in amputation at the wrong level. Perhaps the best example of this is venous gangrene which in its acute stage often looks alarming and dangerous – with swelling, necrosis and blistering. At this stage one may be led to amputate at a relatively high level applying similar principles as in arterial gangrene. This is incorrect. Provided that uncontrolled sepsis is not present, high elevation of the limb combined with thrombolysis or heparin therapy should be continued for as long as possible, as it usually results in most or all of the limb being preserved.

In arterial gangrene there are a number of situations where amputation should not be delayed. These include:

1. Diabetic gangrene with spreading cellulitis, not promptly responding to antibiotics;
2. gangrene or pregangrene associated with severe intractable pain;
3. severe irreversible acute ischaemia involving muscle masses;
4. gangrene in the patient who is toxic, bacteraemic or has deteriorating renal function.

Emergency amputation in these circumstances does not necessarily have to be a definitive, surgically meticulous affair. Particularly in the case of uncontrolled sepsis the preferred option may be a guillotine amputation, for example in the lower calf, to be followed by an elective, carefully fashioned below-knee amputation when the patient's condition has stabilized. This approach is reported to give significantly lower amputation failure rates[3].

Who should perform the operation?

It could be argued that amputation should be performed by a specialist trained in vascular disease, orthopaedics and prosthetics – an improbable combination. Although in some centres amputation surgery has been taken over by the orthopaedic service the great majority of limb ablations are performed by vascular surgeons who then transfer patient care to the limb-fitting and rehabilitation services. It follows that vascular training must include thorough experience of amputation surgery.

When reconstruction is no longer an option, amputation by the vascular surgeon provides continuity of care for the patient through the acute phase. Subsequent transfer of care to other specialists carries the disadvantage that the surgeon is usually unable to see the late results.

Even in those patients referred back to the vascular surgeon because of ischaemia in the other limb, how often do we study our previous handiwork; finding out how long it took to prepare the stump for limb fitting, checking whether the length, shape, texture, wound healing and wound position were ideal? Do we understand how much of a struggle it has been for the patient to mobilize? How often do we appreciate that the deterioration of the other leg is due to strain caused by a faulty stump? There is little incentive for surgeons to revise their techniques.

It may take a long time for the consequences of faulty surgical technique to become apparent: stumps which are too long or too short; floppy stumps with redundant skin due to inappropriate design of flaps; distortion due to the contraction of muscles which were never secured to bone or to opposing muscles; tethering of scar to muscle; inadequately contoured and inadequately covered bone ends, prone to trauma and liable to erosion through skin or scar. In the amputation stump whose blood supply is defective minor differences in technique may produce major differences in healing. The operative technique must therefore be meticulous, accurate and minimally traumatic to tissues. It must also evolve as the study of prosthetics evolves.

So, who should perform amputation surgery? The answer is an experienced and interested surgeon who is prepared to take time and trouble to get it right. The tradition of the fast amputation, speed being equated with surgical skill, dies hard. Like so much of surgery today, as specialization is recognized to lead to better results, it is not appropriate to leave amputation operations to the unsupervised, inexperienced trainee. Unnecessary sacrifice of the knee joint is a very serious mistake.

What level of amputation?

Modern writings correctly stress the importance of preserving the knee joint. This is widely acknowledged to be one of the most important determinants of success of rehabilitation. Claims have been made for a high ratio of below-knee to above-knee amputations; however, in isolation this ratio is not a meaningful piece of information. There are many unanswered questions lurking behind such claims which need to be addressed and to which we will return later.

This issue is at its most important when deciding between below-knee and above-knee amputation, less often in deciding between a foot amputation and a below-knee amputation. The last decade has seen many techniques employed in an attempt to measure the blood supply to potential skin flaps. Have they caught on? It is of interest that in a recent multicentre trial of alternative techniques for below-knee amputation[4] involving sixteen vascular surgeons in ten leading UK centres not one was routinely employing an adjunctive technique to select level or to design flaps. This tells us something either about the practical value of the available methods or the conservatism of the surgeons concerned.

Methods advocated for judging amputation level are listed in Table 16.1. Their very number is an indication that a satisfactory method has yet to be identified.

What should be the attributes of the ideal test? First and foremost it should provide information not just of individual points of measurement but a map of the blood supply over the whole circumference of the limb at the level in question. It should be quick, simple, inexpensive, non-invasive and ideally conducted at the bedside. This

Table 16.1 Methods of evaluating healing potential before amputation

Segmental pressures and pulse volume recording[6,8,9]
Doppler ankle pressures[5,6,8]
Photoplethysmography[8,10]
^{133}Xe clearance[7,11]
Iodoantipyrine clearance[12]
Transcutaneous oxygen[6,7,14–17]
Thermography[12]
Fluorescein fluorometry[6,18]
Skin thermometry[9]
Angiography[8]

last, however is a particular difficulty, since skin blood flow is greatly influenced by changes in ambient temperature. It should not require expensive or inaccessible equipment or extra technical staff. Let us consider each test in turn.

Doppler ultrasound pressures

This simple test, performed as segmental or simply ankle pressures, is part of the routine patient assessment in virtually every vascular unit. Pollock and Ernst[5] studied the correlation between pre-operative Doppler ankle pressures and healing in 18 patients undergoing below-knee amputation. They concluded that satisfactory healing would follow amputation if a pressure of 70 mmHg was present at the ankle or an ankle–brachial ratio of at least 0.3. However, there were two patients in their healed group with pressures well below 70 mmHg, and one in their non-healing group had an ankle pressure of greater than 100 mmHg.

Wagner et al.[6] included ankle Doppler pressure measurement in a comparison of four methods of identifying amputation level in 109 amputations. They concluded that absolute pressure was an unreliable criterion and was not improved by conversion to an ankle/arm ratio.

A battery of tests was studied by Malone and co-workers in 48 patients undergoing 52 major amputations[7]. Neither popliteal artery pressure nor ankle–brachial systolic index proved significantly different between the healed and failed groups.

Van den Broek et al.[8] studied a range of methods, including Doppler pressures, in 55 patients undergoing lower limb amputations. The mean ultrasound pressure was 69 mmHg in the healed group and 51 mmHg in the failed group, these differences not being significant.

Doppler pressure measurements are known to be misleading in diabetic patients, in that spuriously high values are commonly obtained. Gibbons and co-workers[9] studied segmental Doppler pressures in 150 diabetic patients and found that they were falsely high or incorrectly predictive in more than half the cases. In below-knee amputations they were falsely high or incorrectly predictive in more than one-third of cases. Some workers therefore prefer to measure toe pressures[10], but these have not been shown to be substantially more reliable.

Photoplethysmography

This technique is relatively simple, inexpensive and non-invasive. It is really a variant of Doppler pressure measurement in that, when applied to the toe, the photoplethysmograph (PPG) provides a measure of systolic pressure. Bone and Pomajzl, in a series of 30 forefoot amputations (of whom 24, 80%, were diabetic) found the mean value associated with healing (86 + 39 mmHg) was significantly different from the mean value in those not healing (28 + 18 mmHg)[10]. There was better separation of values with PPG than with Doppler ankle pressures.

PPG can also be used at calf level. Van den Broek and colleagues[8] used it to measure skin perfusion pressure both posteriorly and anteriorly on the leg at potential amputation sites. They found significant differences between the healed and failed groups with reasonably good separation as judged by small standard errors, but scattergrams to show overlap of ranges were not provided.

Isotope clearance

One of the established methods of studying skin blood flow is isotope clearance. It requires a gamma camera and the ready availability of radioisotopes. Moore *et al.*[11] studied ^{133}Xe clearance in 45 lower extremities. Ambient temperature was always maintained at more than 25°C and the patient was allowed to equilibrate for 15–30 min before the test. They found that a minimum skin blood flow rate of 2.4 ml/min per 100 g tissue was always associated with healing. Furthermore, there was clear separation in values between healing and non-healing.

This was one of several techniques compared by Malone *et al.*[7] of 52 major lower limb amputations in 48 patients. They failed to demonstrate any significant difference in clearances between healed and failed groups at either below-knee or transmetatarsal level. We must conclude therefore that the method is of doubtful value and is in any case not practical for routine clinical practice in most hospitals.

McCollom *et al.* have described a technique using an alternative radioisotope (iodoantipyrine) and have shown a good correlation with thermography[12]. They report improved amputation results, using a combination of these two methods[13].

Transcutaneous oxygen (Tc*p*O$_2$)

This is also one of the accepted methods for studying skin blood flow and has been applied to a variety of healing problems. It is a simple and non-invasive, although time-consuming, technique which can be performed at the bedside – ideally in a temperature-controlled environment. Readings can be taken at several points around the leg although this makes it even more laborious.

Several authors have shown a high degree of statistical difference in readings between tissues that have healed and the failures[6,7,14–17]. A common finding was that above 40 mmHg almost all stumps healed. The problem is, as shown in Figure 16.2, there is a large overlap between the two groups and some stumps with extremely low Tc*p*O$_2$ values healed.

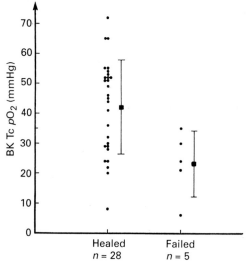

Figure 16.2   Transcutaneous oxygen tension in below-knee amputations, $t=2.51$; $P<0.02$ (from [15] by permission)

Thermography

McCollom *et al.* have correctly emphasized the importance of circumferential blood flow measurements at potential amputation sites[12]. They have employed infrared thermography to map out individual variations in skin blood flow and to design skin flaps accordingly, and have reported impressive figures for below-knee stump healing[13]. Unfortunately thermography equipment capable of providing this type of mapping is not widely available.

Other methods

Other methods reported include fluorescein fluorometry[6,18], skin thermometry[6] and angiographic scoring[8] but none of these methods can be recommended as being dependable predictors of healing, or more particularly as predictors of failure to heal.

Conclusions

It is striking that none of the recommended techniques have been objectively evaluated by controlled trial. Most have been shown to provide an index which correlates with a probability of healing but it is much more difficult reliably to identify those tissues which will fail to heal. When data are presented in scattergram form there is usually a large overlap between the healing and non-healing group (Figure 16.2). It is not surprising that none of these methods has entered routine clinical practice and some authors have concluded that the use of clinical acumen remains the best method[6,19].

Since most vascular surgeons now use below-knee amputation whenever there is a remote chance of healing, and will probably continue so to do, there will always be a proportion of revision operations required. Indeed a certain revision rate is the necessary penalty for maximum preservation of the knee joint. If the number of revisions becomes very small one must suspect that not enough below knee-operations are being attempted or that below-knee amputations are being performed when amputations at foot level would suffice. The aim therefore is to maintain a low revision rate while performing the maximum possible below-knee operations.

One particularly promising approach is that offered by the Dundee group[13], who have sought to map out the cutaneous blood flow and have designed their flaps accordingly. Incidentally, by so doing, they have produced support for the skew-flap method of below-knee amputation[12].

Amputation technique – general principles

Time spent in carefully measuring and marking skin flaps is time well spent. Tissues should be incised with the minimal number of bold, clean cuts. Subcutaneous fat has a tendency to bulge out between the margins of opposing wound edges, but this can be avoided by slightly bevelling the subcutaneous layer at the time of initial skin incision by angling the scalpel blade upwards (see Figure 16.5(c)).

The no-touch technique, much favoured by orthopaedic surgeons, is inappropriate for ischaemic tissues which can be considerably traumatized by instruments. Tissues are handled with fingers, not forceps. Haemostasis using fine absorbable ligature material must be thorough and exact, mass ligatures of bunches of tissue being unacceptable.

Bones are divided with a saw, preferably a power saw, rather than with bone cutters which are apt to crush and splinter. Great care must be taken not to traumatize soft tissue with the saw blade. Bone edges are carefully contoured with file or nibblers so that no sharp edge is presented to overriding tissue. Sawdust and other debris should be washed out of the wound with saline. Oozing from marrow stops eventually, and the use of bone wax is not recommended.

Nerves are drawn down, divided with a single scalpel cut and allowed to retract. Most deep tissues are approximated with fine absorbable sutures, the author's preference being 3/0 vicryl which retains its strength for longer and absorbs with less reaction than catgut. Non-absorbable sutures such as polypropylene are employed for tendons, ligaments or fascia which are to be subject to the action of muscles. For all amputations except those which are grossly infected primary closure is employed over vacuum drain(s). It is vital that skin approximation should be accurate and tension free. Continuous subcuticular sutures or alternated interrupted monofilament sutures and wound tapes are both methods which provide satisfactory results. For below-knee and Syme's amputations a rigid plaster dressing carries advantages, provided that it is applied with careful attention to detail (see below).

Wound infection being a serious consideration, a broad-spectrum antibiotic, whose cover includes clostridia, is begun at the time of the premedication and continued for 48 hours. If an infected synthetic graft is in place it should be entirely removed at the time of the amputation: if it is merely thrombosed it is sufficient to excise the graft as high as possible from the amputation field.

Amputation of digits

It is well-known that successful amputation of ischaemic digits as an isolated treatment can often be achieved in diabetics, but it is rare for this to be the case in non-diabetic atherosclerotics. Concomitant intervention to improve arterial circulation, whether by angioplasty or reconstruction is usually required.

Disarticulation is generally a mistake in the ischaemic toe since healing does not usually occur over an exposed articular surface. Toes should be amputated through the proximal phalanx or through the shaft of the metatarsal.

It is often tempting in the case of a necrotic or septic toe to amputate and leave an unsutured wound which can be dressed and allowed to granulate. If there has been a successful reconstruction this may work, but unless the blood supply is exceptionally good such wounds are slow to heal and often fail altogether. Surgeons should ensure that there is skin cover without tension and, if this cannot be achieved, should consider a more proximal amputation from the start.

If infection or gangrene has reached the base of the toe excision must include the head of the metatarsal – ray amputation. In the author's experience this amputation has a poor healing record, but it has a place when the digit involved is the hallux, and also in diabetics when the remainder of the foot is well perfused. To gain access to the metatarsal head a racquet incision is used, with the handle of the racquet on the dorsum of the foot.

Transmetatarsal amputation

To be successful this amputation usually requires concomitant arterial reconstruction. In diabetics, although digital amputation is often successful without reconstruction, this seldom applies to transmetatarsal amputation because the usual indication for amputation at foot level is sepsis, which typically extends into the deep plantar spaces of the foot making ray or below-knee amputations the more likely options.

Cut the flaps as generously as possible, keeping the knife close to the bone to ensure maximum flap thickness. Remove all tendons and cartilage. Divide the bones with a saw, not bone cutters. File smooth all sharp edges. A few 4/0 absorbable subcutaneous sutures are placed and the skin approximated with fine monofilament and wound tapes. A vacuum drain is brought out through a separate stab.

Other foot amputations

A variety of other foot amputations have occasionally been employed in vascular patients. These include Lisfranc's amputation (forefoot disarticulation between the tarsal and metatarsal bones); Chopart's amputation (forefoot disarticulation at the talonavicular and calcaneocuboid joints) and Pirogoff's amputation (ankle disarticulation with transection of the distal tibia and fibula just above the joint surface). These amputations are not recommended as they seldom heal well and are subject to equinus and equinovarus deformities, so the techniques are not discussed.

Satisfactory healing is also rare after the Syme's amputation, sometimes recommended in diabetics. Even in those patients in whom primary healing is obtained, it may take a very long time to achieve weight bearing and the stump is prone to neuropathy in the long term.

Below-knee amputation

In the author's view the skew flap[20] is the best technique. It heals as successfully as the Burgess type of long posterior flap[4] and provides a stump with better coverage of the bone, a scar which is not positioned over the end of the tibia and a shape more conducive to early limb fitting.

The skew-flap method has been fully described by Robinson[20], but here are some salient technical points. Precise marking of the skin is essential, the junction of the equal anteromedial and posterolateral flaps is sited 1–2 finger breadths lateral to the anterior border of the tibia (Figures 16.3(a,b)). The circumference is measured and divided equally into two to give the width of the flaps and then into four to give the radius of each flap. Also crucial to success is the correct shaping of the gastrocnemius tendon and fascia. It does not correspond to the skin flap but is cut about 5 cm longer and more directly posterior than the skin flap (Figure 16.3(b)). All other muscles are divided at the level of tibial section. As with the long posterior flap method a sliver of gastrocnemius usually has to be taken off each side of the posterior flap to minimize bulk. It is the way in which this myofascial tongue is used to cover the bone end which confers much of the benefit of this amputation (Figure 16.3(d)).

Haemostasis should be thorough, using fine absorbable ligatures. Bone is divided in the same way as for the conventional below-knee technique, the tibia being divided approximately a hand's breadth below the tibial tuberosity – slightly longer in tall individuals – and the fibula 2–3 cm more proximal. If a power saw is available the anterior tibial border can be shaped at the time of division. Otherwise three separate cuts of a tenon saw are used (Figure 16.4(c)) and – very important – the bone ends meticulously rounded and smoothed with a hand file. Sawdust is washed away with saline.

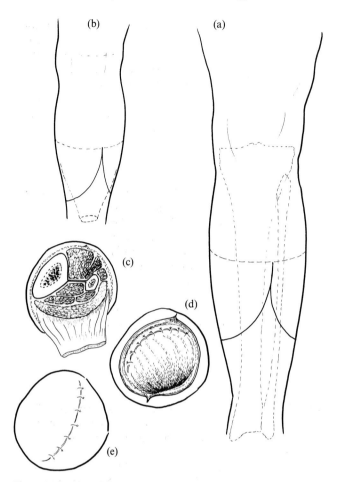

Figure 16.3 Skew-flap amputation.
(a) The flaps meet anteriorly 1–2 finger breadths lateral to the anterior border of the tibia;
(b) posteriorly the skin flap does not correspond to the myofascial flap;
(c) the posterior myofascial flap comprises deep fascia plus gastrocnemius;
(d) it is rotated obliquely forward, over the tibia, and sutured to deep fascia;
(e) the skin suture line does not overlie the bone end

The gastrocnemius tendon and deep fascia are brought obliquely forward and sutured to the anterior periosteum and deep fascia (Figures 16.3(c,d)). Absorbable 3/0 vicryl sutures are used to approximate all layers, the subcutaneous sutures being inverted to bury the knots. For skin closure the author's practice has been to use interrupted 3/0 monofilament alternated with adhesive strips but fine subcuticular sutures are preferred by many and give excellent results. Vacuum drains are brought out on each side, one crossing the bone ends, the other more superficially. They are not anchored to the skin so that they can be removed at 24–48 hours without disturbing the dressing.

Stump dressing

In the author's view a rigid plaster dressing confers great advantages in that it provides security, protection, reassurance, less pain, light support and an ideal position for the knee. Considerable attention to detail in the application is essential.

The method is as follows. About ten gauze swabs are fluffed out, 'boxing glove' style, and positioned towards the back of the end of the stump. Tubular gauze over a thigh-size applicator is then applied in two or three layers, starting at the top of the thigh, twisting over the gauze padding at the end of the stump and taken back up to the top of the thigh. The assistant grasps the top of the gauze medially and laterally and maintains moderate upward traction to impact and shape the padding over the end of the stump until the remaining layers have been applied. As immediate prosthetic fitting is no longer recommended, pressure points do not need to be individually padded, but a layer of orthopaedic wool is applied overall. This is followed by a lightweight synthetic plaster which is carefully moulded using jelly on the gloves. The plaster is moulded inwards on each side above the knee to prevent rotation, as for a walking plaster. The knee is positioned in about 10 degrees of flexion.

A plaster dressing is left undisturbed for a week unless the patient complains of severe pain or runs a high fever, in which case it can be bivalved to allow stump inspection and reapplied if all is well. It does not preclude quadriceps exercises or patient mobilization, and if not too bulky can be inserted into a pneumatic walking aid.

Below-knee amputation with long posterior flap

This well-proven method may be preferred if there is a medial scar or damaged anterior skin. It has been well described in many texts. Many of the technical points described above apply, including bevelling of the subcutaneous fat, the retention of gastrocnemius but not soleus on the posterior flap, the lateral and medial narrowing of the muscle bulk posteriorly, meticulous contouring of the tibia, thorough haemostasis, fine absorbable sutures, vacuum drains and plaster dressing. Figure 16.4 shows how the posterior flap is cut longer than required and contoured to shape at the time of skin closure.

Through-knee amputation

Amputation at knee level is probably underrated[21]. It has been regarded as cosmetically unattractive but modern prosthetics have improved and can accommodate the wide bone end. It may be considered in the wheelchair-bound or bed-ridden patient where a long lever is an advantage, and in the very unfit patient with severe gangrene where an urgent debridement is advisable.

This amputation can be performed quickly, with minimal blood loss, using equal lateral and medial flaps. The patellar tendon is detached from its tibial insertion and sutured with strong non-absorbable sutures to the cruciate ligaments. This brings the skin suture line to lie neatly posteriorly between the condyles. The main disadvantages of this amputation, other than those already mentioned, are the vulnerability of the skin over the condyles and the tendency for prolonged leakage of synovial fluid from the wound. In the author's opinion other amputations around the knee, such as the Gritti–Stokes, have little to commend them in the light of modern advances in prosthetics.

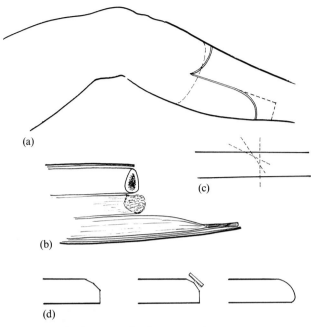

Figure 16.4   The long posterior flap amputation.
(a) Cut the posterior flap longer initially than will be required;
(b) the posterior flap includes gastrocnemius but not soleus;
(c) if a power saw is not available the bone end is shaped with two oblique and one vertical cuts with a hand saw;
(d) smoothing the anterior border of the tibia

Above-knee amputation

By the time a patient comes to above-knee amputation he or she may have been through an arduous sequence of ischaemic events, investigations, failed reconstructions and more distal amputations. Relatively little attention appears to be paid to technique as it is generally assumed that healing will be successful at this level, an assumption which has led many surgeons in the past to elect for this level for the first amputation, sometimes without even considering arterial reconstruction. Regrettably, pressure of work and insufficient resources may be factors in such decisions. Even relatively recent series have reported as many as 70% of amputations at above-knee level[22].

An aggressive policy towards arterial reconstruction may lead ultimately to a higher proportion of above-knee amputations[23] and an increasingly aged population may have a similar effect, since there is little point in risking defective healing by striving to preserve the knee joint in a patient who clearly cannot progress beyond a wheelchair. However, the importance of preserving the knee joint in patients who may rehabilitate successfully is now widely understood.

Perhaps the poor prospects for rehabilitation (around 30% of above-knee amputees walk compared with 75% of below knee-amputees[24]) is another factor which has caused the technical aspects of above-knee amputation to receive minimal attention. Whether full limb fitting is intended or the stump simply destined to function as a

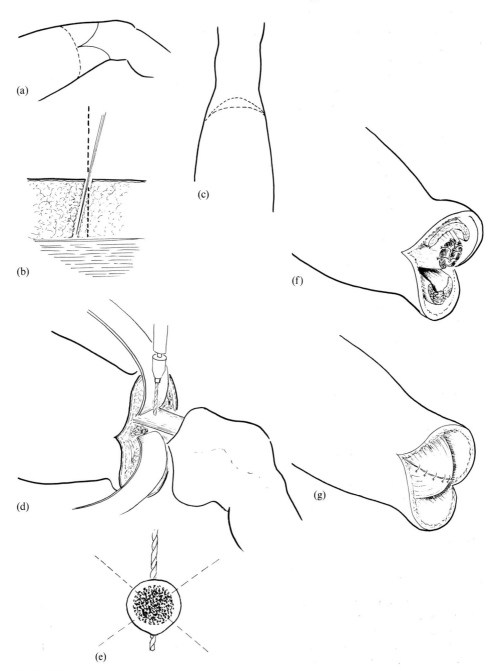

Figure 16.5   Above-knee amputation.
  (a) Anterior and posterior skin flaps;
  (b) bevelling the subcutaneous fat;
  (c) extra convexity on the posterior flap to minimize 'puckering';
  (d, e) drilling the femur in preparation for myoplasty;
  (f) lateral and medial muscle bundles sutured to bone;
  (g) anterior and posterior muscles and deep fascia sutured across the bone end

prop and lever for the wheelchair patient, it should have certain qualities. The stump should be firm, well tapered and as long as can be achieved, consistent with good healing. The bone end should be rounded and well covered with soft tissue. There should be maximum muscle fixation to the distal bone to confer optimal propriocep- tion and leverage. This is achieved by a myoplastic type of stump construction.

The circumference of the leg should be measured and marked to give equal anterior and posterior flaps extended distally to a point one to two finger breadths above the patella (Figure 16.5(a)). Skin and subcutaneous tissue should be incised with a single clean cut, with the knife blade angled slightly upwards as described for below-knee amputations (Figure 16.5(c)).

Muscle retraction and the gutter between the hamstrings causes the middle portion of the posterior flap to retract. This effect can be minimized by cutting an extra convexity on the posterior flap (Figure 16.5(c)). Fascia and muscles are divided in line with the skin incisions and the periosteum raised off the bone, which is then drilled at three points to give six holes for suturing, just proximal to the intended line of division (Figure 16.5(d,e)). It is difficult to drill the femur after it has been divided.

The myoplastic effect is then achieved by suturing the lateral and medial groups of muscles, vastus lateralis and the adductor tendons respectively, to the bone end with non-absorbable sutures. As a second layer the anterior and posterior muscles, quadriceps and hamstrings are sutured to each other over the bone end (Figure 16.5(f,g)). Sutures are placed through fascia rather than fleshy muscle and tension must be avoided. Deep and superficial wide bore vacuum drains are used. The subcutaneous tissues and skin should be closed as previously described, and the stump lightly bandaged.

Amputations at hip level

In vascular patients it is fortunately rare for hip disarticulation or hindquarter amputation to be considered. They are described in standard texts. It is essential to consider very carefully before submitting a patient with advanced vascular disease to these mutilating operations. Mortality is high and complications are frequent, particularly sacral pressure sores. A reasonable quality of life is seldom achieved in these circumstances.

Outcome

Early complications

Space does not allow full discussion of complications, the most serious being delayed healing, stump necrosis, flexion contracture and stump pain. Suffice it to say that careful selection of level combined with application of the technical principles described above should minimize these problems. As far as pain is concerned the avoidance of undue delay when there is severe preoperative pain, psychological support and complete pain control in the early postoperative period are all- important. A stump which remains severely painful is often ischaemic and may require further amputation. For phantom pain electrical transcutaneous nerve stimulation is sometimes successful. The injection of calcitonin, salmon variety, has been advocated[25] but requires testing by controlled trial.

Table 16.2   Reporting the results of amputation surgery: some relevant questions

1. Is the series complete?
2. What are the demographic characteristics of the population?
3. What are the associated diseases, especially diabetes?
4. What proportion of patients with critical ischaemia are referred to vascular specialists?
5. What are the numbers, amputation levels and outcomes of amputations for vascular disease in patients not referred to vascular surgeons?
6. What proportion of patients with critical ischaemia receive no active treatment?
7. What proportion have angiography?
8. What proportion undergo arterial reconstruction?
9. What types of reconstruction are being performed?
10. What are the outcomes of reconstruction?
11. What proportion undergo amputation?
12. How many amputations are performed in total in the entire population?
13. Who performs the amputations?
14. What is the ratio of amputation to reconstruction?
15. What are the numbers and ratios of amputations at each level, including minor amputations?
16. What are the revision rates at each level?

Comparability of results

Few dispute the need to preserve the knee joint whenever possible. Reference has been made to the ratio of below-knee to above-knee amputations as a criterion of quality of practice. Is it a reliable criterion? Table 16.2 lists the questions which should be addressed when presenting the results of amputation. The message is that amputation data need to be considered against a comprehensive, population-based background of referral and selection policies, demographic data and information on all aspects of arterial reconstruction. Without this information statements about amputation ratios are relatively meaningless.

References

1. Bernhard, V. M. (1989) Bypass to the popliteal and infrapopliteal arteries. *Vascular Surgery* (ed. R. B. Rutherford). W. B. Saunders, Philadelphia, pp. 692–704
2. De Weese, J. A. and Robb, C. G. (1977) Autogenous venous grafts ten years later. *Surgery*, **82**, 775–780
3. McIntyre, K. E., Bailey, S. A., Malone, J. M. and Goldstone, J.(1984) Guillotine amputation in the treatment of non-salvageable lower-extremity infections. *Arch. Surg.*, **119**, 450–453
4. Ruckley, C. V., Stonebridge, P. A. and Prescott, R. J. (1991) Skew flap versus long posterior flap in below knee amputation: a multicentre trial. *J. Vasc. Surg.*, (in press)
5. Pollock, S. B. and Ernst, C. B. (1980) Use of Doppler pressure measurements in predicting success in amputation of the leg. *Am. J. Surg.*, **139**, 303–306
6. Wagner, W. H., Keagy, B. A., Kotis, M. M., Burnham, S. J. and Johnson, G. (1988) Noninvasive determination of healing of major lower-extremity amputation: the continued role of clinical judgement. *J. Vasc. Surg.*, **8**, 703–710
7. Malone, J. M., Anderson, G. G., Lalka, S. G., Hagaman, R. M., Henry, R., McIntyre, K. E. and Bernhard, V. M. (1987) Prospective comparison of noninvasive techniques for amputation level selection. *Am J. Surg.*, **154**, 179–184
8. Van den Broek, T. A. Dwars, B. J., Rauwerda, J. A. and Bakker, F. C. (1990) A multivariate analysis of determinants of wound healing in patients after amputation for peripheral vascular disease. *Eur. J. Vasc. Surg.*, **4**, 291–295
9. Gibbons, G. W., Wheelock, F. C., Siembieda, C., Hoar, C. S., Rowbottom, J. L. and Persson, A. B. (1979) Non-invasive prediction of amputation level in diabetic patients. *Arch Surg.*, **114**, 1253–1257
10. Bone, G. E. and Pomajzl, M. J. (1981) Toe blood pressure by photoplethysmography: an index of healing in forefoot amputation. *Surgery*, **89**, 569–574

11. Moore, W. S., Henry, R. E., Malone, J. M., Daly, M. J., Patton, D. and Childers, S. J. (1981) Prospective use of Xenon 133 clearance for amputation level selection. *Arch. Surg.*, **116**, 86–88
12. McCollom, P. T., Spence, V. A., Walker, W. F., Swanson, A. J. G., Turner, M. S. and Murdoch, G. (1985) Circumferential skin blood flow measurements in the ischaemic lower limb. *Br. J. Surg.*, **72**, 310–312
13. McCollum, P. T., Spence, V. A. and Walker, W. F. (1988) Amputation for peripheral vascular disease: the case for level selection. *Br. J. Surg.*, **75**, 1193–1195
14. Katsamouris, A., Brewster, D. C., Megerman, J., Cina, C. and Darling, R. C. (1984) Transcutaneous oxygen tension in selection of amputation level. *Am. J. Surg.*, **147**, 510–517
15. Ratliff, D. A., Clyne, C. A. C., Chant, A. D. B. and Webster, J. H. H. (1984) Prediction of amputation wound healing: the role of transcutaneous pO_2 assessment. *Br. J. Surg.*, **71**, 219–222
16. Dowd, G. S. E. (1986) Predicting stump healing following amputation for peripheral vascular disease using transcutaneous oxygen monitor. *Ann. R. Coll. Surg. Eng.*, **68**, 31–35
17. Wyss, C. R., Harrington, R. M., Burgess, E. M. and Matsen, F. A. (1988) Transcutaneous oxygen tension as a predictor of success after an amputation. *J. Bone Joint Surg.*, **70**, 203–207.
18. Silverman, D. G., Roberts, A., Reilly, C. A., Brousseau, D. A., Norton, K. J., Bartley, E. and Neufeld, G. R. (1987) Fluorometric quantification of low-dose fluorescein delivery to predict amputation site healing. *Surgery*, **101**, 335–341
19. Barber, G. G., McPhail, N. V., Scobie, T. K., Brennan, M. C. D. and Ellis, C. C. (1983) A prospective study of lower limb amputations. *Can. J. Surg.*, **26**, 339–341
20. Robinson, K. P., Hoile, R. and Coddington, T. (1982) Skew flap myoplastic below-knee amputation: a preliminary report. *Br. J. Surg.*, **69**, 554–557
21. Moran, B. J., Buttenshaw, R., Mulcahy, M. and Robinson, K. P. (1990) Through knee amputation in high risk patients with vascular disease: indications, complications and rehabilitation. *Br. J. Surg.*, **77**, 1118–1120
22. Haynes, I. G. and Middleton, M. D. (1981) Amputation for peripheral vascular disease: experience of a district general hospital. *Ann. R. Coll. Surg.*, **63**, 342–344
23. Kazmers, M., Satiani, B. and Evans, W. E. (1980) Amputation level following unsuccessful distal limb salvage operations. *Surgery*, **87**, 683–687
24. Couch, N. P., David, J. K., Tilney, N. L. and Crane, C. (1977) The natural history of the leg amputee. *Am. J. Surg.*, **133**, 469–473
25. Jaeger, H., Maier, Ch. and Wawersik, J. (1988) Calcitonin in the postoperative treatment of phantom limb pains and causalgia. *Anaesthetist*, **37**, 71–76

Chapter 17

Chronic venous insufficiency – should the long saphenous vein be stripped?

Simon G. Darke

Varicose veins affect between 10 and 12% of the adult population[1,2]. Of these most have varicosities of the long saphenous system. In the author's experience 85% of patients referred for treatment had long saphenous varicosities of which in turn, 75% had incompetence at the saphenofemoral junction[3]. Compression sclerotherapy in the presence of groin reflux is associated with an unacceptably high recurrence rate, 63% at three years[4] and 93% at six years[5]. Because most surgeons would therefore agree that a surgical approach is necessary under these circumstances, long saphenous varicosities with saphenofemoral incompetence represent a large surgical workload. It is not surprising that it has doubled in the UK in the last decade[6].

It is unsatisfactory, therefore, that uncertainty still remains about fundamental technical aspects of such a common problem. All would agree that accurate saphenofemoral ligation and division should be undertaken. But should the saphenous trunk also be stripped or excised? The same dilemma to a lesser extent exists for the short saphenous system.

What are the conceptual attractions of performing a simple ligation and preserving the long saphenous trunk? It can be combined with a synchronous local excision of distal varicosities by multiple stabs or alternatively with subsequent compression sclerotherapy. This therapeutic approach represents a lesser procedure. Stripping the saphenous vein necessitates general or regional anaesthesia, and increases bruising in the thigh in the postoperative period. Recovery is more painful and less rapid. Simple groin ligation favours daycase surgery, possibly under local anaesthetic, which in turn may increase convenience for the patient and be more cost-effective in terms of resource management. A further theoretically compelling reason for retaining the saphenous trunk is that it might remain available for future arterial surgery should it become necessary in order either to bypass the coronary arteries or to reconstruct the lower limb. Certainly in the latter situation there is little doubt that vein gives superior results to prosthetic material in bypasses below the knee[7]. In addressing this issue therefore there are a number of points that need to be considered.

What is the likelihood of a patient undergoing varicose vein surgery requiring a bypass at some time in the future? Lofgren[8], in a retrospective enquiry, found that it was uncommon for a patient who had previously undergone stripping to be denied a subsequent bypass. However, it must be conceded that this study was undertaken some time ago and since then the position might have changed somewhat due to the increasing numbers, particularly of coronary artery bypass grafts, that are undertaken in contemporary practice. However, on an *ad hoc* basis it is not very common to encompass a patient for femorodistal grafting in whom the vein has previously been removed for varicose veins. The high vein utilization rate (95%) in reported series of femorodistal bypass bears testimony to this observation[9].

Even if it were retained, is a saphenous vein with associated varicosities and pre-existing groin incompetence an adequate conduit for a bypass? In attempting to answer this, among other questions, we undertook peroperative descending veno-grams at the time of venous surgery to assess the saphenous vein in the thigh. The extent of varicose changes present in 65% of veins were sufficient to render them unsuitable for grafting (see Table 17.1)[10]. Even in the remaining 35% it is difficult to speculate as to what further changes in terms of subsequent varicose dilatation or thrombotic events might have occurred in the future. In contrast to this finding is a recent report by Hammarsten et al.[11], in which 42 patients were randomized to high ligation and stripping or high ligation alone. In both groups this was combined with local avulsions to distal varicosities. At follow-up 52 ± 5 months later, vein mapping by means of real-time high-resolution ultrasound showed that 78% of the preserved saphenous veins would have been suitable for use as an artificial conduit.

Why is there this conflict between our own and Hammarsten's results? Are the methods of assessment or interpretation different? This seems unlikely. One obvious factor may be the extent of saphenous incompetence and varicose changes by which patients were selected for surgery in the two groups. Certainly it is reasonable to believe that in our own patient material these changes may have been extensive. Of the 80 limbs studied 27 were undergoing surgery for associated venous ulceration attributable to saphenous incompetence. It was evident that the morphological changes were more prominent in this group of patients than in those with varicosities uncomplicated by skin change. Even so, would this factor alone explain the differences between the two studies? Perhaps the degree of saphenous incompetence in the Swedish study[11] was nominal. No details are given as to how saphenous 'incompetence' was diagnosed, and in particular whether this was evident on descending venography. However, pre- and postoperative plethysmographic studies performed on their patients did suggest that there were haemodynamic improvements following saphenous ligation.

What then is the practical conclusion about this issue? It must be evident to any experienced surgeon that a proportion at least of long saphenous veins removed for varicose change are totally unsuited for use as an arterial bypass conduit. Equally, some veins when explored with a view to femorodistal bypass (or assessed pre-

Table 17.1   Peroperative descending saphenography in patients with long saphenous incompetence

| | Number of patients | |
	No skin change	Skin ulceration
Number of saphenograms	53	27
Contrast to knee joint	51	24
Contrast to calf	33	17
Varicose long saphenous vein	31	21
Mean length of normal vein seen (mm)	150	160
Mean width of normal vein seen (mm)	6	7
Long saphenous veins with valves	34*	9*
Mean number of valves present	2	2
Direct thigh perforators	46	24
Thigh perforator 'incompetence'	8	7

* Statistically significant, $P < 0.05$

operatively by venography or duplex scanning) are similarly unusable. But is this the case in any patient with demonstrable long saphenous varicosities and sapheno-femoral incompetence? The answer to this is probably 'no', but we do not know to what extent. Clearly there are variable degrees of incompetence and dilatation. The Swedish study[11] provides new and valuable information. Those long saphenous veins assessed to be usable at the time of flush saphenofemoral ligation and left *in situ* remained potentially usable for five years and may have remained so for longer in most limbs.

There are refinements to this argument. Saphenofemoral incompetence may be present but feeding a so-called 'anterior thigh vein' into which the principal or early reflux occurs. There may be relative normality of the long saphenous trunk. It is clearly wrong, therefore, to regard incompetence at groin level as inevitably descending into the long saphenous trunk and that this will be incompetent throughout its length. For instance, in a recent study by Koyano and Sakaguchi[12] the long saphenous was assessed from ankle to groin with Doppler ultrasonic flowmeters. Reverse flow in the saphenous vein was assessed in ascending segments by reflux after manual calf compression. Of the 309 limbs studied, 205 (66%) had flow in the entire vein length from groin to ankle; the remaining limbs however had reverse flow only in some segments of the saphenous vein. Based on this finding, selective stripping was undertaken in these patients. The recurrence rate was comparable to those patients in whom the entire length was removed from groin to ankle. Thus in some patients it was possible to conserve part at least of the long saphenous vein without apparently prejudicing long-term results, and illustrates that relatively localized incompetence may occur in a proportion of veins.

There seems reasonable evidence therefore that in a percentage at least of patients with saphenofemoral incompetence part or all of the long saphenous trunk may be preserved and will remain in a potentially usable state for future grafting. The next question is to what extent a conservationist policy might influence future recurrence of varicose veins and what, if anything, might be done to minimize the risk of recurrence if in fact this risk does exist? At this juncture it is of interest and relevance to consider aspects regarding the incidence of recurrence following varicose vein surgery, factors relating to its development, and the possible role that retaining the saphenous trunk after groin ligation might play. Finally, how common is recurrence and does it therefore represent a significant problem?

Classification and incidence of recurrent varicose veins

It is helpful, not only in terms of investigation and management but also in addressing the specific issue of saphenous stripping, to attempt to identify and classify various types of recurrent varicose veins (Figure 17.1). As a loose definition here we regard recurrence as patients seeking treatment who have had previous surgery for this condition. The following groups can be recognized.

Type I

Recurrence of varicosities without demonstrable incompetence in the saphenous system, long or short (see below).

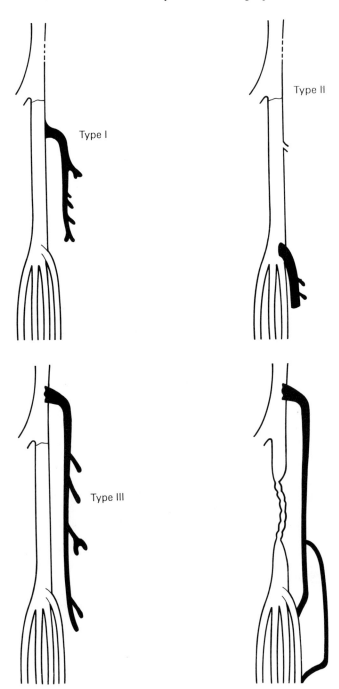

Figure 17.1   Recurrent varicose veins

Type II

'Recurrence' due to evolution or persistence of varicosities derived from incompetence in a second saphenous system, e.g. in the short saphenous system following previous, apparently successful, surgery directed towards the long saphenous system (or vice versa).

Type III

Varicosities derived from recurrence of incompetence in either the saphenofemoral or the saphenopopliteal junction following previous ligation.

To these for completeness might be added a further group, although it is not specifically relevant to the issues debated here. These are patients who develop recurrent 'varicosities' as a consequence of deep vein obstruction from previous deep vein thrombosis. The superficial veins may be valuable collaterals and attempts at surgical removal are often ill advised. Clinical awareness of this possibility is therefore mandatory. Excessive haemorrhage may ensue under these circumstances and the pain and swelling made worse.

In a recent study undertaken by the author an attempt has been made to estimate the extent of recurrence after previous surgery in patients referred for treatment. Of a total of 318 consecutive patients examined over a 13-month period, 76 (24%) had undergone previous surgery directed at one or other saphenous system or both.

Type I Of the 76, 21 (28% of those with recurrences) had recurrent varicosities but no clinical evidence of recurrent saphenofemoral incompetence on unidirectional ultrasound.

Type II Six of the 76 patients had incompetence in the short saphenous system, having previously undergone long saphenous surgery. In one patient the opposite situation pertained. (A total of 9% of recurrences.)

Type 3 Forty-eight patients (63% of recurrences) had recurrent saphenofemoral incompetence; 42 in the long saphenous system and six in the short saphenous system.

Sheppard[13] has reported similar findings in a comparable study of 501 new patients referred for treatment. Recurrence after surgery was present in 28% of the total. Of these recurrences 90% were attributable to further incompetence at the saphenofemoral junction.

These two surveys have assessed the recurrence rate in patients being referred for primary treatment. Of more specific importance is the recurrence rate in patients followed up systematically after surgery. Hobbs[5] reported the failure rate at six years following radical and enthusiastic surgery to be 10%. No breakdown regarding the different types referred to above is given. In a personal series by Royle[14], with a minimum follow up of five years, 18% of 367 patients had sufficiently severe recurrence to warrant further surgery. Lofgren[8], in reporting his experience of 278 patients examined at 10 years following surgery found that 15% of patients had varicosities of sufficient severity to warrant further surgery. After 20 years the proportion had risen to 33%. Berridge and Makin[15] found a recurrence rate of 20% 3–10 years after surgery in 164 patients. Of these 34 patients with recurrence, 24 (71%) had developed recurrent saphenofemoral incompetence, and one recurrent saphenopopliteal incompetence.

These data from a number of centres worldwide illustrate two important points. The recurrence rate after about five years is of the order of 20% and probably increases with time. Recurrent saphenofemoral incompetence plays a major role in the pathogenesis.

Does the retention of the saphenous trunk at the time of initial surgery have any bearing on these facts? Does it increase the risk of recurrence in general, and recurrent saphenofemoral incompetence specifically? There are to my knowledge three published prospective controlled trials that examine the outcome with and without stripping. The first of these, published in 1979 by Jakobsen[5], divided 516 patients with previously untreated varicose veins into three treatment groups in a randomized prospective trial. Group II patients received a radical operation consisting of saphenofemoral or popliteal disconnection extraction of the appropriate saphenous trunk, multiple avulsions of distal varices and ligation of ankle perforators. Group II patients underwent saphenous ligation under local anaesthetic and subsequent compression sclerotherapy. Group III underwent compression sclerotherapy alone. The patients were reviewed at three months at which stage over 95% of groups I and II were satisfactory and 85% in group III. At three years, however, the objective results were satisfactory in 90% of group I, 65% in group II and only 36% in group III. Subjective assessments were essentially the same.

In a second study published by Munn and colleagues in 1981[16], a prospective double-blind trial was undertaken on patients with bilateral symmetrical long saphenous incompetence. The two treatment groups consisted of groin ligation and local excisions in one set, combined in the other with stripping from ankle to groin. Unfortunately of the 100 patients only 57 were available for follow-up between 2.5 and 3.5 years. Fifty-five limbs (48%) of the 114 limbs reviewed had recurrence, of which 34 had not been stripped. (Difference statistically significant, $P < 0.01$.)

The trial already referred to by Hammarsten et al.[11] is in contrast to these findings with no difference at three years between those stripped and not stripped. However, this was with a small trial with a short follow-up, and reference has already been made regarding the severity of saphenous incompetence that existed in these patients. It would be interesting to see what the results were after three years. Finally, to this must be added the observations of Lofgren and Lofgren[17], who concluded that incomplete removal of the saphenous trunk was a common source of recurrence.

On the basis of this limited experience therefore, leaving the long saphenous trunk *in situ* after groin ligation would seem to increase significantly the risk of recurrence. Accepting that this is the case, what are the mechanisms underlying recurrence and what role does the retained long saphenous trunk play in its pathogenesis? Let us look at the three types of recurrence and try to consider this issue further.

Type I

The recurrence in this category is characterized by symptomatic varicosities without evidence of either saphenofemoral or saphenopopliteal incompetence occurring primarily or recurrently. Preoperative varicography has been used to evaluate this form of recurrence and indicates that the principal source is incompetent thigh perforating veins[18]. Type I recurrence was first recognized and reported by Sherman in 1944 who found that it was particularly likely to occur in patients who had been treated by flush ligation alone[19]. Dodd[20] studied 52 limbs, in 40 of which there had been recurrence after previous surgery. At operation he exposed the entire subsartorial canal and found at least one incompetent perforator in 10 of these patients, two in a further 20 patients and as many as three in a final patient. Clearly wide exposure of this nature would not be appropriate in contemporary practice but the data are of interest and relevance in the current debate. Under these circumstances preoperative varicography gives useful information in confirming the cause for the recurrence and as guidance in anatomical terms to dictate operative strategy for its correction[18].

The question that must be asked is whether the failure to remove the long saphenous trunk at the time of the original surgery has increased the risk of thigh recurrence. Reference has already been made to work in which patients were submitted to perioperative retrograde saphenography at the time of definitive surgery[10]. The procedure was undertaken in 80 limbs of 60 patients, in 27 of whom there was ulceration. All had normal deep vein systems on ascending and descending venography. The mean number of valves in the saphenous trunk to the level of the knee was two, but in none of these limbs were competent valves demonstrable. Thigh perforators, which are of particular significance, were present in 87%, and were inferred to be incompetent if they were greater than 3 mm diameter with no identifiable valves and were varicose or directly associated with localized varicosities of the long saphenous trunk[21]. By these rather rigid criteria 15 of the limbs were thought to have contained incompetent thigh-perforating veins, which might represent an underestimate. Furthermore, one has to consider that even if this dynamic state existed at the time of assessment, incompetence might develop in perforators in the ensuing years. The relevant data are summarized in Table 17.1.

Papadakis[22] reported 42 patients, all of whom had previous saphenofemoral ligation for varicose veins predominantly without stripping, studied by ascending venography for recurrent varicose veins. Fifteen had recurrent saphenofemoral reflux (thus type II). However, in 80% of patients at least one incompetent thigh-perforating vein was demonstrated and in 20% more than one was seen. There was no consistency of exact anatomical site of these thigh communicating veins, which supports the findings of Dodd[20].

To leave an incompetent saphenous trunk connected by an incompetent thigh perforator to the deep system would seem, on theoretical grounds at least, to be an inevitable recipe for recurrence. However, it must be conceded that a counter-argument might claim that by removing the major incompetence from the saphenofemoral junction above improvement in valve function below that level could occur.

Type II

This form of recurrence or persistence would not seem to be related to whether or not the saphenous trunk has been stripped and therefore is not relevant to this debate.

Type III

It is perhaps germane at this juncture to digress slightly to address the question regarding the criteria by which saphenofemoral incompetence, occurring primarily or recurrently, might be assessed. The simplest evaluations of course are long-standing, time-honoured, clinical tests, however, (in common with many contemporary workers) the author is of the opinion that a hand-held unidirectional Doppler is essential in the evaluation of the saphenofemoral junction[3,23–27]. Limbs are easily assessed in the outpatient clinic at first presentation. Examination should be by a combination of inspection, standard clinical tests and (as pointed out above) Doppler ultrasound. For this the patient stands immobile facing the examiner and the probe is located over the saphenofemoral junction by moving it medially from the femoral artery signal until the signal ceases. Confirmation of correct position is obtained by manual calf compression which produces an audible signal. On releasing the calf compression no further signal in a normal limb is heard, provided of course both deep and superficial systems are competent. Occasionally a very short (< 1s) refluxing signal may be heard, which is not regarded as significant. If a signal similar to that heard on compression follows the release of compression it is regarded as signifying valvular incompetence. Abolition of refluxing signal by compression of the long saphenous in the thigh manually or by tourniquet confirms saphenofemoral incompetence.

The same principles can only be applied to recurrent saphenofemoral incompetence in a proportion of cases. In some cases it is difficult to insonate over the bizarre varicosities that exist at groin level and in these cases complementary tests should be employed by locating the probe over one of the more distal obvious subcutaneous varicosities and confirming adequate insonation by squeeze and release of the calf. A retrograde signal on patient coughing implies reflux of blood from the deep system into the superficial varicosity (this can be due to a number of anatomical variations which are discussed further below). Firm pressure over the saphenofemoral junction causing abolition of the signal is confirmation that recurrent saphenofemoral incompetence exists.

It is of interest to digress at this juncture to consider the specificity and sensitivity of Doppler evaluation. In the author's experience Doppler can be employed to good effect in assessing both primary and recurrent saphenofemoral incompetence[28]. In this study, undertaken on complex venous insufficiency (patients with ulceration, excessive pain and swelling or both), the results of Doppler ultrasound as performed above were compared with descending venography. The results are shown in Table 17.2.

It will be seen that although there is correlation between these two modalities of assessment in 57% of the total of those with competence (96 of the 145 limbs examined) in 28% it was demonstrable on Doppler alone and in 14.5% on venography alone. For technical reasons it is understandable how saphenous reflux might be missed on descending venography due to low siting of the needle, particularly if there is reflux of the dye into the femoral system. On this basis it is to be expected that venography is specific but lacking in sensitivity. What is more difficult to understand is the small number demonstrated on venography alone. This may be due to technical error with the Doppler. Further resolution of this dilemma is likely to come from duplex scanning, where the long saphenous vein can be imaged with certainty and semi-quantifiable information on reflux demonstrated. For the time being however these data cast some doubt on the sensitivity and specificity of both Doppler ultrasound and venography. It would seem likely that the more tests that are applied the more 'incompetence' will be discovered.

We return now to address the morphology of recurrent saphenofemoral incompe-

Table 17.2 Diagnosis of saphenofemoral incompetence in a study on a total of 145 limbs

Modality of assessment	Number of limbs (%)
Doppler evidence alone	27 (18.6)
Doppler and venographic evidence	55 (38)
Venographic evidence alone	12 (8)
All	96 (66.2)

tence and how this might relate to retention of the saphenous trunk at the time of original surgery. The use of venography enables us to define different kinds of recurrent saphenofemoral incompetence which we will classify III a–d (Figure 17.2). In order to obtain maximum information comprehensive ascending and descending venography should be undertaken.

Type IIIa recurrence
In this type it is apparent that an incomplete or inadequate groin ligation has previously been undertaken[17]. Either a persistent or accessory saphenous vein or a major branch emanating from the saphenofemoral trunk has been missed. There are numerous anatomical possibilities. These in turn communicate with varicosities further down the limb. Recurrence of this nature must be put down to technical error by the original operating surgeon. However, it seems possible that the subsequent repercussions of this situation will be compounded by the persistence of the saphenous trunk to which anastomoses may develop.

Type IIIb recurrence
An incompetent thigh perforator communicates via a persistent saphenous trunk or directly with varicosities lower in the limb. If the valves in the superficial femoral and common femoral veins above this level are incompetent this will be indistinguishable both clinically and on ultrasound from true saphenofemoral incompetence. Usually

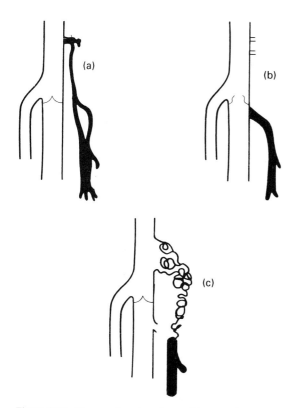

Figure 17.2   Recurrent saphenofemoral incompetence

under these circumstances the perforator is high in the thigh, which really makes its distinction from true saphenofemoral somewhat academic. However, in practical terms it is important because clearly the operative management will require more extensive dissection.

Type IIIc recurrence
This is the most common source of recurrence but has yet to gain wide recognition. It is due to 'neovascularization', characterized by the development of a reconstituted new channel between the common femoral and adjacent veins. The latter may be either the residual unstripped saphenous trunk (with obvious implications to the current debate) or an accessory saphenous trunk or one of its tributaries. This can be readily demonstrated by both ascending and descending venography[28,29] and it is apparent at operation[30].

The histological evolution of neovascularization has been documented in humans[29–31]. These studies show that in the early period following initial saphenous ligation there is organizing thrombus in which numerous small vessels emerge. Within a year these become fewer in number and those that remain enlarge, sometimes coalescing to a single trunk. They develop muscle and elastin in their walls resembling mature veins[30]. These findings have been duplicated in animal experiments[31]. The author has personal anecdotal experience of this phenomenon occurring within 6–9 months of surgery, an observation that has been noted by others[29].

A question which remains unanswered but is of critical importance is what distinguishes those patients in whom this occurs from those who have no subsequent problem? An ongoing study by the author suggests that retention of the saphenous trunk and the coexistence of primary deep incompetence may be critical factors. The author's preliminary and as yet unpublished data show that neovascularization accounts for 75% of Type III recurrences, 63% of these with deep incompetence. However, 48% were found to have a persistent saphenous trunk at least in part, so it would seem that this common form of recurrence can occur even if the saphenous trunk is removed.

Type IIId recurrence
Recurrences may occasionally occur directly from pelvic, principally the internal iliac, veins or via the internal pudendal veins. Similar recurrences can be seen down the veins of the round ligament. Strictly speaking, these are not saphenofemoral but are likely to be interpreted as such in the first instance. These fortunately uncommon cases lead to diagnostic and management difficulties and complex venographic procedures may be required to elucidate the exact morphology.

Summary

Varicosities of the long saphenous system with incompetence of the saphenofemoral junction are common in primary varicose veins. The arguments in favour of performing a groin ligation with preservation of the saphenous trunk are that this represents a lesser procedure and that the vein is retained as a potential conduit should future bypass grafting become necessary. In a proportion of these patients, however, the saphenous trunk, even if conserved, is too varicose to be usable. None the less, in an undetermined percentage of patients it would seem to be possible to retain part or most of the saphenous trunk and this will remain as a potentially useful vessel.

Against this must be assessed the risks of recurrence of varicosities. Varicose veins are a common problem with considerable consequences in terms of resource allocation for health care. Systematic follow-up of patients and review of the 'new' patients referred for surgery show that 20 or 30% develop recurrence of sufficient severity to justify further surgical intervention. The implications of this finding are self-evident.

What prospective randomized studies there are suggest that the recurrence rate is significantly higher if simple ligation alone is undertaken with retention of the saphenous trunk. Furthermore there are theoretical reasons why this might be so. The retained thigh saphenous can be demonstrated to be in communication with the deep system via an incompetent perforator in a significant number of patients; but the principal cause of recurrent varicose veins is due to the reconstruction of the 'saphenofemoral junction' by neovascularization. While this can be observed to occur after the apparent complete removal of the saphenous system in the thigh, it seems likely that retention of the saphenous trunk will facilitate this phenomenon and make its effect more obvious.

What, then, is the answer to the question: 'Should the long saphenous vein be stripped?' The qualified answer to this is 'yes', but a pragmatic approach of selective retention of the saphenous trunk where it appears still usable as a potential bypass conduit is reasonable. This might apply particularly in older patients in whom the time-scale for varicose vein recurrence is that much shorter.

References

1. Coon, W. W., Willis, P. W. III, and Keller, J. B. (1973) Venous thrombo-embolism and other venous disease in the Tecumseh Community Health Study. *Circulation*, **48**, 839–846
2. Widmer, L. K., Hall, T. and Mactin, H. (1977) Epidemiology and sociomedical importance of peripheral venous disease. In *The Treatment of Venous Disorders* (ed. J. T. Hobbs). MTP Press, Lancaster, pp. 3–12
3. Mitchell, D. C. and Darke, S. G. (1987) The assessment of primary varicose veins by doppler ultrasound – the role of sapheno popliteal incompetence and the short saphenous system in calf varicosities. *Eur. J. Vasc. Surg.*, **1**, 113–115
4. Hobbs, J. T. (1974) Surgery and sclerotherapy in the treatment of varicose veins. *Arch. Surg.*, **109**, 793–796
5. Jakobsen, B. H. (1979) The value of different forms of treatment for varicose veins. *Br. J. Surg.*, **66**, 182–184
6. Campbell, W. B. (1990) Varicose veins. *Br. Med. J.*, **300**, 763–764
7. Veith, F. J., Gupta, S. K., Ascer, E., White-Flores, S., Samson, R. H. *et al.* (1986) Six year prospective multicentre randomised comparison of autologous saphenous vein and expanded polytetrafluoroethylene grafts in infra inguinal arterial reconstruction. *J. Vasc. Surg.*, **3**, 104–114
8. Lofgren, E. P. (1985) Treatment of long saphenous varicosities and their recurrence: A long term follow up. In *Surgery of the Veins* (eds J. J. Bergar and J. S. T. Yao). Grune and Stratton, Orlando, pp. 285–299
9. Leather, R. P. and Shah, D. M. (1989) In situ saphenous vein arterial bypass. In *Vascular Surgery*, 3rd edition (ed. R. B. Rutherford). W. B. Saunders, Philadelphia, pp. 414–434
10. Sutton, R. and Darke, S. G. (1986) Stripping the long saphenous vein: peroperative retrograde saphenography in patients with and without ulceration. *Br. J. Surg.*, **73**, 305–307
11. Hammersten, J., Pedersen, P., Claes-Goran, C. and Campanello, M. (1990) Long saphenous vein saving surgery for varicose veins. A long term follow up. *Eur. J. Vasc. Surg.*, **4**, 361–364
12. Koyano, K. and Sakaguchi, S. (1988) Selective stripping operation based on doppler ultrasonic findings for primary varicose veins of the lower limb. *Surgery*, **103**, 615–619
13. Sheppard, M. (1978) A procedure for the prevention of recurrent sapheno femoral incompetence. *Aust. NZ. J. Surg.*, **48**, 322–326
14. Royle, J. P. (1986) Recurrent varicose veins. *World J. Surg.*, **10**, 944–958
15. Berridge, D. C. and Makin, G. S. (1987) Day case surgery: a viable alternative for surgical treatment of varicose veins. *Phlebology*, **2**, 103–108

16. Munn, S. R., Morton, J. B., MacBeth, W. A. A. G. and McLeish, A. R. (1981) To strip or not to strip the long saphenous vein? A varicose veins trial. *Br. J. Surg.*, **68**, 426–428
17. Lofgren, E. P. and Lofgren, K. A. (1971) Recurrence of varicose veins after the stripping operation. *Arch. Surg.*, **102**, 111–114
18. Corbett, C. R., McIrvine, A. J., Astor, N. O., Jamieson, C. W. and Lea Thomas, M. L. (1982) The use of varicography to identify the sources of incompetence in recurrent varicose veins. *Ann. R. Coll. Surg.*, **66**, 412–415
19. Sherman, R. S. (1944) Varicose veins anatomic findings and an operative procedure based upon them. *Ann Surg.*, **120**, 772–784
20. Dodd, H. (1959) The varicose tributaries of the superficial femoral vein passing into the Hunter's Canal. *Postgrad. Med. J.*, **35**, 18–23
21. Thompson, H. (1979) The surgical anatomy of the superficial and perforating veins of the lower limb. *Ann. R. Coll. Surg. Eng.*, **61**, 198–205
22. Papadakis, K., Christodoulou, C., Christopoulos, D., Hobbs, J., Malony, G. M. *et al.* (1989) The number and anatomical distribution of incompetent thigh perforating veins. *Br. J. Surg.*, **76**, 581–584
23. Nicolaides, A. N., Miles, C. and Zimmerman, H. (1981) The non invasive assessment of venous insufficiency. In *Hormones and Vascular Disease* (ed. R. M. Greenhalgh). Pitman, London, pp. 209–234
24. Chan, A., Chisholm, J. and Royle, J. P. (1983) The use of directional doppler ultrasound in the assessment of sapheno femoral incompetence. *Aust. NZ. J. Surg.*, **53**, 399–402
25. McIrvine, A. J., Corbett, C. R. R., Aston, N. O., Sherriff, E. A., Wiseman, P. A. and Jamieson, C. W. (1984) The demonstration of sapheno femoral incompetence: Doppler ultrasound compared with standard clinical tests. *Br. J. Surg.*, **71**, 509–510
26. Hoare, M. C. and Royle, J. P. (1984) Doppler ultrasound detection of sapheno femoral and sapheno popliteal incompetence and operative venography to ensure precise sapheno popliteal ligation. *Aust. NZ. J. Surg.*, **54**, 49–52
27. Sheppard, M. (1986) The incidence diagnosis and management of sapheno femoral incompetence. *Phlebology*, **1**, 23–32
28. Darke, S. G. and Andress, M. R. (1985) The value of venography in the management of chronic venous disorders of the lower limbs. In *Diagnostic Techniques and Assessment Procedures in Vascular Surgery* (ed. R. M. Greenhalgh). Grune and Stratton, London, pp. 421–446
29. Glass, G. M. (1988) Neovascularisation in recurrence varices of the great saphenous vein in the groin, phlebography. *Angiology*, **39**, 577–582
30. Glass, G. M. (1987) Neovascularisation in recurrence of the varicose great saphenous vein following transection. *Phlebology*, **2**, 81–91
31. Glass, G. M. (1987) Neovascularisation in restoration of continuity of the not femoral vein following surgical interruption. *Phlebology*, **2**, 1–6

Chapter 18

Deep vein thrombosis and its sequelae – how can they be averted?

John M. D. Galloway

Over the last 40 years knowledge of deep vein thrombosis (DVT) and its sequelae of pulmonary embolism and venous insufficiency, has been significantly advanced by numerous studies. However, conflicting results in some of these have led to confusion and many clinicians remain ignorant of what can be achieved in prevention and treatment.

The true incidence of DVT is unknown. It has been estimated that pulmonary embolism is about half as common as acute myocardial infarction and three times as common as cerebrovascular accidents[1]. The National Hospital Discharge Survey in the USA[2] suggests this is an overestimate. That study claims that DVT accounts for 10 000 deaths per annum and is a major contributing factor in 22 000 more. One in every hundred adults in the UK will at some time suffer from a venous ulcer[3]. As all pulmonary emboli and most venous ulcers are secondary to DVT, its importance as a cause of morbidity and mortality cannot be overstated. Despite this, venous disease in the eyes of most vascular surgeons remains the poor relation of arterial problems and treatment often suffers in consequence.

Deep vein thrombosis and pulmonary embolism are almost as common in medical as in surgical patients. In a survey from a general hospital[4], pulmonary emboli were found to be present at post-mortem in 63% of surgical patients and 45% of medical patients. Similar findings have been reported twenty years later[5]. In both these studies the absence of prior clinical diagnosis even when embolism was a major contributory cause of death was striking. Many postoperative DVT and pulmonary emboli do not become apparent until some days after discharge from hospital. These patients may come under the care of practitioners other than vascular surgeons, and as the diagnosis is often missed the management and outcome of these problems is extremely variable.

The absence of clinical evidence of venous thrombosis in 50% of patients dying from pulmonary embolism makes it essential that our efforts are directed to prevention at an early stage.

Prophylaxis

Prophylactic measures can be primary or secondary. *Primary prophylaxis* involves prevention of DVT (and consequently embolism); *secondary prophylaxis* is aimed at preventing pulmonary embolism and avoiding or minimizing venous insufficiency where DVT is already established.

Only 30% of thromboembolic events occur in patients following surgery and trauma: elderly patients on medical wards are equally at risk. If prophylaxis is to be effective it must be undertaken in all disciplines and instituted before thrombosis occurs. This means anticipating the event in those at risk.

It is tempting to suppose that any prophylactic measure that reduces DVT will lessen the incidence of pulmonary embolism. This is not necessarily so. A drug might effect a significant reduction in peripheral venous thrombosis without influencing iliofemoral venous thrombosis which is a more important source of pulmonary embolism[6,7]. Therefore, before a new form of prophylaxis can be adopted, it must be shown to decrease, and hopefully eliminate, pulmonary embolism as well as reduce DVT.

Primary prophylaxis

Prophylactic measures are directed at influencing the elements of Virchow's triad (Table 18.1): predominantly pharmacological manipulation of blood coagulability and mechanical manoeuvres to reduce venous stasis. Although doctors have felt powerless to diminish vessel wall changes, the traditional nursing of patients with heels on pillows is designed to reduce pressure damage to the endothelium of the calf veins.

Pharmacological prophylaxis

Oral anticoagulants   The beneficial effects of oral anticoagulants in DVT prophylaxis in hip fractures is well established. They have been shown not only to reduce the incidence of DVT and pulmonary embolism (both fatal and non-fatal), but also to effect a reduction in overall mortality[8]. Despite this, Morris and Mitchell[9] found that only 3% of the 411 orthopaedic surgeons who responded to their postal questionnaire routinely used oral anticoagulant prophylaxis in patients with hip fractures. A higher proportion of respondents (5%) did not consider venous thromboembolism to be a problem, despite the fact that post-mortem studies show that 83% of patients who die from hip fracture have DVT and 10% die as a direct consequence of pulmonary embolism. Morris and Mitchell[10] confirmed these

Table 18.1 DVT prophylaxis

Theoretical benefit	Clinical method	Disadvantages
Prevention of stasis	Compression stockings	Ineffective unless supine
	Early ambulation	Difficult to institute
	Avoiding dependency	Poor patient/staff compliance
Reduction of coagulability	Oral anticoagulants	Haemorrhage
		Laboratory control
	Low dose heparin	Haemorrhage
		Discomfort and inconvenience of injections
	Dextran	Cardiac decompensation
		Unsuitable in medical wards and patients admitted in advance of surgery
	Antiplatelet agents	No evidence of efficacy
Endothelial damage	Elevation of heels in bed	Soleal sinus dependency and stasis

results in a similar study using warfarin. Even more disappointing is the fact that a repeat of this questionnaire four years later still revealed that only 5% of orthopaedic surgeons used anticoagulant prophylaxis in hip fractures – 2% oral anticoagulants and 3% low-dose heparin[11].

Fear of bleeding has contributed to poor acceptance of anticoagulants in these circumstances. Bleeding occurs in 20% of patients on oral anticoagulants, frequently into wounds, puncture sites and the urinary tract and is more likely when the INR (Internal Normalized Ratio) is prolonged[12,13]. It is rarely serious, being fatal in less than 0.1% of patients. Recently minidose warfarin (1 mg daily without laboratory tests) has been shown to be safe and effective in gynaecological practice[14]. Oral anticoagulants are generally unsuitable in neurosurgery and vascular surgery where bleeding is particularly problematic.

Heparin Numerous studies using radioactive fibrinogen uptake scanning have shown that low-dose subcutaneous heparin significantly reduces the incidence of subclinical DVT in the calf and may also reduce proximal vein thrombosis[15,16]. The International Multicentre Trial[17], coordinated by Kakkar, seemed to put its efficacy in prevention of pulmonary embolism in general surgery beyond doubt. However, when one centre originally included in this study (Basle)[50] questioned the figures and conclusions of this trial uncertainty was engendered. Reappraisal of the figures of the trial, excluding the Basle cases, confirmed the original conclusions[18] and later the Basle group published evidence supporting the efficacy of subcutaneous heparin[19] but despite all that doubts have lingered. Several studies with small numbers of patients have suggested that low-dose heparin is ineffective in elective and emergency orthopaedic surgery[20]. As a result many surgeons still remain unconvinced and fail to adopt routine prophylaxis[11].

As postoperative pulmonary embolism is uncommon (3%) and fatal embolism is rare (0.8%) in general surgery it would require a trial with several thousands of patients to detect a 50% reduction in mortality[21]. It might need 100 000 patients to show that this produced a similar reduction in overall mortality when pulmonary embolism only accounts for 20% of postoperative deaths. It is unlikely that such a study will ever be carried out.

It is against this background that the overview of all known properly randomized trials of subcutaneous low-dose heparin was published[22]. Findings are shown in Table 18.2. It was concluded that prophylactic subcutaneous heparin was effective in

Table 18.2   Results of overview of all randomized trials of low-dose heparin prophylaxis in surgery

Condition	Available	Heparin DVT/ emboli	%	Available	Control DVT/ emboli	%
DVT						
General surgery	3966	355	8.95	3396	760	22.38
Orthopaedics	635	151	23.77	619	294	47.49
Urology	129	18	13.95	129	53	41.1
Total	4730	423	8.94	4144	1107	26.7
Pulmonary emboli						
Non-fatal	7879	105	1.3	7239	147	2.0
Fatal	7307	19	0.26	6777	55	0.81

Adapted from [22]

reducing DVT by at least two-thirds in general, orthopaedic and urological surgery. This not only applied to peripheral venous thrombosis but also to proximal thrombosis and was confirmed where venography was used. (Here the numbers were much smaller but identical figures emerged.) Further, they confirmed the findings of the International Multicentre Trial that pulmonary embolism odds were reduced by 47% and that in fatal pulmonary embolism odds were even more markedly reduced by 64%. These results applied to orthopaedic as well as general surgery. Finally, prophylactic subcutaneous heparin produced a reduction in overall postoperative mortality in all forms of surgery ($P < 0.02$). This overcomes the problem, raised by Mitchell[23] that a decision that death is due to pulmonary embolism is subjective, because, although a pathologist may say what a patient died *with*, he cannot tell what a patient died *of*. Although haemorrhagic complications were more common (2% increase in excessive bleeding) they were not of a major nature and they did not contribute to mortality. Bleeding was not significantly different when heparin was given 12-hourly as compared with 8-hourly.

These conclusions are almost identical to those of the 1986 Consensus Development Conference on Prevention of Venous Thrombosis and Pulmonary Embolism[24]. From this one can only echo Sherry[25] and say: 'One is forced to the conclusion that there is a very high probability that the difference in fatal pulmonary embolism between the two groups is real'.

To be effective low-dose subcutaneous heparin must be started before thrombosis is initiated since it works by accelerating antithrombin III inhibition of factor X activation, which is early in the coagulation process. Because of the cascade effect (producing increasing quantities of coagulants) much larger doses of heparin are required for it to act as an antithrombin. To start subcutaneous heparin postoperatively is not sensible. Clearly if patients are admitted to hospital some days in advance of surgery heparin must be commenced on admission. In all major studies medication was continued for seven days postoperatively. This need not prolong hospital stay for patients find self-administration quite easy.

The introduction of low molecular weight heparin, claimed to be as effective in DVT and pulmonary embolism prophylaxis, with fewer haemorrhagic complications and requiring one daily injection only, will clearly have great advantages[26]. Controlled studies in general surgery[27] and orthopaedics[28] seem to confirm its value in reducing DVT.

Dihydroergotamine (0.5 mg) when combined with heparin may enhance its efficacy, but as it has been associated with serious vasospastic changes resulting in amputations and some deaths[29], caution must be exercised especially in patients with lower limb trauma.

Dextran   Dextran 70 in 5% dextrose 500 ml given at the time of operation and once during each of the next two days has been used extensively in DVT prophylaxis, particularly following hip arthroplasty. Some evidence suggests that it does not prevent calf vein thrombosis and therefore shows up poorly in ^{125}I fibrinogen scan studies. However, it does reduce proximal vein thrombosis and significantly lowers the incidence of pulmonary embolism[19].

Bleeding following dextran is less than that with heparin[19]. There are problems in using dextran in patients admitted several days in advance of surgery and in patients with cardiac decompensation because of the need for daily infusions. It may be that, as peripheral venous thrombosis still occurs despite using dextran, venous insufficiency will be a greater long-term problem with this form of prophylaxis. To date there is no evidence that this is the case.

Mechanical prophylaxis

The importance of blood stasis in the causation of venous thrombosis is generally accepted. Dependency and immobility, as occurs in the operating theatre, increase this. It is particularly marked in the valve pockets of the femoral vein and the soleal sinuses, where stasis may persist for up to 30 minutes in the average adult, and is prolonged by advancing age. McLachlin *et al.*[30] showed that a foot uptilt of 15 degrees would prevent these changes and advocated this posture as the norm in the recovery room and in the early postoperative period; regrettably very few surgeons have adopted this simple manoeuvre. The results of studies (Browse *et al.*[31]) in which leg elevation was confined to the period of the operation alone may have persuaded many surgeons that it had little effect. Elevation was achieved by pads under the heels, a method encouraging soleal sinus dependency and stasis. The case against elevation therefore remains unproven.

Compression stockings have found much greater acceptance. Numerous fibrinogen scanning studies have confirmed the efficacy of such stockings in preventing peripheral venous thrombosis. It is tempting to assume that they will reduce the incidence of pulmonary embolism also, but there is no proof for this, and it is incorrect to label such stockings 'antiembolic'. The compression applied by such stockings is only protective in the supine position.

Many other mechanical methods, such as pneumatic compression and electrical stimulation of the calf muscles, have been advocated, but although some of these are effective they are also inconvenient and therefore not routinely adopted. However, in high risk patients undergoing surgery in which bleeding is particularly dangerous, e.g. neurosurgical operations, such measures may be of value.

Probably the most important method of prophylaxis is early ambulation but it is the most difficult to institute. Nurses in all specialties sometimes regard 'early ambulation' as progress from the bed to sitting in a chair, and seem to take comfort in the fact that the patient is wearing antithrombotic stockings, which in this position are ineffective.

Perhaps as important as understanding the methods of DVT prophylaxis and adopting one's own policy is the need to encourage the whole team, junior doctors, nurses, physiotherapists etc. to implement it. Recent studies indicate that in less than 70% of patients under my care is my prescribed regime for DVT prophylaxis fully implemented (Table 18.3). They may miss out on antithrombotic stockings, or elevation in the postoperative period. Perhaps more frequently, they do not receive heparin until several days after admission or miss the immediately preoperative and/ or postoperative, and arguably most important, heparin doses. Few patients miss out on all of these but many miss out on some. To improve the rate of conformity it is important to limit the exclusion criteria and to accept that all others will receive the whole package unless otherwise stipulated. All patients over 40 years of age undergoing surgery of other than the most minor type and patients under 40 in high risk groups (Table 18.4) should have prophylaxis. Although hard evidence is lacking,

Table 18.3 Author's prophylactic regime

Subcutaneous heparin*
Antithrombotic stockings
Foot elevation postoperatively
Early ambulation

* Seven days postoperative

Table 18.4   Risk factors for DVT

Age
Congestive cardiac failure
Operation
Pregnancy and delivery
Malignancy
Obesity
Previous thromboembolism
Trauma to lower limb and pelvis
Oral contraceptives
Hormone replacement therapy

it seems prudent that patients on the contraceptive pill or on hormone replacement therapy should have these stopped for six weeks before elective operations, and if surgery has to be undertaken urgently, they should be given full prophylaxis.

It was formerly considered that patients undergoing vascular surgical operations were at too great a risk from bleeding to receive heparin prophylaxis and that the risks of thromboembolic complications were low. In fact vascular surgical patients seem to be at an increased risk of thrombosis, especially in view of the frequency of distal dissection down the calf and further down the profunda femoris artery, with division of accompanying veins. In vascular surgery I follow the same regime as for other operations but omit the immediate preoperative heparin dose substituting intraoperative intravenous heparin.

Finally it is important to remember that no form of prophylaxis absolutely prevents thromboembolic complications and that any patient who develops suspicious features must be fully investigated.

Secondary prophylaxis

Secondary prevention of pulmonary embolism and the postphlebitic syndrome is essentially the management of established DVT. It is critical that the diagnosis of DVT is soundly established before therapy is instituted, as all forms of treatment are associated with significant morbidity and mortality. Equally, it must be started urgently to minimize thrombus propagation.

Diagnosis of DVT

Clinical diagnosis of DVT is difficult. In one series[32] 50% of patients referred with DVT and with clinical manifestations considered to be compatible with the diagnosis did not in fact have evidence of DVT on phlebography. The subsequent course of the patients who did not have DVT on phlebography, and were therefore not treated, confirmed the diagnostic accuracy of this investigation. Furthermore, massive pulmonary embolism can result from non-occlusive and, therefore, clinically undetectable iliofemoral thrombosis[7].

None the less it is essential to try to make a clinical diagnosis of DVT. Routine daily examination of the legs on the ward can be rewarding. Calf tenderness raises an index of suspicion though it is often due to superficial thrombophlebitis (when a cord-like tender vein is often palpable), a muscle strain or tendo-achilles injury.

Ankle oedema is widely regarded as a sign of DVT and is claimed to be the only sign which has been shown to indicate the presence of DVT [33,34]. However, the latter group specifically described and measured swelling *above* the ankle and did not mention oedema. Since clinical oedema is excess extracellular fluid in the subcutaneous tissues (the tissues beneath the deep fascia cannot be indented by finger pressure), it would be surprising if it was caused by limited calf vein thrombosis deep to the fascia. Subcutaneous oedema at the ankle is more often the result of dependency or superficial thrombophlebitis. It is also seen in association with synovial rupture of the knee (Baker's cyst rupture), another cause of calf tenderness easily confused with DVT.

In more extensive iliofemoral occlusion subcutaneous (pitting) oedema is rarely of severe degree. Marked oedema reflects lymphatic obstruction and usually indicates associated malignant disease, most commonly lymphoma, carcinoma of prostate, bladder or ovary.

Skin discoloration is common in extensive iliofemoral venous occlusion, giving rise to phlegmasia alba dolens or caerulea dolens but in those circumstances the diagnosis is rarely in doubt. It must be remembered that when swelling extends up to the groin crease the iliac veins are always occluded. When gangrene develops it may be difficult to be sure if the cause is primarily arterial or venous occlusion. In venous gangrene peripheral pulses may be impalpable due to low cardiac output from fluid sequestration and also because tissue pressure exceeds the critical closing pressure of the peripheral arterioles. A useful sign in such circumstances is pulp tension in the toes, especially the great toe. In arterial embolism loss of pulp volume with wrinkling of the skin occurs within 30 min of occlusion. In venous gangrene the pulp is full and round. Unexplained low grade pyrexia, especially, in the postoperative period may be the sole pointer to DVT. Whereas significant pyrexia may be indicative of associated pulmonary embolism.

Although the diagnosis of DVT is difficult, clinical vigilance and a high index of suspicion are often rewarded.

Investigations
Unless there are strong contraindications 7500 u of heparin should be given intravenously immediately on suspicion of DVT or pulmonary embolism, but it must be recognized that this is a precautionary measure. It is not acceptable to continue anticoagulants solely on the basis of a clinical diagnosis. If the diagnosis is subsequently refuted by objective tests no harm has resulted from a single dose of heparin, if it is confirmed the heparin will give some protection while definitive treatment is being instituted. At this stage the appropriate site for carrying out this treatment should be considered: it should usually be in a hospital with full resuscitative and investigative facilities, so that major pulmonary embolism can be adequately dealt with, should it occur. A large number of investigations are available and their advantages and disadvantages are listed in Table 18.5.

Bilateral ascending phlebography is the most useful test in practice, not only confirming or refuting the diagnosis but providing information about the site, size and extent of thrombosis, and giving some indication of its propensity for embolizing. Phlebographic technique must be standardized[35] and carried out by a radiologist who is determined to show the deep venous system from foot to vena cava. It is not sufficient to say 'failure to fill veins in calf – DVT can be assumed'. The diagnostic criteria for thrombosis on phlebography are the presence of a filling defect in the contrast medium on more than one film (to exclude 'poor mixing' defects), or if a vein is completely occluded dye must be seen above and below the occluded segment and in the veins around it. Only if these criteria are fulfilled is it safe to accept that a

Table 18.5   Methods of investigation of DVT

Investigation	Advantages	Disadvantages
Phlebography	Positive diagnosis Result immediately available	Expensive Invasive
[125]I fibrinogen scanning	Excellent for mass screening	Expensive May take several days for result Poor for major veins
Thermography	Simple	Expensive Uncertain accuracy
Ultrasound	Cheap and quick Useful in pregnancy	Can miss large non-occlusive thrombi Operator-dependent
Duplex scanning	Accurate	Expensive Not available in many hospitals Operator-dependent
Plethysmography	Relatively cheap	Cannot detect non-occlusive thrombi Not readily available in many hospitals

negative phlebogram means there is no thrombosis. It is essential that in all cases phlebograms are bilateral, for a patient may have symptoms from occlusive thrombus in a minor vein on one side, while harbouring a totally asymptomatic, but much more dangerous non-occlusive iliofemoral thrombus on the other. The risk of phlebography causing DVT, skin necrosis or anaphylaxis has been largely abolished with the advent of non ionic iso-osmolar contrast media.

[125]I fibrinogen scanning, although very useful as a screening test and in assessment of methods of prophylaxis, is of no value in the clinical setting. *Doppler ultrasound* has the advantage of simplicity, and is particularly useful in pregnancy, where phlebography is contraindicated. It is especially important to establish the diagnosis because of the increased risks of anticoagulants at this time. *Duplex scanning* may in time replace phlebography, but at present it is not routinely available in a large number of hospitals. The equipment is improving and operator experience is growing. The possibility of a non-invasive gold standard investigation is exciting. For the present phlebography remains that gold standard. Because *thermography* and *plethysmography* do not detect many non-occlusive major vein thromboses they have found little favour in the UK.

No *blood tests* are of diagnostic value. However, it is important to take blood for activated partial thromboplastin time (APTT) before the first dose of heparin is given as subsequent dosage will depend on this estimation.

Investigation for associated conditions

It has, rightly, been emphasized that DVT is frequently associated with malignancy, which may sometimes be occult. For this reason many clinicians undertake extensive investigations to try to discover malignant disease, including upper and lower gastrointestinal endoscopy, and CT scanning. Such investigation is perhaps rarely justified. When malignancy is associated with DVT it is usually clinically obvious and when it is not the condition is characteristically untreatable, e.g. carcinoma of the pancreas. The exceptions to this are cases of iliofemoral occlusion associated with marked oedema where the underlying cause may be carcinoma of prostate or ovary. Pelvic examination will often establish the diagnosis and pelvic B-mode ultrasound will confirm it. As both these lesions are amenable to treatment by hormone manipulation and chemotherapy with lasting symptomatic benefit their detection can prove worthwhile.

Treatment of acute DVT

Thrombectomy

Although at one stage venous thrombectomy was considered the treatment of choice[36], long-term follow-up has shown that the incidence of venous insufficiency despite surgical intervention increases with the years. Unless thrombectomy results in complete clearance postoperative pulmonary embolism is common and may be fatal[36]. Complete clearance is only possible in isolated iliofemoral thrombosis, an uncommon situation except in patients on a high-dose oestrogen contraceptive pill. Because of this thrombectomy has been abandoned except in special circumstances (see below). When it is undertaken phlebographic monitoring is essential[37].

It has been suggested that thrombectomy should be combined with an arteriovenous fistula between the long saphenous vein and the superficial femoral artery[38,39]. The resulting high flow rate increases postoperative patency and long-term phlebographic follow-up shows that this difference is maintained. These workers may have been looking at a particularly favourable group of patients, with very localized disease, because two-thirds of their controls had a patent femoropopliteal segment on follow-up phlebography.

However, there is still significant late stenosis and rethrombosis and another Swedish group[40] found only eight of 19 iliac veins to be normally patent three years after thrombectomy. They also recorded postphlebitic symptoms and objective evidence of valvular dysfunction in 11 patients, some of whom had a patent iliofemoral segment. This confirmed earlier Scandinavian experience of thrombectomy (without arteriovenous fistula) in which, although venous patency was preserved in 20% of patients, none had normal valvular function on plethysmography[41].

Eklof minimizes the dangers of embolism in relation to thrombectomy, but in his own randomized series 23% of patients treated surgically developed further embolism (on routine lung perfusion scan) compared with 15% in those treated with anticoagulants alone[38]. This difference may be even greater given the fact that they accepted lower heparin doses and lower APTT levels than controlled studies suggest are optimal[42].

Thrombolysis

Thrombolysis has also been used extensively but is associated with the same problems as thrombectomy and is accompanied by more bleeding complications. There is no convincing evidence that late venous insufficiency is reduced[43]. Recent experience in the treatment of acute myocardial infarction using a single large dose of fibrinolytic agent may indicate the way forward. Recombinant tissue plasminogen activator (rt–PA), it is claimed, will be more effective and cause fewer haemorrhagic complications. Sherry[25] has sounded a note of caution here but we await full-scale studies.

Even effective thrombolysis may not prevent venous insufficiency. Thrombosis usually starts in the depth of the valve pockets. It is well organized and has virtually destroyed the cusp before it is large enough to cause symptoms by encroaching on the lumen of the vein[44]. The only way to prevent venous insufficiency may be to prevent DVT.

Anticoagulants

The aim of anticoagulation is to prevent propagation of thrombus and to allow its early retraction and organization so that an adequate lumen is restored. Valve function is rarely retained.

Anticoagulation with intravenous heparin remains the sheet anchor of treatment of DVT. When properly controlled[42] it will prevent pulmonary embolism and produce rapid resolution of leg symptoms. To obtain maximum benefit in preventing clot extension a plasma heparin level of 0.3 u/ml is required. This is regularly achieved when the APTT is maintained at twice the patient's own pretreatment level. The dose must be adjusted daily according to the APTT level. Poor response usually indicates poor control. In one series (Fennerty et al.[45]) about one third of APTT results were ignored by the supervising clinician, often when they were dangerously high or ineffectually low. The average dose required will be 40 000 u in 24 hours but there is wide interpatient variability. It would appear that continuous infusion for 10 days is optimal though there have been no controlled studies to confirm this. Because of the risk of heparin-induced thrombocytopenia the platelet count should be monitored after six days.

Oral anticoagulants should be introduced on the sixth day and administered concurrent with heparin until an INR of 1.5–2 has been achieved[46]. The optimum time for continuing oral anticoagulants is probably six months, particularly if there has been associated pulmonary embolism. Walker[47] has suggested that full-dose subcutaneous heparin is as effective, or more effective, than heparin by i.v. infusion in the treatment of DVT and pulmonary embolism. This has not been our experience, and dosage adjustment has proved difficult.

Although in most cases of DVT the above regimen is the treatment of choice, there are three circumstances in which this must be modified:

1. After total failure to obtain relief of symptoms in iliofemoral venous thrombosis, and in the situation of impending venous gangrene, urgent venous thrombectomy is indicated.
2. When pulmonary embolism has occurred despite adequate anticoagulation. Some form of barrier to embolism is indicated. If on phlebography thrombosis is evident below iliac level then superficial femoral vein ligation (immediately below the common femoral origin) should be carried out. This is coupled with common femoral thrombectomy if thrombus protrudes into the common femoral vein. If thrombus is found above this level then an IVC filter of the Greenfield type is inserted[48]. Our experience is similar to that of Greenfield in that these filters do not seem to occlude probably because they act as shredders, breaking emboli up into small particles which travel peripherally in the lung and are lysed. In the long

term nearly half the patients require graduated compression for venous insufficiency and 15% develop ulceration. This more probably reflects the severity of the original thrombosis than an effect of the filter. Filters are not entirely without problems, however, as recent experiences of migration and caval penetration by the Gunther filter, necessitating its withdrawal, have highlighted.

3. Where venography reveals large non-occlusive iliofemoral thrombus which appears poorly attached urgent thrombectomy is indicated to prevent massive pulmonary embolism.

In all these circumstances anticoagulant therapy must be continued.

Pulmonary embolism

The diagnosis of pulmonary embolism is often easily made on clinical grounds from a history of pleuritic chest pain and/or haemoptysis. However, there are other less obvious presentations. Unexplained pyrexia, tachycardia, dysrhythmia, breathlessness, tachypnoea and syncopal attacks, especially in the postoperative or postpartum period, should alert the clinician to look for pulmonary embolism. Massive pulmonary embolism with acute right heart failure can occur without warning.

Chest X-ray and ECG may provide useful pointers to diagnosis which should be confirmed by perfusion lung scan using technetium-labelled macroaggregated albumin or by pulmonary angiography. Pulmonary scanning, however, has limitations: only 75% of suggestive scans are confirmed by pulmonary angiography. Nevertheless, if the scan is normal angiography never shows embolism, which makes it a good minimally invasive test. Treatment of pulmonary embolism depends on its size. In major embolism immediate cardiopulmonary resuscitation is required. The diagnosis should be established by lung scan and/or pulmonary angiography as soon as possible. Thrombolytic therapy is then the treatment of choice unless it is contraindicated because of bleeding risks. In these circumstances, or where the patient is still shocked after an hour, pulmonary embolectomy, preferably on cardiopulmonary bypass, should be carried out through a median sternotomy. Where cardiopulmonary bypass is not available the operation can still be carried out with inflow or caval occlusion to achieve a 70% survival rate[49]. Following successful pulmonary embolectomy or lysis it may be prudent to insert an IVC filter as secondary fatal embolism may occur in up to 20% of patients. When pulmonary embolism is less severe attention must be directed to the causative DVT which should be investigated and treated as described earlier.

Prevention of post-phlebitic venous insufficiency

There is no good evidence that post-phlebitic venous insufficiency can be prevented by any form of long-term treatment. However, it is common experience that minor degrees of venous insufficiency respond better to graduated compression than do more severe degrees. For this reason it is my practice to insist that patients wear below-knee graduated compression stockings for 18 months following DVT. At that time if there is any clinical evidence of venous insufficiency or evidence of popliteal or perforator reflux on Doppler they are advised to wear below-knee graduated compression stockings on a lifelong basis in the hope of preventing the misery of venous ulceration.

A small number of patients experience recurrent spontaneous DVT. In these circumstances it is important to exclude deficiency of antithrombin III protein C or S, and to look for evidence of endothelial plasminogen activator deficiency. In all of these conditions long-term oral anticoagulant therapy is indicated. There remains another small group of patients who, despite all investigations, have no apparent cause for recurrent thrombosis. Empirically these patients may also require long-term anticoagulant therapy or some of them will eventually die from pulmonary embolism.

Summary

DVT and pulmonary embolism remains a major cause of morbidity and mortality despite the vast increase in our knowledge of aetiology, prevention and treatment. Post-mortem surveys in general hospitals undertaken after a 30-year interval have shown little change in mortality[5,8].

Prophylaxis therefore remains the only way to change this dismal picture. Adequate methods of prophylaxis *are* available. Only by understanding and systematic implementation of well tried and tested methods by all members of the healthcare team will these unnecessary deaths be prevented. DVT prophylactic policies must be adopted in *all* hospitals just as antibiotic policies have become routine.

References

1. Dalen, J. E. and Alpert, J. S. (1975) Natural history of pulmonary embolism. *Prog. Cardiovasc. Dis.*, **17**, 259–270
2. Gillum, R. F. (1987) Pulmonary embolism and thrombophlebitis in the United States. 1970–1985. *Am. Heart J.*, **114**, 1262–1264
3. Callam, M. J., Ruckley, C. V., Harper, D. R. and Dale, J. J. (1985) Chronic ulceration of the leg: extent of the problem and provision of care. *Br. Med. J.*, **2**, 1855–1856
4. Morrell, M. T. and Dunhill, M. S. (1968) The post-mortem incidence of pulmonary embolism in a hospital population. *Br. J. Surg.*, **55**, 347–352
5. Sandler, D. A. and Martin, J. F. (1989) Autopsy proven pulmonary embolism in hospital patients: are we detecting enough deep vein thrombosis? *J. R. Soc. Med.*, **82**, 203–205
6. Gibbs, N. M. (1957) Venous thrombosis of the lower limbs with particular reference to bed-rest. *Br. J. Surg.*, **45**, 209–236
7. Mavor, G. E. and Galloway, J. M. D. (1967) The iliofemoral venous segment as a source of pulmonary emboli. *Lancet*, **i**, 871–874
8. Sevitt, S. and Gallagher, N. G. (1959) Prevention of venous thrombosis and pulmonary embolism in injured patients. *Lancet*, **ii**, 981–989
9. Morris, G. K. and Mitchell, J. R. A. (1976) Prevention and diagnosis of venous thrombosis in patients with hip fractures. *Lancet*, **ii**, 867–869
10. Morris, G. K. and Mitchell, J. R. A. (1976) Warfarin Sodium in prevention of deep vein thrombosis and pulmonary embolism in patients with fractured neck of femur. *Lancet*, **ii**, 869–872
11. Morris, G. K. (1980) Prevention of venous thromboembolism. *Lancet*, **ii**, 572–574
12. Mant, J. J., O'Brien, B. D., Thong, K. L., Hammond, G. W., Birtwhistle, R. V. and Grace, M. G. (1977) Haemorrhagic complications of heparin therapy. *Lancet*, **i**, 1133–1135
13. Forfar, J. C. (1979) A 7 year analysis of haemorrhage in patients on long-term anticoagulant treatment. *Br. Heart J.*, **42**, 128–132
14. Poller, L., McKernan, A., Thomson, J. M., Elstein, M., Hirsch, P. J. and Jones, J. B. (1987) Fixed minidose warfarin: a new approach to prophylaxis against venous thrombosis after major surgery. *Br. Med. J.*, **2**, 1309–1312
15. Nicolaides, A. N., Dupont, P. A., Desai, S., Lewis, J. D., Douglas, J. N. *et al.* (1972) Small doses of subcutaneous sodium heparin in preventing deep venous thrombosis after major surgery. *Lancet*, **ii**, 890–893

16. Gallus, A. S., Hirsh, J., O'Brien, S. E., McBride, J. A., Tuttle, R. J. and Gent, M. (1976) Prevention of venous thrombosis with small, subcutaneous doses of Heparin. *J. Am. Med. Ass.*, **235**, 1980–1982
17. International Multicentre Trial (1975) Prevention of fatal post-operative pulmonary embolism by low doses of heparin. *Lancet*, **ii**, 45–51
18. International Multicentre Trial – Reappraisal of Results (1977) Prevention of Fatal post-operative pulmonary embolism by low doses of heparin. *Lancet*, **i**, 567–569
19. Gruber, U. F., Saldeen, T., Brokop, T., Eklof, B., Erikson, I. *et al.* (1980) Incidence of fatal post-operative pulmonary embolism after prophylaxis with dextran 70 and low-dose heparin: an international multicentre study. *Br. Med. J.*, **1**, 69–72
20. Evarts, C. M. and Alfidi, R. J. (1973) Thromboembolism after total hip reconstruction; failure of low doses of heparin in prevention. *J. Am. Med. Ass.*, **225**, 515–516
21. Yusuf, S., Collins, R. and Peto, R. (1984) Why do we need some large, simple trials? *Stat. Med.*, **3**, 409–420
22. Collins, R., Scrimgeour, A., Yusuf, S. and Peto, R. (1988) Reduction in fatal pulmonary embolism and venous thrombosis by perioperative administration of subcutaneous heparin. *New Eng. J. Med.*, **318**, 1162–1173
23. Mitchell, J. R. A. (1979) Can we really prevent post-operative pulmonary emboli? *Br. Med. J.*, **1**, 1523–1524
24. Consensus Conference. (1986) Prevention of Venous Thrombosis and Pulmonary Embolism. *J. Am. Med. Ass.*, **256**, 744–749
25. Sherry, S. (1985) Tissue plasminogen activator. Will it fulfill its promise. *New Eng. J. Med.*, **313**, 1014–1017
26. Kakkar, V. V., Lawrence, D., Bentley, P. G., Detlas, H. A., Ward, V. P. and Scully, M. F. (1978) A comparative study of low doses of heparin and a heparin analogue in the prevention of post-operative deep vein thrombosis. *Thrombosis Research*, **13**, 111–115
27. Kakkar, V. V. and Murray, W. J. G. (1985) Efficacy and safety of low-molecular-weight heparin (CY216) in preventing post-operative venous thrombo-embolism; a co-operative study. *Br. J. Surg.*, **72**, 786–791
28. Turpie, A. G. G., Levine, M., Hirsh, J., Carter, C. J., Jay, R. M. *et al.* (1986) A randomized controlled trial of a low-molecular-weight heparin (enoxaparin) to prevent deep-vein thrombosis in patients undergoing elective hip surgery. *New Eng. J. Med.*, **315**, 925–929
29. Wiesmann, W., Peters, P. E., Irsken, U. and Schwering, H. (1987) Diagnosis and treatment of ergotism following Heparin–DHE thrombosis prophylaxis. *Fortschr. Rontgenstr.*, **147**, 446–449
30. McLachlin, A. D., McLachlin, J. A., Jory, T. A. and Rawlings, E. G. (1960) Venous stasis in the lower extremity. *Ann. Surg.*, **152**, 678–685
31. Browse, N. L., Jackson, B. T., Mayo, M. E. and Negus, D. (1974) The value of mechanical methods of preventing post-operative calf vein thrombosis. *Br. J. Surg.*, **61**, 219–223
32. Hull, R., Hirsh, J., Sackett, D. L., Taylor, D. W., Carter, C. *et al.* (1981) Clinical validity of a negative venogram in patients with clinically suspected venous thrombosis. *Circulation*, **64**, 622–625
33. Browse, N. L., Burnand, K. G. and Lea, Thomas, M. (1988) *Diseases of the veins* Edward Arnold, London
34. McLachlin, J., Richards, T. and Paterson, J. C. (1962) An evaluation of clinical signs in the diagnosis of venous thrombosis. *Arch. Surg.*, **85**, 58–64
35. Lea Thomas, M. (1982) *Phlebography of the Lower Limb.* Churchill Livingstone, Edinburgh
36. Mavor, G. E. and Galloway, J. M. D. (1969) Iliofemoral venous thrombosis. *Br. J. Surg.*, **56**, 45–59
37. Mavor, G. E. and Galloway, J. M. D. (1967) Radiographic control of iliofemoral venous thrombectomy. *Br. J. Surg.*, **54**, 1019–1022
38. Eklof, B., Einarsson, E., Plate, G. (1985) Role of thrombectomy and temporary arteriovenous fistula in acute iliofemoral venous thrombosis. In *Surgery of the Veins* (eds J. J. Bergan and J. S. T. Yao). Grune and Stratton, New York, pp. 131–144
39. Plate, G. (1989) Thrombectomy with temporary arteriovenous fistula in acute iliofemoral venous thrombosis. In *Controversies in the Management of Venous Disorders* (eds B. Eklof, J. E. Gjores, O. Thulesius and D. Bergquist) Butterworths, London, pp. 127–139
40. Zetterquist, S., Hagglof, R., Jacobsson, H., Johansson, J., Johansson, H. *et al.* (1985) Long-term results of thrombectomy with temporary arterio-venous fistula for ilio-femoral venous thrombosis. In *Phlebology 1985* (eds D. Negus and G. Jantet). John Libbey, London, pp. 488–490
41. Johansson, E., Nordlander, S. and Zetterquist, S. (1973) Venous thrombectomy in the lower extremity – clinical, phlebographic and plethysmographic evaluation of early and late results. *Acta Chir. Scand.* **139**, 511–516
42. Hirsh, J., Genton, E. and Hull, R. (1981) *Venous Thromboembolism.* Grune and Stratton, New York

43. Kakkar, V. V., Paes, T. R. F. and Murray, W. J. G. (1985) Does thrombolytic therapy prevent the post-phlebitic syndrome? In *Phlebology 1985* (eds D. Negus and G. Jantet). John Libbey, London, pp. 487

44. Paterson, J. C. and McLachlin, J. (1954) Precipitating factors in venous thrombosis. *Surg. Gynecol. Obstet.*, **98**, 96–100

45. Fennerty, A. G., Thomas, P., Blackhouse, G., Bentley, P., Campbell, I. A. and Routledge, P. A. (1985) Audit control of heparin treatment. *Br. Med. J.*, **2**, 27–28

46. Hirsh, J. and Levine, M. N. (1987) The optimal intensity of oral anticoagulant therapy. *J. Am. Med. Ass.*, **258**, 2723–2726

47. Walker, M. G., Shaw, J. W., Thomson, G. J., Cumming, J. G. and Thomas, M. L. (1987) Subcutaneous calcium heparin versus intravenous sodium heparin in treatment of established acute deep vein thrombosis of the legs: a multicentre prospective randomised trial. *Br. Med. J.*, **2**, 1189–1192

48. Greenfield, L. J. (1985) Results of catheter embolectomy and Greenfield Filter insertion. In *Surgery of the Veins* (eds J. J. Bergan and J. S. T. Yao). Grune and Stratton, New York, pp. 479–486

49. Clark, D. B., Abrams, L. D. (1972) Pulmonary embolectomy with venous inflow-occlusion. *Lancet*, **i**, 767–769

50. Gruber, U. F., Fridrich, R., Duckert, F., Torhorst, J. and Rem, J. (1977) Prevention of fatal post-operative thrombo-embolism by dextran 40, low doses of heparin, or xantinol nicotinate. *Lancet*, **i**, 207–210

Chapter 19

How do I audit my general/vascular surgery?

Denis C. Wilkins

Like many surgeons, I and my colleagues have struggled against the vagaries of bureaucracy, high workload and depleted budgets to introduce some form of audit into our surgical practices. This chapter is an account of how we have tried to evolve this audit. It is not an exhaustive treatise on surgical audit and emphasis is laid on the steps that we have found particularly difficult or feel are important. Despite the fact that we are all convinced of the benefits which will accrue from regular audit, one is struck by the effort it has taken to come such a relatively short way. However, the new National Health Service reforms have injected a much needed dose of financial and management interest into this discipline and it is hoped that we will now begin to see more widespread, systematic and detailed surgical audit carried out. For others who are just starting, I hope that our experiences may be of some interest.

What is audit?

The definition of medical audit is deceptively simple:

> 'Medical audit can be defined as the systematic, critical analysis of the quality of medical care, including the procedures used for diagnosis and treatment, the use of resources, and the resulting outcome and quality of life for the patient.'[1]

This can be depicted diagrammatically, as in Figure 19.1.

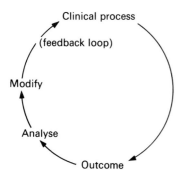

Figure 19.1

This apparent simplicity is confounded by several factors. First, although the assessment of outcome, including the subsequent quality of life, is highly desirable, and must be the ultimate yardstick of medical or surgical care, it can be extremely difficult and expensive to measure[2]. The current European trial which is aimed at assessing the value of carotid endarterectomy is an example of the complexities and expense involved. There has been increasing interest recently in measuring quality of life both before and after medical treatment, but it is still not widely assessed although there are now several indices available. Perhaps the best known of these indices is the 'Rosser' index[3], which comprises a matrix constructed from eight degrees of disability ranging from nil to unconsciousness along one margin and degrees of distress ranging from none to very severe along the other. At each point on this matrix may be derived a fraction which, when multiplied by the expected survival in years, will give a figure expressed in 'Quality Adjusted Life Years' or 'QUALYs'. Because anything other than short-term outcome is difficult to measure, most surgical audit confines itself to this and to various aspects of the medical process. While audit of this type is adequate for many common procedures such as hernias and cholecystectomies which are well defined endpoints, expensive vascular surgeons will increasingly feel the need to ensure that the longer term results of their work are well documented in terms of QUALYs and their costs!

A further aspect of medical audit, to which we should pay particular attention, is the ability to produce change as a result of deficiencies identified during audit. This is termed 'closing the feedback loop' and unless it can be reliably achieved as a matter of routine audit becomes an expensive waste of time. The Royal College of Surgeons, in their guidelines for surgical audit (*Guidelines to Clinical Audit in Surgical Practice*[4]), have suggested that an 'audit of the audit' be carried out periodically in order to gauge what changes have been effected. We found this exercise very salutary in that many of the recommendations and further studies mooted during audit meetings had not been implemented. During a six-month period we found that twenty actions had been agreed by our audit group which consisted of ten firms, of which only 25% were actually taken up. For the most part, this lack of action was attributable to a paucity of time and resources, but it is clearly part of the audit process that should be kept under regular scrutiny.

Why audit?

A wise old surgeon once said to me 'You know, surgery is just like cricket; unless you keep track of the score, it loses much of its interest!'. No doubt this is true, but it is not the only good reason to institute a regular review of one's work. Much has been written recently regarding the benefits of medical audit. For a review of the whole topic of surgical audit, the reader is referred to the excellent monograph by Pollock and Evans[5]. The series of papers appearing currently in the *British Medical Journal* entitled 'Audit in Practice' is another source of ideas and information. No doubt we shall soon see the emergence of yet another specialist medical journal, perhaps entitled *Medical Audit Review*! However, I can best describe one of the benefits of surgical audit by giving an illustration.

Shortly after we instituted our regular weekly audit meetings some years ago, it became apparent from a series of presentations of mishaps and near misses that patients were sometimes suffering an inordinate delay in getting to theatre for their emergency surgery. Accordingly, the prospective collection of more detailed information regarding times of admission, times of theatre bookings, actual times of surgery, availability of anaesthetic support, etc. was instituted. Analysis of this information revealed a clear case for providing a regular afternoon emergency operating session and anaesthetist. Discussions ensued, the theatre session was negotiated, and a subsequent audit showed the position to have improved markedly[6]. Another recurring problem concerned the treatment of ruptured abdominal aortic aneurysms: again, from several presentations at audit meetings it was apparent that patients were not always being transferred directly to the operating suite once diagnosis was suspected. After discussion local guidelines were agreed, the general level of awareness of the problem was raised and these patients are now seen to be receiving a much improved service. The foregoing are but two illustrations of the sorts of benefit that can be achieved by auditing at a very basic level. Larger, more sophisticated databases can no doubt be used to draw more far reaching conclusions. For example, the Lothian audit in Scotland showed that emergency surgery for aortic aneurysms carried a much higher mortality when carried out by general surgeons than when performed by vascular surgeons. As a result, it was recommended that all such cases were transferred to centres where a vascular surgeon was available. The recent *Confidential Enquiry into Peri-operative Deaths* is another example.

The benefit that regular audit is held to provide for the quality of surgical care and the efficiency with which it is delivered is generally well known, but there are other very good reasons why we should audit. Medicine and surgery are becoming increasingly divided into specialized compartments and it can be very difficult to keep up with the rapid advances in adjacent specialties. If the format of an audit meeting is correct, it can provide an excellent forum at which colleagues can educate each other. Looked at from the point of view of training, systematic review by a firm of its clinical activity can quickly demonstrate the strengths and weaknesses of its training programme. We should also not overlook the fact that medical audit imposes upon us the discipline of data collection. In the 'new-look' National Health Service, information will be all-important. Those who do not have data on their clinical throughput will surely find themselves at a grave disadvantage when compared to those who have. Perhaps I could give another example. Some years ago, and in response to a budget deficit, managers proposed that the male surgical ward of the hospital where I then worked be closed during August, as it was 'a quiet month'. With the help of data from the audit system, this argument was successfully refuted, not only for the previous year but for the previous three years, and the consequences of such a closure were clearly demonstrated. This sort of scenario is seen increasingly nowadays and demonstrates how the gathering and 'ownership' of relevant information can be of great importance to the clinician.

Data gathering

It goes almost without saying that adequate, accurate data is a prerequisite for surgical audit. We found the setting up of systematic data collection such a difficult business that it deserves discussion in some detail.

Organization of data gathering

Fundamental principles must be borne in mind: the data must be accurate, timely and relevant.

CLINICAL WORKSHEET   INPATIENT EPISODE

Surname: ....   Unit No: ....   Date: ....

Forename: ....   D.O.B.: ....   Time: ....

Address: ....   Sex: ....   Own GP: ....

           ....   Ref GP: ....

Post Code: ....   Hospital: ....   Ward: ....

Telephone: ....   Consultant: ....

NHS / PRIVATE (please circle)

METHOD OF ADMISSION (please circle) -   1. W.L.   2. Booked   3. Planned   4. Other not Immed   5. A/E   6. Emergency GP
7. Emergency Bed Bureau   8. Emergency OPD   9. Emergency DOM   10. Other Immed   11. MAT.A/N   12. MAT. P/N   13 Inst.Oth Dist.
14. Born in Hosp.   15. Born outside Hosp.   16. N/K   17. Other Hospital in District:...

SOURCE OF ADMISSION   (please circle)   1. Uusual Res.   2. Temp Res.   3. Penl Est.   4. Special Hosp.   5. NHS Other Dist Gen.
6. NHS Other Dist. Maternity.   7. NHS Other Dist MI.   8. LA Res.   9. Born in/on way Hosp   10. Other Non NHS.   11. Other.
11a. Other unit in Hospital.   11b. NHS Other Hosp. this District.

DIAGNOSIS DETAILS

ADMITTING DIAGNOSIS/SYMPTOMS
(eg cholelithiasis or undiagnosed abdominal pain)

PREVIOUS SIGNIFICANT MEDICAL HISTORY

FINAL DIAGNOSIS   1.   1.

SECONDARY DIAGNOSES   2.   2.
(ie diabetes, hypertension
myocardial ischaemia)   3.   3.

ASA GRADE:
(see below for classification)

NON OP. MANAGEMENT
(eg Arteriography, Ercp Etc)

OPERATION DETAILS

(If more than one operation on different dates please attached a separate sheet)   BUPA
DATE: ....   DURATION: ...., mins.   THEATRE: ....   classification

PROCEDURE 1.

              2.

              3.

	TICK		TICK		TICK
EMERGENCY		IN SESSION		REFERRED FOR SURGERY ONLY	
URGENT		OUT SESSION			
ELECTIVE					

Personal (Unsupervised)
Surgeon   ....   Supervised
Assistant 1   ....   Assistant 2   ....
Anaesthetist: ....   Anaesthetic Type: ....

COMMENTS ON OPERATION (if appropriate)

American Society Of Anaesthesiology Classification   BUPA Classification
Class 1   No organic, physiological, biochemical or psychiatric disturbances   1. Minor
Class 2   Mild/moderate systemic disturbance caused either by condition to be treated surgically or other disease.   2. Intermediate
           EG, mild diabetes, anaemia, slightly limiting heart disease, obesity.   3. Major
Class 3   Severe systemic disturbance, eg, severely limiting organic heart disease, severe diabetes with vascular   4. Major +
           complication, angina   5. Complex Major D
Class 4   Severe, already life threatening, systemic disorders, eg organic heart disease with cardiac insufficiency,   6. Complex Major C
           advanced degrees of pulmonary, hepatitic, renal or endocrine insufficiency   7. Complex Major B
Class 5   Moribund patient who has little chance of survival, eg ruptured abdominal aneurysm profound shock.   8. Complex Major A

COMPLICATIONS

If applicable:

1	2
3	4
5	6
7	8
9	10

DISCHARGE   DETAILS

Date of discharge [| |]

Method of Discharge :   *(please circle)*
1. On medical advice   2. By self/relative   3. MH Trib/Court   4. Died   5. Stillbirth   6. Sent on leave

If died was post-mortem required: Yes/No   *(please circle)*

If died GP contacted   Yes/No/Not available   *(please circle)*

Histology :   To hand [   ]   Awaited [   ]   None [   ]   To be included in Discharge Summary [   ]

Destination on Discharge :   *(please circle)*

1. Usual Res   2. Temp Res   3. Penal Est   4. Spec. Hosp   5. NHS Hosp Other Dist
6. NHS Hosp Other Dist MAT   7. NHS Hosp Other Dist. MI 8. LA Res   9. Non NHS Hosp

10. Other Hosp. in Dist. .... 11. Other Unit in Hosp. ....

Drugs given on discharge:

	Drug	Dosage		Drug	Dosage
1			7		
2			8		
3			9		
4			10		
5			11		
6			12		

Information Given
1. Patient informed   2. Patient NOT informed   3. Relatives seen and informed   4. Relatives seen and NOT informed.
5. Diagnosis NOT yet known

Future Plans: FU in .... weeks. Clinic. Location .... Consultant ....

BRIEF HISTORY - SUMMARY OF PROGRESS AND COMMENTS

INVESTIGATIONS -

TREATMENT AND PROGRESS -

Figure 19.2   Example of worksheet for data input

Experts in the burgeoning specialty of information technology will tell you that to be accurate, data should be collected as close to the point at which they are generated as possible, 'close' meaning not only physically but also in time. Assuming that a computerized system of some sort will be used for storage and analysis of the data, certain constraints are placed upon where the data are gathered and where entered into the computer. It would be ideal, for instance, to collect and enter data into such a system from the patient's bedside, from the operating theatre or even from the consulting room. However, in practice there is bound to be a compromise between what is ideal and what is practical. For inpatient care, therefore, one should look at the points where data streams converge within a short time of the inpatient episode – the 'railway termini' of data routes. Clearly, the ward station or the medical secretary's office would fit the bill. Since the poor medical secretary spends most of the day entering data at an unforgiving keyboard, it seems logical to utilize this pre-existing pathway. For inpatient care, therefore, we elected to use a worksheet to collect data during each inpatient episode, vascular or general surgical, and then to enter it into the system at the secretary's office. The closer the medical secretary's office is to the wards and the more concentrated the inpatient work is on one ward, the better this sort of system will work. It is amazing how files can become lost or distorted along a corridor and down two flights of stairs. There is also the very practical consideration of support for the harassed medical secretary. However efficient the system, if data are to be collected accurately and quickly, medical staff must be on hand to facilitate and answer queries.

Data are entered onto the clinical worksheet in four stages. The initial stage comprises admission details such as patient identification, source of admission, mode of admission, etc. and is generally completed by the ward clerk or admitting nursing staff. The second stage covers medical history, clinical details and primary and secondary diagnoses. This section is completed by the admitting physician – usually the house officer. The third section contains operative details, if appropriate, and is completed by the operating surgeon. Finally, the fourth section provides for discharge information and a brief resumé of the case which may be completed by the house officer or senior house officer. The worksheet is then presented to the medical secretary at, or preferably just before, the time of discharge; the data are entered into the word processor/computer where they are then stored and a discharge summary generated either for the patient to take home or to be sent directly to the general practitioner, depending on preference. A few hospitals have systems where, instead of worksheets and medical secretaries, data are entered into the computer data bank from the ward. We have taken the view that with the high turnover of medical staff, the medical secretary is much more likely to provide a consistent level of expertise necessary to operate the system satisfactorily. An example of the worksheet that we have adopted as a modified version of our regional standard, is shown in Figure 19.2. We have not yet started to collect clinical data on outpatient attenders, but this must soon be addressed.

This worksheet has served our needs for several years but herein lies another important point. There would probably be little argument among surgeons regarding a common core of data comprising main diagnoses, operations, complications, etc. However, it can be guaranteed that each of us will differ when it comes to detail. Moreover, data needs are bound to vary from time to time and in response to specific projects. At an early stage we invested in a desk-top publishing software package which has proved to be of enormous benefit. It is run by our administrative (*not medical*) secretariat and for a relatively modest outlay it has served the need for instant worksheets and many other occasional forms throughout the hospital. In this way, we have the means to modify the data sets that are collected from time to time, and the ability to make them relevant.

What data?

Some years ago the two of us who then had a vascular interest at the hospital, attempted to compile a comprehensive list of the data to be collected during each inpatient episode so as to achieve a satisfactory audit of our work. As the list grew, the realization dawned upon us that the chances of routinely collecting such data, given our limited resources, was virtually nil. In practice it became obvious to our somewhat harrassed and overworked teams that, at least in the early stages, the amount of data to be collected and stored had to be kept to a minimum. Our initial approach was also flawed in that we should have posed the questions first, and worked out the data items from these rather than vice versa. Using this approach, and keeping the questions extremely simple, we progressed to a point where a useful basic data set comprising diagnoses, operations, complications and deaths, together with a certain amount of logistic data can now be routinely collected. If one is too ambitious regarding the quantity of data to be collected routinely, then the whole system is likely to break down.

Audit assistants

Inevitably, the processs of audit will raise more questions than it can satisfactorily answer immediately. Also, each surgeon is likely to have his or her own area of special interest as, for example, with vascular surgery. There is no reason why more detailed data sets cannot be collected to cover these points, either sporadically or systematically, and depending on circumstance. We have, for instance, designed a *pro forma*, separate from the worksheets, which will provide us with an adequate data bank on risk factors in patients undergoing aortic surgery. As the amount of data could not be collected, entered into the computer and analysed within our existing resources, a part-time, unqualified research assistant was financed on the support given to carry out some pharmaceutical trials. Specific audit projects, some involving aggregated data, clinical trials and research projects became possible. Now that specific Health Service monies have become available, 'audit assistants', 'analysts' or research assistants are likely to become much more commonplace.

Data storage

We have covered organization and data collection, but what of storage, processing and retrieval? Here again, it took us some time to realize that we should not be starting with a computer system to which we tailor our data collection. Rather, we should ask the questions, collect the appropriate data and then look around for a system that would perform the task satisfactorily. This proved to be very time-consuming and frustrating. We learned to beware the computer enthusiast and the computer salesman. The expression 'No, it doesn't at the moment, but it will ...' struck terror into our hearts! The detailed evaluation of individual systems is beyond the scope of this article but there are several major points that are worth making. There is also a small book issued by the West Midlands Health Authority[7] which gives much useful advice. It is extremely difficult to determine the finer points of a system from the manufacturer's description and sales rep's demonstration and we found that there was no substitute for 'hands on' experience of a system on a trial before deciding upon purchase.

It seemed to us pointless that we should be faced with entering data already collected elsewhere in the hospital. We therefore made an early decision to specify a system which was either integral or could be interfaced with the main hospital computer system. Apart from the advantage of avoiding duplicating data entry regarding registration details, it also meant that the office terminal would give the medical secretary access to all other facilities such as the Patient Administration System, Master Patient Index, Laboratories, etc. Secondly, we felt that the system should be flexible so that it could be set up to take the data that we wished, rather than that predetermined by the programmers. In particular, the thorny subject of classification and coding raised its ugly head, and it is worth discussing this in a little more detail. Whatever system is used, it should place minimal extra work on either the medical or the secretarial staff. Apart from adopting a user-friendly coding system, this can best be realized by avoiding duplicate entries as we have mentioned, keeping keystrokes and screen changes to an absolute minimum and by making sure that expert training and technical assistance is readily available. The importance of this last stipulation cannot be over-emphasized. The size of the manufacturing company, its track record and its proximity are extremely important in this respect. Eventually, and after trying several systems, we chose one that had been developed to our own specification by a software company who also held the Facilities Management contract for the hospital. This had the advantage that they were able to provide superb technical and training support. Our system consists of a personal computer which interfaces with software on the main hospital computer, providing access via one terminal not only to enormous computing power, but also to all the other hospital systems.

Coding and classification

Computers store and sort words and phrases by converting them first into codes comprising letters and/or figures. Encoding, therefore, from the written word (such as diagnosis or operation) is a necessary step in data handling. During evaluation, it quickly became apparent that many of the audit systems worked well until the point at which the diagnosis or title of an operation had to be entered. Some systems required medical staff to translate medical terms into the International Classification of Disease, Ninth Revision (ICD (9)) of Office or Population Census Surveys, Fourth Revision (OPCS (4)) codes using a book. The medical secretary then entered the digits at the appropriate point on the screen. Other systems required the medical terminology of the worksheet/houseman to match that of the machine before it was accepted for coding. For the purposes of audit and as our organization has been arranged, three factors seemed to us to be important. First, when the point is reached at which a diagnosis or an operation has to be entered into the computer, there must be no interruption to secretarial work while different screens, books or medical staff are being searched! Secondly, the classification into which the terms are encoded must be sufficiently discriminating for satisfactory audit to be carried out. For example, a code which covers the whole of biliary calculous disease without discriminating between the different variants is unlikely to be satisfactory. Thirdly, it is not, in our view, acceptable that medical staff should have to work out the codes from the various classifications of diagnoses etc., for each inpatient episode, which seemed to us to be an inappropriate use of medical staff time. With these points in mind, we specified a system that encodes automatically from the written medical word into ICD (9) or OPCS (4). Where this coding system is not sufficiently discriminating for audit, then an extra letter has been added. Using this approach, a large part of the hospital coding department's work may be automated and speeded up if the appropriate computer links are made. Inevitably, classifications and their codes will change: it is likely, for instance, that the Read classification will be adopted by the Department of Health when it has been agreed by the appropriate committees[8]. With software such as ours it will be a relatively straightforward task for the coding department to recode against the same medical dictionary that we use now.

Introduction of data gathering systems and training

This can be conveniently divided into two consecutive phases. The first phase concerns the 'paper' exercise up to the point of data entry into the computer. The questions concerning which data, who completes which parts of the worksheets and how they arrive at the secretary's office, how one fits outlying wards and operating lists into the system, etc. all need sorting out. Until this aspect is working satisfactorily there is not much point in inputting data. Once data collection is running smoothly then the second phase should follow on expeditiously – namely, the introduction of computerized data capture. Some surgeons and their secretaries who managed this without any initial extra resources have had to face the turmoil where work piles up as the secretary tears her hair out at the keyboard of an unyielding machine. Much the best way is to invest in a 'training' secretary, preferably a medical secretary, who takes on the training role for the department or even the whole hospital. During the introductory phase of the computer system, which may last a week or two, the trainer shares the office and its workload with the 'pupil' secretary so that activities do not grind to a full stop. Once things are working smoothly, the 'training' secretary retires gracefully and moves on to the next 'pupil'. This arrangement has worked very well for us.

Verification and 'mini audit'

We had now arrived at the stage where data sets had been specified, collected routinely and stored in a data bank on computer, a system set up to run as part of the day-to-day service without any greatly increased involvement of consultant staff. The houseman and the operating surgeon were made responsible for data collection from which discharge summaries were routinely produced. As a further check on the quality of the data produced, our firm now spends half an hour during a weekday lunchtime going through the previous week's discharge summaries. These sessions have become an enjoyable part of our routine where we review a considerable amount of our work and data, and also tie up any loose ends, discuss points that have arisen and review the work projected for the week to come. It is essential to build some form of verification procedure into a data collection system and for us this seems to work well. Incidentally, apart from medical members of the firm and the medical secretary, the coding clerk responsible for surgery attends and we check the number of discharges and deaths as recorded by the ward against the number of discharge summaries produced during a given period. We find that 85% of discharge summaries are sent on the day of discharge and our overall total data capture for inpatient episodes is now 98%. This compares with a period of 8–10 weeks for discharge summary production before the system was introduced and an overall discharge summary and coding default rate in excess of 10% – even twelve months after discharge! Interestingly, the accuracy of coding, albeit on ICD (9) and OPCS (4) classification has improved dramatically as it has been brought under more direct medical staff supervision.

Enquiries

The first step in the transformation of 'data' into 'information' comes with the institution of an enquiry on the computer. The ease and sophistication of these enquiries varies according to the computer system and its software. It should be one of the criteria against which such a system is purchased. It is likely that certain of these enquiries such as the number of patients admitted and discharged during a given period, together with their diagnoses, operations, complications, length of stay, etc. will be required every two weeks or so for the purpose of audit meetings. It should be possible to produce this enquiry by one or two keystrokes. Entry into this part of the system can, if required, be protected by password but it seems reasonable that the medical secretary should produce this as a routine.

Other regular enquires such as those used to assess training of junior staff are desirable. When a member of the team leaves, it should be possible to provide him or her with a printout of all the operations performed or assisted at – rather along the lines of the log books produced by the Royal Colleges of Surgeons. More difficult to obtain, but none the less crucial are the *ad hoc* enquiries that are required on an occasional basis, for instance 'how many inguinal hernias have been repaired over a given period and how many complications have occurred?' 'How many abdominal aortic aneurysms have been repaired during a given period and what are the details of urgency, age, mortality etc'. For most systems this is a task requiring some time and training. It is certainly not a task that can be left to an overworked medical secretary but it is well within the capabilities of our 'audit assistant' or 'analyst'. Here again, it is important to have ready access to technical help until the intricacies and subtleties of the system have been mastered.

One other type of enquiry is worthy of mention, and that is the 'browsing' facility. Here one can merely call up data specified according to broad limits of date, age, etc. and browse through them as they scroll up the screen. This is a useful facility when searching for the patient whose name you cannot quite remember! Having enquired, the system will produce the data in tabular form. It is possible with a little time and patience to download these tables into another piece of software where further analysis can be carried out. Results can then be subjected to statistical analysis or expressed as charts, etc. This is an extremely useful facility and, again, it is something that should be borne in mind when selecting a system. *Supercalc* is one such popular system but there are several other very good packages readily available.

Security

Entry into a system is usually governed via a password. The complexity of the password and the frequency with which it is changed is a matter of personal preference. The 'stand alone' supporter will argue strongly against the 'integrated' enthusiast that their system is more secure and vice versa. It is clearly important to have a definite policy regarding access. We have had one episode of hacking by an unauthorized member of the junior medical staff who was showing off to his colleagues, but this was without malicious intent and produced no lasting damage. Apart from the fear of unauthorized inspection of confidential data, medical staff have a paranoia that management will secretly take databases for their own machiavellian purposes and without prior consent. All I can say is that it seems so extraordinarily difficult and time-consuming to provide links to other modules within a hospital system that I cannot see this being a problem. Nevertheless it would seem a wise move, if one does have an integrated audit system, to specify in writing who has access to what data on the central computer system.

How does one audit?

I suppose that the most informal sort of medical audit is held at any lunch table when two or more doctors get together! However, medical audit in the true sense requires a more systematic approach. As with data collection, we have seen a gradual evolution of the methods of audit within our unit, our hospital and our region. The method chosen must depend on local circumstances but however small the unit, and however limited the resources, the important task is to get audit going in some form or other. The position in which general/vascular surgeons find themselves, demonstrates nicely the problems of audit experienced by members of large and small specialties.

Ten or more years ago, our hospital surgical meetings were extremely poorly attended partly because they were held at the end of the day and partly because of the exigencies of clinical work. Even so, people were hardly at their best at this time of day which the meetings seemed to reflect. We persuaded the administration to provide us with a high roughage breakfast and changed the meeting time to 07.30 every Wednesday. Despite much initial weeping and wailing attendance went up to very nearly 100% of available staff and the meetings were generally agreed to be much more successful. When we decided to institute regular audit meetings within the department of general surgery, we used this meeting on alternate weeks. All the figures on mortality and morbidity for each of the ten surgical firms (seven general surgeons, two urologists and one thoracic surgeon) were reviewed. The chairmanship was changed for each meeting and *all* complications and *all* deaths were shown in the one hour available. This time proved insufficient and so to coincide with the formation of our surgical directorate and the imposition of service cutback within the hospital, we took the opportunity to dedicate one half-session each week to a formal surgical audit meeting. Individual timetables were not readily altered and so, not to disadvantage any particular firm by holding these meetings at a fixed time each week, this half-session was allocated on a rolling programme – that is to say on Monday morning during the first week, on Monday afternoon in the second week, on Tuesday morning in the third week and so on. The anaesthetic department quickly followed suit as did most of the other surgical specialties. Attendance is mandatory and is monitored. All the work of each of the surgical firms is collected from the audit computers by the departmental secretary and is presented in the form of diagnoses, length of stay, operations, deaths and complications by overhead projection. Junior staff involvement in the discussions tended to be poor until they were persuaded to sit in the front two rows and to lead those discussions.

At the end of each session, the chairman agrees any conclusions that have been reached and minutes them, together with a brief and anonymous record of the cases discussed. Audit of the audit is held at the end of each six-month period, when a session is devoted to an analysis of what was proposed and what has been achieved from the meetings. A report is sent to the District Hospital Medical Audit Committee. This analysis has shown overall attendance rates for both consultant and junior medical staff during the past two years to be 60%.

The laudable intention to stimulate audit projects and research studies has not met with as much success as we would have wished, but there have been some very interesting and worthwhile conclusions drawn from those projects that have reached fruition. To give but one example, as a result of discussion at several audit meetings, we examined the treatment of carcinoma of the head of the pancreas causing biliary obstruction. Our aggregated figures for the treatment and survival of this miserable condition showed no advantage of laparotomy and bypass surgery over endoscopic insertion of a biliary stent. We believe that as we appoint further audit assistants and the task becomes easier, our project rate will improve.

From the foregoing it can be appreciated that the form of our audit meetings is still evolving. There is a definite tendency for meetings to become stereotyped and dull, but to mitigate this we are instituting regular case-note review meetings in which one firm will randomly select notes from another firm and review them for quality of notekeeping and case management in general. Perhaps a bottle of wine given to the team doing the best 'demolition' job or, alternatively, 'putting up the best defence' will add further impetus. For some years, we have also held combined meetings with other specialties – particularly anaesthetists and physicians. These meetings are held once or twice per year and cases are selected in advance by the joint chairman from the previous six months' clinical material. If possible, we try to select cases with a common theme such as morbidity associated with central venous cannulation, management of haematemesis, inflammatory bowel disease, etc. It is difficult to measure objectively the success of these meetings, but they have resulted in local consensus guidelines being drawn up for such conditions as haematemesis.

In a large district general hospital there is no difficulty in finding a group of sufficient size and common interest with which to hold audit meetings and peer review, but unfortunately this does not hold true for minority specialties such as vascular surgery or urology. Although presentations are regularly made at general surgical audit meetings, there is no real peer review. This can only be rectified by setting up an audit group on either a regional or subregional basis. In our region, several non-surgical specialties are presently working on audit in this way and it seems possible that this will be the format for vascular audit in the future.

Audit meetings of one sort or another with peer review are clearly the mainstay of our surgical audit but other methods should not be neglected. One measure of outcome is 'patient satisfaction'. This may be criticized as a poor indicator of overall quality of care but one can say that if patient dissatisfaction is high then there is certainly something wrong. We have tackled this in two ways. First, each patient on our ward receives a questionnaire which is returned anonymously on discharge (Figure 19.3). Where a patient is incapable of completing the form (i.e. is a child or incapacitated adult) the next of kin does so on their behalf. Batch analysis of the

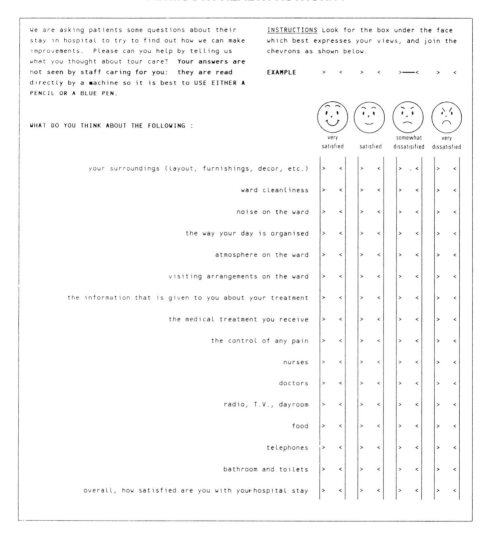

Figure 19.3   Assessment of 'patient satisfaction' – a questionnaire completed anonymously on discharge is an excellent way of receiving feedback from patients on the quality of care they have received in hospital

forms using an optical scanner is straightforward and inexpensive. We find, not surprisingly, that quality of food and amount of noise on the wards give rise to more dissatisfaction than anything else. This sort of continuous audit of quality must surely be a potent weapon against overcrowding and understaffing in the future.

The other method that we have used for assessing patient satisfaction is postal surveys. Straightforward surgical conditions lend themselves to this type of approach. We have just completed one survey for varicose veins treated surgically over a period of ten years using a standard questionnaire (Figure 19.4). Of a total of 480

VARICOSE VEINS SURVEY 1990

NAME ....

DATE OF BIRTH ....

ADDRESS......................................

       ....

       ....

Please answer the following questions:

1. Aproximately how long ago was your surgery?...........................

2. Was it for one leg/both legs? ....

3. Was it for recurrent varicose veins? ....

4. Were there any problems in the immediate post operative period(i.e.before you were seen again in the clinic).
   Please list:
              ....
              ....
              ....
              ....

5. Were you satisfied with communications and explanation of procedure? Yes/No

6. Are you satisfied with the overall results of your surgery? Yes/No

   If No,would you please itemise:

   a. Scarring satisfactory/unsatisfactory?
      If unsatisfactory,please detail ....
      ....

   b. Leg(s) still ache? Yes/No
                         Better/Worse than before operation

   c. Varicose veins have recurred? Yes/No
                                    Better/Worse than before operation

   d. Skin symptoms(itching,tenderness) persist? ....
      ....

   e. Other-please specify ....

7. Have you had to have further treatment elsewhere for your varicose veins since discharge from my care? ....
   If you care to,please specify.

Figure 19.4 A postal questionnaire, such as this one helps assess long-term patient satisfaction and pinpoints requirements for long-term follow-up

questionnaires, 359 patients replied. The overall level of substantial dissatisfaction with the result was 20%. Dissatisfied patients were offered a further outpatient appointment and from there further treatment, if appropriate. Several facts emerged. One of the most striking was that the overwhelming majority of dissatisfied patients were from the group who had undergone surgery for recurrent varicose veins. One middle-aged patient had developed crippling pains in her legs some months after her surgery which she attributed to her original varicose veins. She was found, at the audit review, to be suffering from claudication which was amenable to percutaneous angioplasty! Crude figures regarding the outcome of inguinal hernia surgery can also be obtained relatively easily in this way – I wonder how many of us have any real idea of our hernia recurrence rate? Finally, we should not neglect the value of self-audit. The mere acquisition and perusal of the data pertaining to one's own clinical work can be very enlightening, especially if 'norms' from other people's results are readily to hand for comparison!

Conclusions

There is a saying 'Good judgement is the result of experience; but let us not forget that experience is often the result of previous *bad* judgement'. One of the main aims of surgical audit is to make the best possible use of previous surgical experience. Surgical audit may take many forms, but common to each of them is the need for accurate, timely and relevant data. The setting up of an efficient clinical data gathering and processing system is a great challenge but it must be given top priority if audit is to take place at other than a very superficial level. Time should be set aside for regular meetings, although the size and composition of audit groups will vary according to local circumstances. A member of the medical staff should be given the responsibility of supervising the evolution of the audit process and an audit assistant, whose task is to collate information for meetings and special projects, is also required. The assessment of long-term outcomes is but poorly addressed at present and needs to become a routine part of the clinical and audit process. This is particularly germane to an expensive specialty such as vascular surgery. Finally, and most importantly, a careful record should be kept of recommendations arising from surgical audit meetings, and the subsequent fate of these recommendations should be kept under regular review in order to ascertain that change is being achieved. Without this, much of the justification for an expensive and time-consuming process is lost.

References

1. NHS Review White Paper *Working for Patients*, Working Paper No. 6 Command 555, HMSO, 1989
2. Blair, D. (1990) Outcome measures needed. *Br. Med. J.*, **299**, 1361
3. Kind, P., Rosser, R. and Williams, (1982) A valuation of quality of life: some psycometric evidence. In *The Value of Life and Safety* (ed. M. W. Jones-Lee). Elsevier/North-Holland, Amsterdam, pp. 159–170
4. The Royal College of Surgeons of England (1989) *Guidelines to Clinical Audit in Surgical Practice*
5. Pollock, A. and Evans, M. (1989) *Surgical Audit 1989*, Butterworths, London
6. Wyatt, M. G., Houghton, P. W. J. and Brodribb, A. J. M. (1990) Theatre delay for emergency general surgical patients: A cause for concern? *Ann. R. Coll. Surg. Eng.*, **72** (4) 236–238
7. Tindall, R., Kennedy, S., Naylor, S. and Pajak, F. (1990) *Computers in Medical Audit*. Royal Society of Medicine Services, London
8. Chisholm, J. (1990) The Read clinical classification. *Br. Med. J.*, **300**, 1092

Appendix

In this section will be found evidence of research activities undertaken by the Joint Vascular Research Group UK.

Communications

1 Wolfe, J. H. N., for the Joint Vascular Research Group UK (1985). *Defining the outcome of critical ischaemia. A one-year prospective study.* Vascular Surgical Society of Great Britain and Ireland, London

2 Wolfe, J. H. N., for the Joint Vascular Research Group UK (1986). *Is critical ischaemia a useful definition? A one-year prospective study.* Second International Vascular Symposium, London

3 Wolfe, J. H. N., for the Joint Vascular Research Group UK (1986). *Critical ischaemia or limb salvage?* European Cardiovascular Society, Brighton

4 Wolfe, J. H. N., for the Joint Vascular Research Group UK (1986). *Critical ischaemia: factors influencing outcome.* European Cardiovascular Society, Brighton

5 Wolfe, J. H. N., for the Joint Vascular Research Group UK (1988). *The definition of critical ischaemia – is this a concept of value?* International Symposium on Limb Salvage and Amputation for Vascular Disease, London

6 Lamont, P. M., for the Joint Vascular Research Group UK (1988). *Femoro-popliteal versus femoro-distal bypass graft for limb salvage in patients with an 'isolated' popliteal segment.* European Society of Vascular Surgery, Rotterdam

7 Ruckley, C. V., for the Joint Vascular Research Group UK (1988). *Is there any advantage of skew-flap rather than Burgess below-knee amputation?* International Symposium on Limb Salvage and Amputation for Vascular Disease, London

8 Lamont, P. M., for the Joint Vascular Research Group UK (1988). *Femoro-popliteal versus femoro-distal bypass graft for limb salvage in patients with isolated popliteal segment.* Vascular Surgical Society of Great Britain and Ireland, Leeds

9 Ruckley, C. V., Stonebridge, P. A., Prescott, R. J., Darke, S. G., Harris, P. L., Bell, P. R. F., Clyne, C. A. C., Wolfe, J. H. N., Chant, A. D. B., Hamer, J. D., Perry, P. M., Barros D'Sa, A. A. B. and Wilkins, D. C. (1989). *Skew-flap versus long posterior flap in below-knee amputation.* Vascular Surgical Society of Great Britain and Ireland, Dundee

10 Wolfe, J. H. N., for the Joint Vascular Research Group UK (1989). *Objective*

assessment of the ischaemic leg: a three-year prospective study. Association of Surgeons of Great Britain and Ireland, Edinburgh

11 Ranaboldo, C., Barros D'Sa, A. A. B., Bell, P. R. F., Perry, P. M. and Chant, A. D. B. (1990). *A prospective carotid patch/non-patch study.* Vascular Surgical Society of Great Britain and Ireland, Tripartite Meeting of the British, Canadian and Dutch Vascular Surgical Societies, London

Abstracts

1 Wolfe, J. H. N., for the Joint Vascular Research Group UK (1986). Defining the outcome of critical ischaemia: A one-year prospective study. *Br. J. Surg.*, **73**, 321

2 Lamont, P. M. and Darke, S. G., for the Joint Vascular Research Group UK (1989). Femoro-popliteal versus infracrural bypass grafting for limb salvage in patients with an 'isolated' popliteal segment. *Br. J. Surg.*, **76**, 413

3 Darke, S. G., Lamont, P. M., Chant, A. D. B., Barros D'Sa, A. A. B., Clyne, C. A. C., Harris, P. L., Ruckley, C. V. and Bell, P. R. F. (1990). Femoro-popliteal versus femoro-distal bypass grafting for limb salvage in patients with an 'isolated' popliteal segment. *J. Vasc. Surg.*, **11**, 613

4 Ruckley, C. V., Stonebridge, P. A., Prescott, R. J., Darke, S. G., Harris, P. L., Bell, P. R. F., Clyne, C. A. C., Wolfe, J. H. N., Chant, A. D. B., Hamer, J. D., Perry, P. M., Barros D'Sa, A. A. B. and Wilkins, D. C. (1990). Skew-flap versus long posterior flap in below-knee amputation. *Br. J. Surg.*, **77A**, 346–347

5 Ranaboldo, C., Barros D'Sa, A. A. B., Bell, P. R. F., Perry, P. M. and Chant, A. D. B. (1991). A prospective carotid patch/non-patch study. *Br. J. Surg.* (in press)

Papers

1 Darke, S. G., Lamont, P. M., Chant, A. D. B., Barros D'Sa, A. A. B., Clyne, C. A. C., Harris, P. I., Ruckley, C. V. and Bell, P. R. F. (1989). Femoro-popliteal versus femoro-distal bypass grafting for limb salvage in patients with an 'isolated' popliteal segment. *Eur. J. Vasc. Surg.*, **3**, 203–207

2 Ruckley, C. V., Stonebridge, P. A. and Prescott, R. J., for the Joint Vascular Research Group UK (1991). Skew-flap versus long posterior flap in below-knee amputations: A multicentre trial. *J. Vasc. Surg.* (in press)

Chapters

1 Wolfe, J. H. N., for the Joint Vascular Research Group UK (1988). The definition of critical ischaemia – is this a concept of value? In *Limb Salvage and Amputation for Vascular Disease* (eds R. M. Greenhalgh, C. W. Jamieson and A. N. Nicolaides) London, Saunders

2 Ruckley, C. V., for the Joint Vascular Research Group UK (1988). Is there any advantage of skew-flap rather than Burgess' below-knee amputation? In *Limb Salvage and Amputation for Vascular Disease* (eds R. M. Greenhalgh, C. W. Jamieson, A. N. Nicolaides) London, Saunders

Completed trials/studies

1 Critical ischaemia study: Three year follow-up
2 *In situ* vein graft proximal versus distal implantation study
3 A trial of skew flap versus long posterior flap in below-knee amputations
4 Carotid endarterectomy patch versus non-patch trial
5 Comparative study of polytetrafluoroethylene (PTFE) versus human umbilical vein (HUV) in femoropopliteal bypass
6 A study of the use of 'heparin' versus 'no heparin' in aortic aneurysm

Current trials and studies

1 Popliteal artery aneurysm study
2 Comparative study of unilateral iliofemoral bypass graft versus femorofemoral crossover bypass graft
3 Unsealed versus collagen-sealed aortic bifurcation graft study
4 The use of the Miller vein cuff in PTFE femorodistal grafts

Proposed projects

1 Trial of the use of Iloprost as an adjunct to femoropopliteal bypass
2 Comparative study of femoral angioplasty versus surgery for long segment superficial femoral artery occlusion

Current members of JVRG UK

Roger N. Baird, Bristol*
Aires A. B. Barros D'Sa, Belfast*
Jonathan D. Beard, Sheffield
Peter R. F. Bell, Leicester*
W. Bruce Campbell, Exeter
John Chamberlain, Newcastle-upon-Tyne
Anthony D. B. Chant, Southampton*
Charles A. C. Clyne, Torquay
Simon G. Darke, Bournemouth*
John M. D. Galloway, Hull
Peter L. Harris, Liverpool*
Michael Horrocks, Bristol
Crawford W. Jamieson, London*
D. Paul Lieberman, Glasgow
Roger Marcuson, Salford*
John A. Murie, Edinburgh
Simon Parvin, Bournemouth
P. Michael Perry, Southampton*
C. Vaughan Ruckley, Edinburgh*
Denis C. Wilkins, Plymouth*

Colin C. Wilmshurst, Torquay
John H. N. Wolfe, London

* Founder members

Venues of JVRG UK meetings

1983   Southampton, London
1984   Lancaster, Birmingham
1985   Edinburgh, London
1986   Torquay, London
1987   London, Newcastle-upon-Tyne
1988   Bristol, Leeds
1989   Leicester, Dundee
1990   Kirkby Lonsdale, London
1991   Belfast

Index

Abdominal aortic aneurysms, 62–8
  contained rupture, 63, 64 (fig.)
  gallstones associated, 68
  incidence, 62
  inflammatory, 65–7
  malignant disease associated, 68
  mortality of rupture, 62–3
  mycotic, 67
  operation, 67–8
    anaesthesia, 67
    prosthesis, 68
  small, 64
    asymptomatic, 64
Above-knee amputation, 202–4
Algodystrophy, 81
Allopurinol, 86
Amoxycillin/clavulanic acid (Augmentin),
    79, 161
Anastomotic aneurysm, 79–80
Angiography, 2
Angioplasty, 116
Angiotensin I, 101
Angiotensin II, 101, 106
Angiotensin-converting enzyme inhibitors,
    106
Ankle vascular pressure, 2
Anterior spinal artery, 53
Antibiotics, prophylactic, 161
Anticoagulants, oral, 220–1, 228–9
Antiplatelet therapy, 152
Aortic bifurcation graft, 116, 119–20
Aortic surgery, elective, complications,
    70–81
  acute limb ischaemia, 74–6
  algodystrophy, 81
  anastomotic aneurysm, 79–80
  anuria, postoperative, 72
  aortoenteric fistula, 79
  bleeding, 73
  cardiac, 70–1
  gastrointestinal, 73

Aortic surgery, elective, complications (*cont.*)
  graft infection, 78–9
  nerve injury, 80–1
  perigraft seroma, 77 (fig.), 81
  pulmonary, 71–2
  renal artery occlusion/embolization, 72
  renal failure, 72
  sexual dysfunction, 80
  spinal cord ischaemia, *see* Spinal cord
    ischaemia
  trash buttock, 74
  trash foot, 74, 75 (fig.)
  ureteric injury, 72–3
  wound, 76, 77 (fig.)
Aortofemoral bypass, 124
Aortoenteric fistula, 79
Aortoiliac endarterectomy, 116, 118–19
Arteriovenous shunt, 147–9
Artery of Ademkiewicz, 76
Audit, 237–47
  data gathering, 235–9
  introduction of data gathering
    systems/training, 241
  meetings, 243–5
  mini audit, 241–2
  patient satisfaction questionnaire,
    244–5
  postal survey, 245–7
  verification, 241–2
  worksheet for data input, 236–7 (table)
Audit assistants, 239
Augmentin (amoxycillin/clavulanic acid), 79,
    161
Autogenous vein, 161
Axillofemoral bypass, 120–1,124

Bacterial adherence to prosthetic materials,
    159–60
Bacterial aortitis, 67
Below-knee amputation, 199–201
  long posterior flap, 201

Below-knee amputation (*cont.*)
    stump dressing, 200–1
Bilateral ascending phlebography, 225–6
Biogel gloves, 160
Blood flow velocity, 145–6

Calcium channel blockers, 54
Calf muscles, electrical stimulation, 223
Carotid artery disease, clinical vascular
        laboratory studies, 3
Captopril, 106
    renal scintigraphy, 106
Captopril-enhanced diethylenetriamine
        penta-acetic acid scan, 103
Carotid body, 31–2
    hyperplasia, 32
    pathophysiology, 32–3
Carotid body tumour, 33–45
    clinical diagnosis, 34–5
    investigation, 35–7, 38 (fig.)
    irradiation treatment, 38
    pathology, 33–4
    recurrent, 43
    surgical treatment, 38–44
        complications, 44–5
        results, 44–5
Carotid endarterectomy, 21–9
    decision pathway, 26 (fig.)
    empirical approach, 25–6
    follow up, 29
    investigation, 27–8
    operation, 28–9
    patient selection, 26–7
    theoretical rationale, 22–4
Carotid sinus syndrome, 35
Causalgia, 81
Cefotaxime, 161
Cefuroxime, 161
Cephalosporins, 79
Cephazolin, 161
Chemodectoma, 31
Cholesterol, 15–16
Cigarette smoking, 13–14
Clinical vascular laboratory, 1–10
    carotid artery disease, 3
    data storage, 10
    equipment, 3–7
    finance, 10
    peripheral occlusive diseases of legs, 2–3
    personnel, 8
    reporting, 9–10
    siting, 7–8
    training of technicians/nurses, 8–9
    vasospastic disease, 3
    venous thromboembolic disease, 3

Coeliac axis, 85
Colonic ischaemia, 73
Common ostium shunt, 147
Completion angiogram, 136, 138 (fig.)
Compression stockings, 223
Computer, 239–43
    browsing facility, 242
    coding/classification, 240–1
    data storage, 239–40
    enquiries, 242
    security, 243

Dacron grafts, 159–60
Deep vein thrombosis, 219–30
    diagnosis, 224–5
    investigation, 225–6
        for associated conditions, 226–7
    prevention of post-phlebitic venous
        insufficiency, 229
    prophylaxis, 219–45
        mechanical, 223–4
        primary, 220–34
        secondary, 224–5
    recurrent spontaneous, 230
    risk factors, 224 (table)
    treatment, 227–9
        anticoagulants, 228–9
        thrombectomy, 227
        thrombolysis, 227–8
Dextran, 222
Diabetes mellitus, 14–15
    blood flow in foot, 178
    peripheral neuropathy, 177–8
    reconstructive arterial surgery, 186
Diabetic foot, 15, 177–88
    amputation, 187
    clinical presentation, 179–82
    infection, 179
    investigation, 182–3
        angiography, 183
        transcutaneous oxygen measurements,
            182–3
    local treatment, 186–7
    lumbar sympathectomy, 185
    transluminal angioplasty, 183–5
Digital subtraction angiography, 104–5
    intra-arterial, 104
Digits amputation, 198
Dihydroergotamine, 222
Doppler flow velocimeter, 3–4
Duplex scanner, 3, 4–5
Duplex ultrasonography, 103–4

Enalapril, 106
Eye-foot syndrome, 15

Familial hypercholesterolaemia, 16
Femorodistal bypass, 127–53
  arteriovenous shunt, adjuvant, 147–9
  assessment, 127–36
    completion angiogram, 136, 138 (fig.)
    dependent Doppler, 130
    inflow, 129–30
    intraoperative, 131–6
    of procedure, 136
    pressure generated runoff, 130–1
    resistance assessment, 133–6
    vein mapping, 131, 132 (fig.)
  choice of graft, 141–2
  choice/exposure of distal recipient artery,
    142–4
  choice of proximal recipient artery, 144
  common ostium shunt, 147
  distal anastomosis technique, 144–5
  distal graft failure, 145–7
  endothelial seeding of prosthetic grafts,
    150–1
  length of graft, 144
  patency rates, adjuvant measures, 147
  pharmacology, adjuvant, 152–3
  postoperative period, 6, 137–40
    early monitoring, 137–9
    late monitoring, 139–40
  preanastomotic shunt, 147
  preoperative selection, 127–9
  venous interposition grafts, patches, cuffs,
    149–50, 151 (fig.)
Femorofemoral bypass, 120, 124
Femoropopliteal graft, postoperative
  surveillance, 6

Gangrene:
  big toe, 128 (fig.)
  foot, 15, 128 (fig.); see also Diabetic foot
  legs, 2, 3
Gelatin sponge, 161
Glomus jugulare tumour, bilateral, 33
Glycocalyx, 156, 160

Heparin, 221–2, 228
High-density lipoprotein, 15
Hip level amputation, 204
HIV infection, 81
Horner's syndrome, 35, 45
Human umbilical vein graft, 142
Hypercholesterolaemia, familial, 16
Hypertension, 101–2
  essential, 102
  renovascular, 102
  surgical treatment, 106–8
Hypertriglyceridaemia, 16

Hypoxanthine, 86

Iliac artery occlusive disease, 116–24
  angioplasty, 116
  aortic bifurcation graft, 116, 119–20
  aortobifemoral bypass, 124
  aortoiliac endarterectomy, 116, 118–19
  axillofemoral bypass, 120–1, 124
  best option, 124
  femorofemoral bypass, 120
  surgical treatment indications, 117–18
  unilateral iliofemoral bypass, 121
Iloprost, 135, 152
Infarction of bowel, 85–6
Inferior mesenteric artery, 73, 85, 90
Intercostal artery re-implantation, 54
Intestinal ischaemia, 85-96
  acute, 86–9
    causes, 86
    clinical experience, 89
    diagnosis, 87
    management, 87–9
    recognition, 86–7
  chronic, 90–6
    causes, 90
    clinical experience, 95–6
    diagnosis, 90–1
    postoperative care, 95
    presentation, 90
    treatment, 92–5
  infarction, 85–6
  pathophysiology, 85
Intravenous urography, 103
Isoenzyme CPK-BB, 86

Lazy loop, 93–5
Left renal vein ligation, 72
Leiomyosarcoma, 174-5
Lipids, 15–16
Lipoproteins:
  (a), 16
  high density, 15
  low density, 15
Lisfranc's amputation, 199
Liver enzyme elevation, 86
Long saphenous vein incompetence, 207–9
  saphenography, 208
  stripping, 217
Low-density lipoprotein, 15
Lower limb amputation, 190–205
  above-knee, 202–4
  below-knee, 199–200
    long posterior flap, 201
    stump dressing, 200–1
  Chopart's, 199

Lower limb amputation (*cont.*)
  comparability of results, 205
  complications, early, 204
  decisions, 191–5
    what level, 194–5
    when, 193
    whether to amputate, 191–2
    who decides, 192–3
    who operates, 193–4
  digits, 198
  healing potential evaluation, 194–7
    angiographic scoring, 197
    Doppler ultrasound, 195
    fluorescein fluorometry, 197
    isotope clearance, 196
    photoplethysmography, 195
    skin thermometry, 197
    thermography, 197
    transcutaneous oxygen, 196
  hip level, 204
  Lisfranc's, 199
  Pirogoff's, 199
  results reporting, 205 (table)
  skew-flap, 199–200
  Syme's, 198, 199
  technique, 197–8
  through-knee, 201
  transmetatarsal, 198–9

Mesenteric ischaemia, acute non-occlusive, 86
Miller Cuff, 149, 151 (fig.)
  Wolfe modification, 149, 152 (fig.)
Multiorgan failure, 86
Multiple tumour syndrome, 33

Neck bruits, 24
Netilmicin plus methicillin, 161

Omentum, 161
Oral anticoagulants, 220–1, 228–9
Oxidized cellulose haemostatic sponge, 161
Oxygen-derived free radicals, 54, 86

Papaverine, 54
Paraganglioma, 33
  catecholamine-secreting, 33
Paralytic ileus, 73
Patient satisfaction questionnaire, 244–5
Percutaneous angioplasty, 92
Percutaneous transluminal angioplasty, 107, 108
Peripheral vascular disease:
  risk factors, 11–17
    age, 11–13

Peripheral vascular disease (*cont.*)
  risk factors (*cont.*)
    cholesterol, 15–16
    cigarette smoking, 13–14
    diabetes mellitus, 14–15
    Framingham study, 11
    haematological, 16
    modification, 16–17
    sex, 11–13
  vascular laboratory tests, 2–3
Persantin, 152
Phlegmasia alba dolens, 225
Phlegmasia caerulea dolens, 225
Phonoangiography, 3
Photoplethysmography, 4
Pirogoff's amputation, 199
Platelets, 152
Plethysmography, 3
Pneumatic compression, 223
Polytetrafluoroethylene grafts, 159–60, 161
Popliteal aneurysm, 165–72
  asymptomatic, 171–2
  diagnosis, 166
  incidence, 166
  investigation, 166–7, 168 (fig.)
  symptomatic, 167–71
    group 1: acute thrombosis, 168–9
    group 2: chronic thrombosis, 169
    group 3: acute embolism, 169
    group 4: chronic embolism, 169
    group 5: local symptoms, 169
    group 6: rupture, 169
Popliteal artery, 165
  cystic adventitial disease, 174
  entrapment, 173–4
  trauma, 172–3
  tumours, 174–5
Postal survey, 245–7
Povidone-iodine, 160
Preanastomotic shunt, 147
Pressure generated runoff, 130–1
Prostaglandins, 54
Pulmonary embolism, 229
Pulse-generated runoff, 3, 5

Quality adjusted life years, 234

Reflex sympathetic dystrophy, 81
Renal artery aneurysm, 100, 102, 105 (fig.)
  macroaneurysm, 101
  microaneurysm, 101
  rupture, 102–3
  surgical treatment, 111
Renal artery disease, 100–11
  atheroma, 100

Renal artery disease (*cont.*)
   fibromuscular dysplasia, 100, 107 (fig.)
   functional tests, 105–6
      captopril renal scintigraphy, 106
      divided renal vein renin studies, 105
   investigation, 103–5
      digital subtraction angiography, 104–5
      duplex ultrasonography, 103–4
      intravenous urography, 103
      radioisotope studies, 103
      screening tests, 103
   occlusion, 102, 108 (fig.)
   surgical treatment, 103
   trauma, 100
Renal failure, 102, 109–11
   percutaneous transluminal angioplasty,
      110–11
Renal artery stenosis, 100, 101 (fig.), 109
      (fig.)
Renin, 101
Reperfusion injury, 86
Rest pain, Doppler studies, 2
Rosser index, 234

Segmental plethysmography, 2
Seroma, 81, 156
Sexual dysfunction, post-aortic surgery, 80
Skew-flap amputation, 199–200
Small bowel ischaemia, 73
Sonogram analysis, 4
Spinal cord ischaemia, 76
   treatment, 53–4
      cerebrospinal fluid drainage, 53
      mechanical, 53
      neurophysiological monitoring, 54
      operative technique modification, 53
      pharmacological methods, 54
Streptokinase, 185
Sudeck's atrophy, 91
Superficial femoral artery occlusion, 76
Superior mesenteric artery, 85, 86–9
Supra-oxide dismutase, 54
Surgical sepsis, 155–62
   incidence, 155

Surgical sepsis (*cont.*)
   microbiology, 155–7
   origin of infection, 157–8
   prevention, 160–2
   risk factors, 158–60
Syme's amputation, 198, 199
Sympathetic dystrophy, reflex, 81

Taylor patch, 149, 150 (fig.)
Thoracoabdominal aneurysms, 50–60
   bleeding, 55
   classification, 51 (fig.)
   investigation, 55–7
   renal ischaemia, 54
      rupture frequency, 50–1
      spinal cord ischaemia treatment, *see*
         Spinal cord ischaemia surgery, 51–2,
         57–60
      results, 55
   visceral ischaemia, 54–5
Thromboplastin Activator, 185
Through-knee amputation, 201
Tibial artery calcification, 182, 183 (fig.)
Transmetatarsal amputation, 198–9
Traysol, 55
Treadmill, 4
Trash buttock, 74
Trash foot, 74, 75 (fig.)

Unilateral iliofemoral bypass, 121

Vacuum drains, 161
Varicose veins, 207–17
   compression sclerotherapy, 207
   Doppler velocimeter analysis, 4
   recurrent, 209–17
Vasospastic disease, clinical laboratory
      studies, 3
Vein mapping, 131, 132 (fig.)
Venous insufficiency, chronic, 207–17
Venous thromboembolic diseases, clinical
      vascular laboratory studies, 3

Waveform analysis, 2